Food Processing and Its Impact on Phenolic and other Bioactive Constituents in Food

Food Processing and Its Impact on Phenolic and other Bioactive Constituents in Food

Editors

Jan Oszmianski
Sabina Lachowicz-Wiśniewska

MDPI • Basel • Beijing • Wuhan • Barcelona • Belgrade • Manchester • Tokyo • Cluj • Tianjin

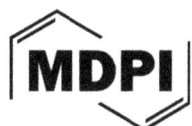

Editors

Jan Oszmianski
Departament of Fruit,
Vegetable and Plant
Nutraceutical Technology
Wroclaw University of
Environmental and
Life Sciences
Wrocław
Poland

Sabina
Lachowicz-Wiśniewska
Department of Health
Sciences
Calisia University
Kalisz
Poland

Editorial Office
MDPI
St. Alban-Anlage 66
4052 Basel, Switzerland

This is a reprint of articles from the Special Issue published online in the open access journal *Molecules* (ISSN 1420-3049) (available at: www.mdpi.com/journal/molecules/special_issues/food_phenols).

For citation purposes, cite each article independently as indicated on the article page online and as indicated below:

LastName, A.A.; LastName, B.B.; LastName, C.C. Article Title. *Journal Name* **Year**, *Volume Number*, Page Range.

ISBN 978-3-0365-4460-1 (Hbk)
ISBN 978-3-0365-4459-5 (PDF)

© 2022 by the authors. Articles in this book are Open Access and distributed under the Creative Commons Attribution (CC BY) license, which allows users to download, copy and build upon published articles, as long as the author and publisher are properly credited, which ensures maximum dissemination and a wider impact of our publications.

The book as a whole is distributed by MDPI under the terms and conditions of the Creative Commons license CC BY-NC-ND.

Contents

About the Editors vii

Leila Arfaoui
Dietary Plant Polyphenols: Effects of Food Processing on Their Content and Bioavailability
Reprinted from: *Molecules* **2021**, *26*, 2959, doi:10.3390/molecules26102959 1

Jan Oszmiański, Sabina Lachowicz, Paulina Nowicka, Paweł Rubiński and Tomasz Cebulak
Evaluation of Innovative Dried Purée from Jerusalem Artichoke—In Vitro Studies of Its Physicochemical and Health-Promoting Properties
Reprinted from: *Molecules* **2021**, *26*, 2644, doi:10.3390/molecules26092644 37

Hichem Bensaada, María Fernanda Soto-Garcia and Juan Carlos Carmona-Hernandez
Antioxidant Activity of Polyphenols, from *Mauritia flexuosa* (Aguaje), Based on Controlled Dehydration
Reprinted from: *Molecules* **2022**, *27*, 3065, doi:10.3390/molecules27103065 49

Shanshan Qu, Soon Jae Kwon, Shucheng Duan, You Jin Lim and Seok Hyun Eom
Isoflavone Changes in Immature and Mature Soybeans by Thermal Processing
Reprinted from: *Molecules* **2021**, *26*, 7471, doi:10.3390/molecules26247471 59

Dorota Żyżelewicz, Joanna Oracz, Martyna Bilicka, Kamila Kulbat-Warycha and Elżbieta Klewicka
Influence of Freeze-Dried Phenolic-Rich Plant Powders on the Bioactive Compounds Profile, Antioxidant Activity and Aroma of Different Types of Chocolates
Reprinted from: *Molecules* **2021**, *26*, 7058, doi:10.3390/molecules26227058 75

Ewa Pejcz, Sabina Lachowicz-Wiśniewska, Paulina Nowicka, Agata Wojciechowicz-Budzisz, Radosław Spychaj and Zygmunt Gil
Effect of Inoculated Lactic Acid Fermentation on the Fermentable Saccharides and Polyols, Polyphenols and Antioxidant Activity Changes in Wheat Sourdough
Reprinted from: *Molecules* **2021**, *26*, 4193, doi:10.3390/molecules26144193 99

Anna Muzykiewicz-Szymańska, Anna Nowak, Daria Wira and Adam Klimowicz
The Effect of Brewing Process Parameters on Antioxidant Activity and Caffeine Content in Infusions of Roasted and Unroasted Arabica Coffee Beans Originated from Different Countries
Reprinted from: *Molecules* **2021**, *26*, 3681, doi:10.3390/molecules26123681 109

Hanna Kowalska, Jolanta Kowalska, Anna Ignaczak, Ewelina Masiarz, Ewa Domian and Sabina Galus et al.
Development of a High-Fibre Multigrain Bar Technology with the Addition of Curly Kale
Reprinted from: *Molecules* **2021**, *26*, 3939, doi:10.3390/molecules26133939 129

Aurita Butkevičiūtė, Mindaugas Liaudanskas, Darius Kviklys, Dalia Gelvonauskienė and Valdimaras Janulis
The Qualitative and Quantitative Compositions of Phenolic Compounds in Fruits of Lithuanian Heirloom Apple Cultivars
Reprinted from: *Molecules* **2020**, *25*, 5263, doi:10.3390/molecules25225263 149

Aurita Butkevičiūtė, Mindaugas Liaudanskas, Kristina Ramanauskienė and Valdimaras Janulis
Biopharmaceutical Evaluation of Capsules with Lyophilized Apple Powder
Reprinted from: *Molecules* **2021**, *26*, 1095, doi:10.3390/molecules26041095 165

Monika Hanula, Arkadiusz Szpicer, Elżbieta Górska-Horczyczak, Gohar Khachatryan, Grzegorz Pogorzelski and Ewelina Pogorzelska-Nowicka et al.
Hydrogel Emulsion with Encapsulated Safflower Oil Enriched with Açai Extract as a Novel Fat Substitute in Beef Burgers Subjected to Storage in Cold Conditions
Reprinted from: *Molecules* **2022**, *27*, 2397, doi:10.3390/molecules27082397 . . . . **179**

Kalina Sikorska-Zimny, Paweł Lisiecki, Weronika Gonciarz, Magdalena Szemraj, Maja Ambroziak and Olga Suska et al.
Influence of Agronomic Practice on Total Phenols, Carotenoids, Chlorophylls Content, and Biological Activities in Dry Herbs Water Macerates
Reprinted from: *Molecules* **2021**, *26*, 1047, doi:10.3390/molecules26041047 . . . . **207**

About the Editors

Jan Oszmianski

Jan Oszmiański, Professor Dr., Retired Professor, completed his Ph.D. degree at Agricultural Academy August Cieszkowski in Poznań in the area of enzymatic transformations of phenolic compounds in model systems and fruit extracts, and subsequently carried out postdoctoral research at the Wroclaw University of Environmental and Life Sciences in the area of polyphenolic compounds and functional food. His main research interest is in phenolic compounds, the isolation and qualitative and quantitative determinations of polyphenols, and chromatography techniques such as UV-VIS and HPLC-MS-MS. He is a member of the committee of Food Sciences and Nutrition of the Polish Academy of Sciences.

Sabina Lachowicz-Wiśniewska

Sabina Lachowicz-Wiśniewska, Doctor, Assistant Professor, completed her Ph.D. degree at Wrocław University of Environmental and Life Sciences under the direction of Professor Jan Oszmiański in the area of natural product technology and chemistry. Nowadays, she carries out postdoctoral research at the Calisia University in the Kalisz Microbiota Research Team under the direction of Professor Ireneusz Kapusta in the area of prebiotic functional food and the bioavailability of their bioactive compounds for the prevention of oxidative stress and inflammation. Her past research is in the general area of functional food, and pharmaceutical and medicinal plant chemistry, with over 74 peer-reviewed scientific papers covering research field such as: (i) the production of innovative functional food designed to have health-promoting properties; (ii) the bioavailability and digestibility of bioactive compounds in the simulated digestive system by in vitro method; (iii) the determination of antioxidant, anti-diabetic, anti-obesity, and anti-inflammatory potential; and (iv) the identification and assessment of the health-promoting properties of bioactive compounds from plant materials based on chromatographic techniques. Research collaborations have been established within Dekaban Fundation with Prof. Anubhav Pratap Singh (Faculty of Land and Food Systems (LFS), University of British Columbia), Prof. Antonio J. Meléndez-Martínez in the Food Colour and Quality Laboratory, Universidad de Sevilla and also with many European research centers.

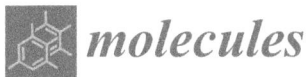

Review

Dietary Plant Polyphenols: Effects of Food Processing on Their Content and Bioavailability

Leila Arfaoui

Department of Clinical Nutrition, Faculty of Applied Medical Sciences, King Abdulaziz University, P.O. Box 80324, Jeddah 21589, Saudi Arabia; larfaoui@kau.edu.sa; Tel.: +966-0126401000 (ext. 41612)

Abstract: Dietary plant polyphenols are natural bioactive compounds that are increasingly attracting the attention of food scientists and nutritionists because of their nutraceutical properties. In fact, many studies have shown that polyphenol-rich diets have protective effects against most chronic diseases. However, these health benefits are strongly related to both polyphenol content and bioavailability, which in turn depend on their origin, food matrix, processing, digestion, and cellular metabolism. Although most fruits and vegetables are valuable sources of polyphenols, they are not usually consumed raw. Instead, they go through some processing steps, either industrially or domestically (e.g., cooling, heating, drying, fermentation, etc.), that affect their content, bioaccessibility, and bioavailability. This review summarizes the status of knowledge on the possible (positive or negative) effects of commonly used food-processing techniques on phenolic compound content and bioavailability in fruits and vegetables. These effects depend on the plant type and applied processing parameters (type, duration, media, and intensity). This review attempts to shed light on the importance of more comprehensive dietary guidelines that consider the recommendations of processing parameters to take full advantage of phenolic compounds toward healthier foods.

Keywords: plant polyphenols; food processing; phenolic content; bioavailability; bioaccessibility

1. Introduction

Recent progress in nutrition and medicine has metamorphosed the way healthcare is conceived and delivered. An international technology-driven revolution is driving this rapid change from traditional healthcare to precision medicine by establishing unprecedented research programs and networks that prioritize diseases' prevention and health promotion mainly through lifestyle and diet-based approaches [1]. A recent emerging area of precision nutrition focusing on bioavailable and metabolizable proportions of ingested foods with claimed health benefits has been developed. In this context, plant-derived polyphenols have been associated with several health benefits and are considered bioactive dietary compounds [2]. Polyphenols are the largest group of dietary antioxidants known for their ability to scavenge free radicals, donate hydrogen atoms, electrons, or chelate metal cations [3]. Because of these mechanisms, they have protective and preventive effects against several non-communicable diseases (NCDs), including cardiovascular diseases (CVDs), cancer, and diabetes [4].

However, the health implications of dietary polyphenols are determined by their bioavailability to a great extent, which is defined as the fraction of polyphenols released from the food matrix, metabolized, absorbed, and able to impose its bioactivity on the target cells or tissues [5]. Several factors influence polyphenol bioavailability, including the initial content in foods, food matrix, gut microbiota, and food processing [6]. In fact, most fruits and vegetables are not usually consumed raw. Instead, they go through industrial or domestic processing steps (e.g., cooling, heating, drying, fermentation, etc.) that affect their content, bioaccessibility, and bioavailability.

The main purpose of food-processing techniques is to transform raw ingredients into food, or to transform food into other end-products suitable for human or animal consumption. Some specific objectives include extending the shelf life of ingredients and products by inactivating pathogens or contaminating microorganisms, enhancing the bioavailability of otherwise inaccessible nutrients, enabling variety in flavor, texture, or aroma of certain foods, and improving the nutrient profile [7]. Domestic and industrial processing affect phenolic compounds' content, antioxidant capacity, bioaccessibility, and bioavailability in different ways. While many food-processing techniques may lead to phenolic compounds' degradation, some others enhance their absorption and bioavailability [8,9]. The final polyphenol content and bioavailability in processed food depend, therefore, on factors such as the nature of the process, duration of treatment, and food matrix subjected to the processing technique [10].

Since dietary polyphenol consumption has been increasingly proposed as an effective measure in the primary prevention and management of NCDs, it is imperative to consider the effect of food processing on their content and bioavailability. This review aims to summarize the effects of the most common food-processing techniques, either domestic or industrial, on dietary polyphenol content, bioaccessibility, and bioavailability. To introduce the topic, a glance at polyphenol types, sources, health implications, and the concepts of bioavailability and bioaccessibility is provided.

2. Polyphenol Types and Sources

The largest antioxidant group present in the human diet is that of phenolic compounds, with more than 8000 different structures identified to date [11]. Plants produce these secondary metabolites in response to ultraviolet light or pathogen attacks [12]. The molecular structure is based on one or several aromatic rings and at least one hydroxyl (phenol) group. They can either have a simple structure (such as in the case of phenolic acids) or a complex structure (such as in the case of flavonoids).

Based on their molecular structure, phenolics are divided into five main groups: phenolic acids, flavonoids, stilbenes, coumarins, and tannins [9]. As phenolic acids and flavonoids were mostly investigated in studies reporting the association between food processing and polyphenol content and bioavailability, these two classes are discussed in greater detail.

2.1. Phenolic Acids

Phenolic acids are non-flavonoid polyphenols, and their typical representatives are hydroxybenzoic acids (e.g., gallic, *p*-hydroxybenzoic, vanillic, and syringic acids) and hydroxycinnamic acids (e.g., ferulic, caffeic, *p*-coumaric, chlorogenic, and sinapic acids). They exist in bound or free form in fruits and vegetables. Grains and seeds are particularly rich in bound phenolic acids, which are released after acid or alkaline hydrolysis or enzymatic reactions [11]. Good sources of phenolic acids are fruits (apples, cherries, berries, and their products, such as wine), vegetables (broccoli, lettuce, and tomatoes), legumes, cereals, and coffee beans [13].

2.2. Flavonoids

Flavonoids are a large group of polyphenols that typically contain two aromatic rings linked by a heterocycle. Their subclasses are distinguished by structural differences based on this heterocycle [14]. These subgroups include anthocyanins, flavan-3-ols, flavones, flavanones, and flavonols [11].

Flavones, flavonols, and flavanones are widely distributed in plants. Flavones and their derivatives flavonols, as well as their acylated products, represent the largest polyphenol subgroup [15]. Quercetin and kaempferol are, for example, the most commonly found flavonol aglycones, and they alone have approximately 300 different glycosidic combinations [15]. The most relevant flavone sources are citrus fruits, parsley, lettuce, and grapes, while flavanones are mostly present in citruses and products based on them [13]. Among all flavanones, hesperidin and naringenin are typical representatives. Good dietary sources of flavonols include plums, apples, onions, and blueberries, with kaempferol and quercetin being the main representatives [13].

Flavanols are a very complex group of polyphenols, which include compounds ranging from monomeric flavan-3-ols to polymeric proanthocyanidins. Proanthocyanidins are the precursors of anthocyanidins, which are produced under acidic conditions as a result of polymeric chain cleavage [11]. The most commonly identified monomeric flavanols in dietary sources are catechin, epi(gallo)catechin, and their gallates [13]. Catechins are mainly present in tea, grapes, red wine, cocoa, and chocolate [13].

Anthocyanidins are compounds responsible for the red, blue, and purple pigments in fruits and vegetables, flower petals, and some grain varieties, such as black rice. As they are mainly present as glycosides, they are commonly referred to as anthocyanins. Among the 31 currently known anthocyanidins, the most frequently identified in plants are cyanidin, delphinidin, and pelargonidin [16]. In fact, 90% of the structure of anthocyanins is based on these compounds and their derivatives [16]. Several factors influence the color of anthocyanins, such as pH and degree of hydroxylation. Depending on these factors, these phenolic compounds can either give blue, red, or purple colors to plants [11]. A wide range of plant-based foods are good sources of these phenolics, with grapes, red wine, berries, and some vegetables being typical representatives [13].

These diverse polyphenol sources and types discussed above are valuable, and therefore it is worth investigating their bioavailability and health benefits in light of the scientific literature available so far.

3. Polyphenols' Health Benefits Related to Chronic Diseases

Oxidative stress and inflammation are common pathways that drive the progression of many NCDs. As polyphenols impair these processes [17], incorporating higher doses of these compounds into the human diet may be a suitable tool for primary prevention, lowering the incidence and delaying the onset of several chronic diseases, including cardiovascular diseases, cancer, obesity, and neurological disorders (Figure 1).

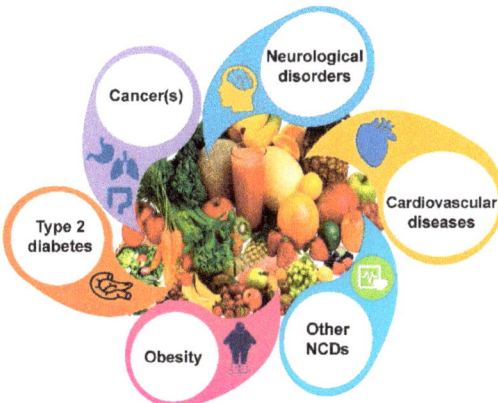

Figure 1. Main health benefits of polyphenols related to chronic diseases.

3.1. Polyphenols Consumption and Their Effects on Obesity

Animal, in vitro, and human studies have shown that dietary anti-inflammatory and antioxidative compounds may increase thermogenesis and energy expenditure, and decrease inflammation and oxidative stress, thereby facilitating weight loss and/or reducing the rate of metabolic conditions [18]. Some polyphenols with anti-obesity properties are tea catechins, specifically epigallocatechin-gallate (EGCG). In vitro studies on isolated EGCG or green tea extracts have reported their potential to inhibit preadipocyte differentiation, decrease adipocyte proliferation, and induce apoptosis. They also suppress lipogenesis and promote lipolysis and beta-oxidation processes [19]. A preclinical animal study has reported that EGCG and green tea extract facilitate weight loss by lowering adipose mass in mice fed a high-fat diet [20]. Other polyphenols with anti-obesity properties include anthocyanins, compounds with great antioxidant [21] and anti-inflammatory potential [22]. Few human clinical trials have assessed the obesity-related effects of anthocyanin-rich foods; however, the available data suggest that black soybean and red orange juice may effectively reduce markers of inflammation and metabolic disease in overweight people [23,24].

3.2. Polyphenols Consumption and Their Effects on Cardiovascular Diseases

Oxidative stress has been linked to endothelial dysfunction, which triggers the onset of early atherosclerosis and CVD. Thus, strategies that aim to reduce oxidative stress and inflammation may be promising to combat CVD-related disorders. In addition, polyphenols can increase NO synthase activity [25], which in turn positively affects flow-mediated dilatation (FMD). Human trial data suggest that oligomeric proanthocyanidins are an efficient dietary intervention for improving plasma lipid profiles and anti-atherogenic components of plasma, as observed in 70 hyperlipidemic subjects [26]. A 6-week supplementation with 162 mg of onion peel quercetin per day was reported to improve hypertensive patients' systolic blood pressure [27]. However, a daily dose of 100 mg quercetin for 12 weeks did not affect blood pressure in 72 healthy overweight and obese subjects, whereas it positively affected endothelial function measured as FMD and circulating endothelial progenitor cell counts [28]. When the findings from randomized controlled trials (RCTs) of polyphenol supplementation were meta-analyzed, it was concluded that polyphenols could exert beneficial effects on LDL-c, HDL-c, FMD, and both systolic and diastolic pressure, thus supporting their implications in primary CVD prevention [29].

3.3. Polyphenols Consumption and Their Effects on Type 2 Diabetes (T2D)

Polyphenols and polyphenol-rich products can also ameliorate the risk of T2D. Polyphenols are involved in attenuating postprandial glycemic responses, fasting hyperglycemia, and improving insulin secretion and sensitivity. These implications might be explained by their ability to inhibit the digestion of carbohydrates and intestinal glucose absorption, stimulate insulin secretion, modulate the liver-related release of glucose, and trigger both gene expression and cell signaling pathways [30]. Many studies have investigated the efficacy of polyphenol supplementation at the onset of T2D. One meta-analysis of observational studies found that a diet rich in polyphenols (specifically flavonoids) may serve as a tool to prevent the onset of T2D [31]. Regarding specific food groups, tea consumption was reported to be inversely associated with the onset of T2D. A dose–response meta-analysis of cohort studies suggests that consuming 4–6 cups of tea per day may decrease T2D risk by up to 15% [32]. Other polyphenol-rich food groups linked with a reduced risk of T2D include fruits, specifically berries and yellow vegetables [33,34].

3.4. Polyphenols' Consumption and Their Effects on Cancer

Polyphenol supplementation can hamper cancer progression, probably because of their involvement in cancer cell apoptosis. They were also shown to modulate cell cycle signaling and promote cell defense systems [35]. Epidemiological studies have shown that dietary polyphenol intake is linked with lower cancer incidence. For example, one Canadian case-control study observed that high dietary flavonoid consumption could reduce lung cancer occurrence [36], while a Korean study confirmed a similar relationship with gastric cancer [37]. Clinical trials also support the notion that polyphenol compounds may exert beneficial effects on disease progression [38,39]. A meta-analysis of 165 prospective and case-control studies did not confirm the association between total flavonoid intake and cancer risk. However, the subgroup analysis confirmed that a higher intake of some flavonoid classes could lower the risk of some cancers, specifically colon, lung, and stomach ulcers [40].

3.5. Polyphenols' Consumption and Their Effects on Neurological Disorders

Finally, the antioxidant properties of polyphenols are important for improving brain health and function. By scavenging free radicals, they facilitate the reduction of brain cell damage [41]. Using animal models with neurocognitive dysfunction, it has been observed that physiological doses of flavonoids may reduce the accumulation of neuropathological proteins and improve synaptic plasticity [41]. Observational studies and RCTs suggest that dietary polyphenols, such as those present in berries, grapes, cocoa, and green tea, may modulate processes related to cognitive health [42]. It was also reported that resveratrol supplementation could enhance both cerebrovascular function and cognition in postmenopausal women, implying that this polyphenol's presence in the diet may improve cognitive function in this specific population [43]. A meta-analysis study found that polyphenol consumption (that is, those present in Ginkgo biloba, resveratrol, and soy isoflavones) did not significantly affect the scores reflecting global cognitive functions; however, they improved those scores related to verbal learning, memory, and executive functions, while not affecting attention-related scores [29].

4. Bioavailability of Polyphenols

Along with the polyphenol content in foods and their distribution in plants, bioavailability is an essential factor that directly influences and determines the biological function of polyphenol-rich-food consumption. A distinction between bioaccessibility and bioavailability should be made. Bioaccessibility refers to the fraction that mobilizes from the food matrix and reaches the gastrointestinal system, undergoing digestion, absorption into intestinal epithelial cells, and metabolic changes in the intestine and liver [44]. This definition does not include their utilization in target cells or tissues, such as in the case of bioavailability [45]. Bioavailability refers to a fraction released from the food matrix, subjected to digestion, absorption, metabolism in the liver and intestine, and its further distribution to target tissues and cells where it imposes its bioactivity and exerts positive health-related effects. It is complicated to measure bioactivity owing to practical (and ethical) issues; therefore, bioavailability definitions today do not include bioactivity [46].

4.1. Bioavailability and Bioaccessibility Assessment

As seen in the previous section, evaluating bioaccessibility is usually carried out by using in vitro methods that simulate digestion, and in some cases, the simulation of uptake by Caco-2 cells is also included [47]. By contrast, bioavailability is measured in vivo as the change in plasma levels (in humans or animals) of that specific compound after an acute or chronic administration of the food matrix containing the investigated compound [48].

According to published literature, analyses of bioavailability and bioaccessibility of polyphenols have been carried out by using both in vitro and in vivo models. The most utilized in vitro method is the static gastrointestinal model, and several modifications have been applied to it, such as the addition of experiments that simulate the oral phase during digestion or colonic fermentation. One of the models that allow the implementation of colon fermentation experiments is the dynamic gastric model, which has been frequently applied to study polyphenol bioavailability. In addition to in vitro models, in vivo assessments have been performed in rats, pigs, and dogs, and the number of clinical trials in humans has been rapidly increasing during the last decade [49].

4.2. Factors Influencing Polyphenols' Bioavailability

It is challenging to conduct bioavailability studies because several different factors influence it (Figure 2). Some of them are external, such as environmental factors (rainfall, sun exposure, soil type, etc.) or the degree of ripeness. The composition of the food matrix and the interaction between polyphenols and other dietary components (proteins, fat, carbohydrate, and fiber), as well as the tendency of polyphenols to build complexes with proteins, should be considered when assessing their bioavailability [10].

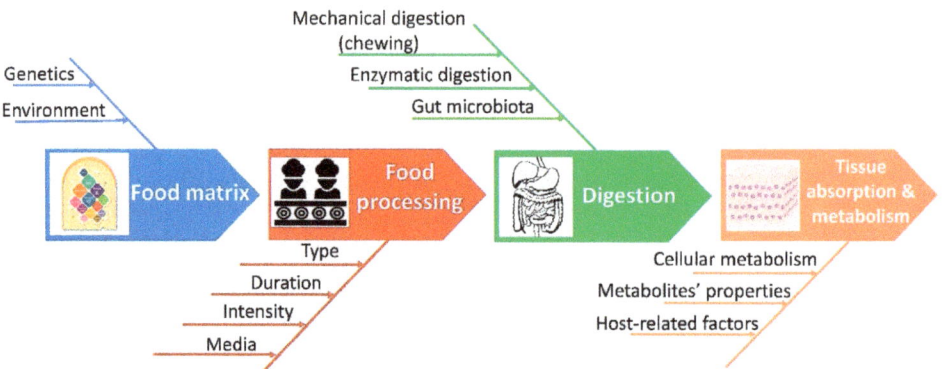

Figure 2. Main factors affecting dietary plant polyphenols content and bioavailability.

The chemical structure of a specific polyphenol determines its fate during digestion in a significant manner. Dietary polyphenols mostly exist as polymers or glycosides, containing a glycone part (the sugar group) and an aglycone part (the polyphenol). Most phenolic compounds resist acidic conditions during gastric digestion [50], and as they cannot be absorbed in their native form (except for anthocyanins), the intestinal enzymes or the colonic microbiota hydrolyze them prior to absorption. Thus, the degree of absorption of polyphenols in the intestine greatly depends on the chemical structure and the type of sugar present in the glycosylated form [10].

The host that ingests food containing polyphenols also influences their metabolism. Specifically, there are two important factors: the intestinal factors and the systemic factors. In fact, the ingested polyphenols undergo several biochemical changes in the small intestine mainly through glycoside hydrolyzation to allow their absorption [10]. The non-absorbed fraction of polyphenols will transit to the colon, where they are transformed by the colonic microflora into other bioactive phenolic metabolites, followed by structural modifications mainly in the liver prior entering the blood stream [34,51–53]. Besides the intestinal factors, these biochemical transformations of polyphenols in the digestive tract and the type and proportions of their derivative metabolites depend also on the host systemic factors, such as gender, age, presence of pathologies, and genetics [10].

Finally, the processing techniques applied in domestic or industrial settings influence the final polyphenol content in the food and thus its bioavailability (Figure 2). The studies investigating these processing-related effects are discussed in the fifth section of this review.

4.3. Polyphenols' Metabolism Pathway during Digestion

Some phenolic compounds are absorbed in the small intestine and those that are not are metabolized in the colon, where glycosides are hydrolyzed into aglycones and further degraded into simple phenolic acids [51,54]. These changes depend on their chemical structure. For example, anthocyanidins are highly unstable and are absorbed as glycoside-anthocyanins [55]. As they are highly susceptible to gastric conditions, a very low amount of anthocyanins is bioavailable (approximately 0.1% of the intake) [56]. It is generally observed that those phenolics that are absorbed in the colon have lower bioavailability rates than those that undergo these processes in the intestine [50]. The bioavailability of proanthocyanidins is determined by the degree of polymerization. Most of these phenolics pass through the small intestine to the colon, where the colon microbiota modifies them [57]. Those with a lower degree of polymerization undergo more intense modifications, while those with a higher degree form complexes with macromolecules that disables their further modifications and absorption [58]. Diverse phenolic acids and flavan-3-ols are produced by the reactions between proanthocyanidins and the colonic microbiota, and these products undergo further absorption in the colon [58]. In the case of phenolic acids, the small intestine absorbs one part, and the colon absorbs the other [14].

After absorption by epithelial cells, phenolic acids or colonic metabolites reach the liver through the portal vein, and they undergo conjugation processes described as phase II metabolism (methylation, sulfation, and glucuronidation). Some conjugation processes occur in the small intestine; however, the majority occurs in the liver [10]. Almost all plasma phenolics are products of phase II metabolism, and these metabolites determine the biological activity of ingested dietary polyphenols [45]. These extensive metabolic changes produce several metabolites from a single polyphenol. Therefore, the compounds that reach the target cells and tissues where they impose their bioactivity are very different from the original form present in food, chemically, biologically, and in many other ways.

5. Food-Processing Techniques and Their Effects on Polyphenols Content and Bioavailability

Vegetables and fruits are a main source of phenolic compounds. For example, several fruits as apple, berries are very rich in polyphenols with more than 200 mg per 100 g of fresh fruits [59]. However, the content and the bioavailability of these phenolic compounds are influenced by the food-processing technique(s) applied. For instance, and since many food-processing methods involve heat treatment, it is believed that higher temperatures may lead to detrimental changes in fruits and vegetables in terms of their nutritional profile; however, some studies observed quite the opposite [8]. A detailed analysis of 161 polyphenols and their food-processing changes reported that domestic cooking induced notable losses in polyphenols, with great variability between the foods. It was also observed that the food that was investigated was often a more important factor than the process employed, thus highlighting the importance of the food matrix [60]. Many other factors influence the fate of polyphenolic compounds during food processing, and these relationships are briefly presented in the following subsections, depending on the type of food-processing technique used at both industrial and domestic sittings (Appendix A Tables A1 and A2).

5.1. Thermal Processing

5.1.1. Heat Treatment

Heat treatments are commonly applied in food processing in both domestic and industrial settings. These treatments include boiling, frying, steaming, baking, stewing, and roasting in traditional, microwave, and steam ovens. Heat is also utilized in other traditional transformation processes such as toasting, coffee roasting, drying, canning, pasteurization, and sterilization.

The fate of polyphenols during thermal processing largely depends on the method applied. The heat ruptures cell walls, enabling the bound phenolics to mobilize to other parts of the plant, enhancing their availability [61]. However, at the same time, they are more prone to oxidation, and some are more or less thermostable.

Studies applying thermal treatments have shown that boiling causes the most detrimental polyphenol composition changes in treated samples. Steaming and frying can preserve higher amounts of these compounds. The underlying reason might be that phenolics are water-soluble, and during the boiling process, they leak into the surrounding medium (water). As heat treatment decomposes the tissue, it enables the migration of cellular components and nutrients into the boiling water [62]. It has been proposed that polar media (water) might be responsible for higher losses due to polyphenol solubility in water, while nonpolar media (oil) would extract lower amounts of lipid-insoluble polyphenols [63].

The detrimental effects of boiling were observed in the case of onions and asparagus. A 60 min boiling process led to a 20.6% and 43.9% loss in overall flavonol content in onions and asparagus, respectively. Notable changes were also observed in the antioxidant capacities [64]. This was confirmed in another study, in which boiling for 1 h induced 53% and 44% degradation of quercetin diglucoside and monoglucoside in onion bulbs, respectively, while boiling for 30 min, frying, and roasting (in microwave and oven) caused less severe changes [65]. The higher degradation of quercetin derivatives might have occurred because of the difference in the surrounding medium, where water as a polar medium led to a higher extraction of these compounds than oil and air. However, this study also points to the polyphenol class being an important determinant—in the case of anthocyanins (cyanidin 3-glucoside, cyanidin 3-laminaribioside, and cyanidin 3-(6″-malonylglucoside) and cyanidin 3-(6″-malonyl-laminaribioside), frying caused the most severe effects, followed by boiling and roasting [65].

Water volume can also influence the degree of polyphenol alteration during heat treatment. Cooking in smaller volumes resulted in higher phenolic content in zucchini (specifically rutin), beans (rutin and quercitrin), and carrots (chlorogenic acid). Accordingly, cooking in smaller water volumes yielded lower phenolic concentrations in the surrounding water than cooking in larger volumes [66].

Musilova et al. explored variety as an influencing factor that modulates the relationship between food processing and polyphenol alterations. Four sweet potato varieties were subjected to four different heat treatments (boiling, steaming, microwaving, and baking). In general, heating had adverse effects on phenolic acid levels. Boiling was shown to have the most detrimental effect: it lowered the levels of chlorogenic acid by 29% (in the 414-purple variety from Slovakia), neochlorogenic acid by 69% (in the 414-purple variety from Croatia), and trans-ferulic acid by 29% (in the Beauregard variety from Croatia). In contrast, all these treatments increased the levels of total polyphenols, total anthocyanins, and total antioxidant activity, mostly in all analyzed samples [67].

Different boiling periods yielded different polyphenol profiles in foods. For example, blanching (short-interval boiling) of kale leaves led to a 51% decrease in polyphenol content (phenolic acids, flavones, flavonols, and anthocyanins), the lowest of which was observed in the case of caffeic acid (28%) and the highest in ferulic acid (55%). However, cooking for a longer time caused more severe damage, resulting in a 73% decrease in the total polyphenol content [68].

Chumyam et al. highlighted the role of the medium in their study by comparing the utilization of water as a medium (in the case of boiling and steaming) and no medium (in the case of microwaving). All procedures were conducted in 5, 10, and 15 min. All treatments significantly increased antioxidant capacity and total phenolic content in purple skin eggplant compared with raw samples. Boiling yielded samples with the lowest levels of total polyphenols [69]. Of all the methods investigated, 10-min microwaving resulted in the highest total phenolic level and highest antioxidant capacity. In addition, 10-min microwaving proved to be the best method for enhancing the antioxidant capacity of eggplant fruits [69]. The authors proposed that phenolic and antioxidant compounds activated by microwaving remained in eggplant fruits, while cooking by boiling and steaming caused their leakage (either directly or indirectly) into water.

High-temperature regimes are also applied to preserve food by inactivating enzymes and pathogen microbes, with sterilization and pasteurization as two commonly applied treatments. In white beans, sterilization significantly decreased the total polyphenol content after 4 and 12 months of storage (by 30 and 46%, respectively). However, these findings may be biased by the effects of storage. This was also observed in condensed tannins; after 12 months of storage, the concentration of these compounds was lower by 30% [70]. Pasteurization of apple juice by conventional high-temperature/short-time treatment also led to notable losses in total polyphenols (by 32.3%). However, pasteurization with pulsed electric field treatment reduced their levels by only 14.9% [71].

Studies have also assessed the effects of thermal processing treatments on the bioavailability of dietary polyphenols. Domestic cooking of cherry tomatoes increased the bioavailability of naringenin and chlorogenic acid in five test subjects [72]. Mechanical and heat treatments applied during tomato sauce production also enhanced the plasma concentration and urinary excretion of naringenin glucuronide. This was observed in a randomized controlled trial in which eight healthy volunteers ingested either tomato sauce or raw tomatoes [73]. These data confirm that heat treatment enhances the mobilization of polyphenol bioactive compounds from the food matrix, making them more bioavailable.

The type of heat treatment is an important determinant of polyphenol bioavailability. When cassava samples were subjected to different cooking methods, the highest total phenolic content was observed in steaming, followed by microwaving and boiling. These cooking methods similarly affected their availability in the subjects, although with only slight differences, steamed samples showed a 74.5% bioavailability, while boiled and microwaved samples obtained similar values (72.9% for boiled and 72.7% for microwaved samples) [74]. Streaming was the best heat method, probably due to the indirect exposure to the polar medium (water); thus, the polyphenols were retained to a higher degree in the plant.

The form in which phenolics are present is a well-recognized factor, as observed in carrots when exposed to heating in a microwave oven for 12 min. Although it did not affect anthocyanin bioavailability, it increased the relative urinary recovery of non-acylated anthocyanins without affecting the acylated anthocyanins. The authors proposed that the acylation of anthocyanin derivatives is an important factor when investigating their bioavailability [75].

Finally, Rodriguez-Mateos et al. [76] investigated how baking affected the content and bioavailability of blueberry polyphenols, namely anthocyanins, procyanidins, and phenolic acids. This RCT involving 10 healthy subjects used a baked product containing blueberries, an unprocessed blueberry drink, and a matching control baked product. Processing induced no significant changes in the total polyphenolic content; however, it significantly lowered the amounts of anthocyanins (−42%), increased the levels of chlorogenic acid (23%), and significantly enhanced the concentrations of flavanol dimers and trimers (36 and 28%, respectively). By determining the plasma levels of 22 metabolites assessed individually after ingestion of the test products, the authors observed that the blueberry baked product induced mainly an increase in four metabolites (m-hydroxyphenylacetic, ferulic, isoferulic, and hydroxyhippuric acids) and a decrease in four others (hippuric, benzoic, salicylic, and sinapic acids) compared with the blueberry drink, without affecting the bioavailability of the total phenolic levels [76].

5.1.2. Canning

Canning is a process that aims to produce commercially sterilized and microbiologically safe products by applying heat treatment. Canned food products can be produced by using retorts, pasteurizers, or heat exchangers. The main aim of heat treatment is to eliminate pathogens or microorganisms that can cause contamination, while metal containers, glass jars, and retort pouches are used to prevent spoilage by new microorganisms. After heating, the canned product is cooled and stored at room temperature to maintain the stability and integrity of both the food and the container/jar used [77].

Canning is reported to reduce total phenolic and flavonoid contents, mostly because phenolic compounds leach into the surrounding medium (brine or syrup) [78]. This extensive leaching results from the applied heat treatment, which disintegrates the cells and tissues, enabling the migration of polyphenols into the medium.

There is also a difference in how the canning process is carried out and the corresponding conditions. One study examined the differences in the effects of domestic and industrial canning on apricots. Thermal processing imitating industrial conditions induced a higher loss of total phenolics (13–47%), while domestic processing led to lower losses (2–33%). This is proposed to be the consequence of the difference in temperature regimes, the more intensive one being employed in industrial processing. Procyanidins were similarly affected: the loss in domestic treatments was 2.4%, and that in industrial treatments was 44%. Phenolic acids (hydroxycinnamic acids, 3-O-caffeoylquinic acid, and 5-O-caffeoylquinic acid) exhibited a significant decline in both thermal processes; however, the greater loss was observed in industrial canning [79].

Interestingly, it has also been reported that canning may lead to the production of some desirable compounds that are not naturally present in raw foods. Investigation of canned peanuts showed that the retorting process damaged some phenolic compounds (resveratrol, caffeic acid, and catechin); however, genistein (a phytoestrogen belonging to the class of soy isoflavones), which was not measured in raw, was quantified in the canned peanut [80].

5.1.3. Drying

Drying is a preservation process that aims to reduce the moisture content of food by using heat and mass transfer [81]. As fruits and vegetables are prone to microbial and biochemical spoilage due to their high water content (which can be more than 80%), drying reduces the water activity and makes a stable end-product with an extended shelf life. Some of these methods include vacuum-drying, solar-drying, air-drying, and freeze-drying.

Since drying involves heat treatment, the temperature regime affects the degree of degradation of dietary polyphenols, as observed in jujube fruits. Jujube fruits were subjected to different drying procedures: vacuum–microwave (480, 120 W), hot air (70, 60, and 50 °C), and combined methods such as pre-drying and finish-drying (60 °C + 480/120 W). Freeze-drying (the control treatment) was the most efficient method for preserving total phenolic content, while hot-air-drying caused the greatest loss in these compounds; the highest losses were observed after applying the highest temperature. The polyphenol content was less affected when the methods were combined. Similarly, antioxidant activity was the highest in freeze-dried samples; high air temperature (60 or 70 °C) caused detrimental changes to antioxidant compounds [82]. In cocoa beans, total polyphenol content decreased with an increase in temperature, with the highest decrease being observed at 60 °C, and the lowest at 40 °C. These detrimental processes may be the result of oxidation and cellular destruction. Moisture content in beans can also be another limiting factor, as it affects the volatility of these compounds and the degree of polyphenol solution [83].

However, the variability of the effects caused by drying is also influenced by the variety and polyphenol class. One study assessed how two drying treatments—one involving air-drying at 55 °C and the other at 75 °C—affected two apricot cultivars. Interestingly, chlorogenic and neochlorogenic acid contents were observed to increase in the higher temperature regime (in one cultivar), and catechin levels showed the same trend in both cultivars. The authors proposed that polyphenol oxidase remained active to a great extent and that its activity affected the higher production of these two phenolic acids. However, the flavonol content decreased proportionally with the increase in temperature, as well as the content of epicatechin [84].

In some cases, the lowest temperature was not the best solution for retaining high polyphenol levels in the samples but optimizing the temperature and drying period. In a study on cocoa beans at three temperature regimes (drying at 60, 70, and 80 °C), the maximum concentration of total phenolics was reported to be in samples that were dried at 70 °C, and their levels decreased as the heating procedure was prolonged [85]. In another study, the researchers subjected several berry fruits (raspberry, boysenberry, redcurrants, and blackcurrant fruit) to drying at 50 °C for 48 h, 65 °C for 20 h, or 130 °C for 2 h until a moisture content below 15% was reached. Drying at 65 °C was the best method in terms of the total polyphenol content and radical scavenging activity. Higher temperatures and longer regimes proved to be detrimental to the polyphenols in berries. Specifically, anthocyanin levels were similar in berries dried at 50 and 65 °C. However, temperatures above 100 °C caused the most detrimental effects on all the analyzed parameters [86].

According to the available literature, drying procedures may be used to obtain products with more bioavailable polyphenols. However, the final effect depends on the specific polyphenol class or the individual compounds investigated and the temperature regime. Kamiloglu et al. investigated the effect of home processing on the availability of total phenolics and flavonoids in tomatoes by employing an in vitro gastrointestinal digestion model. They observed that oven drying (70 °C for 36 h) yielded a two-fold higher bioavailability of total polyphenols; however, this was not the case with total flavonoids [87]. In another study, Kamiloğlu and Capanoglu (2013) observed that an 8 d sun-drying procedure at 30 °C positively affected the bioaccessibility of chlorogenic acid, while adversely affecting rutin and anthocyanins (cyanidin-3-glucoside (C3G) and cyanidin-3-rutinoside) in yellow and purple figs, which were undetectable after in vitro digestion [88]. Finally, when conventional hot-air-drying in an oven (60 °C for 24 h) was compared with freeze-drying, the authors observed that oven-drying induced more favorable changes in pumpkin flour. The oven-dried samples had higher phenolics, bioaccessible phenolics and phenolic acids, and antioxidant activities [89].

5.2. Cold Processing

Freezing is a preservation technique that leads to the formation of water crystals and ice below the freezing temperature, thus slowing down biochemical and physicochemical reactions. Consequently, it stops the activity of most pathogenic microorganisms and enables longer shelf life of foods [90].

Chilling or cooling also reduces microbial and biochemical alterations in foods to maintain stability but to a lesser degree (the temperature range is between −1 and 8 °C). Cooling decreases the initial temperature of the food product and maintains its quality for a longer period [90].

The literature mainly points to these low-temperature regimes as non-invasive methods for preserving polyphenols in foods, as observed by Korus and Lisiewska, who concluded that freezing of either blanched or cooked kale leaves did not induce notable changes while freezing decreased the polyphenol levels by 3% and their antioxidative activity by 7% [68]. In addition, freezing at −30 °C of fresh red raspberries did not alter their antioxidant capacity or phenolic levels, measured as total phenolics, anthocyanins, lambertianin C, sanguiin H-6, and ellagic acid [91]. However, in some cases, these techniques can even enhance the content of polyphenols, such as in maqui fruits in which cooling (5 °C) and freezing (−20 °C) increased the total polyphenol concentration. The frozen samples had higher levels of anthocyanins, and the changes were variable. In addition, the freezing technique was better in terms of preserving these antioxidants, as they were present in these samples even after six months of storage [92].

One of the most important factors that affect the degree of dietary polyphenol preservation during food freezing is the freezing rate, as observed in a study that reported that slow-frozen strawberries had lower levels of monomeric anthocyanins than quick-frozen ones [93]. Similarly, Poiana et al. observed that individual quick freezing had no significant effect on polyphenolic compounds (total phenolic content, total monomeric anthocyanins) in three berries: blueberry, red raspberry, and blackberry [94]. The proposed mechanism is based on the nature of crystal formation. Freezing is a process that leads to the formation of ice crystals, making solutes (such as anthocyanins) localized and relocating the water molecules in the cell structure. Quick freezing induces the formation of smaller crystals, and consequently, the cells undergo less damage during the freezing process. The thawing process will also lead to a lower phenolic loss in quick-frozen samples because less water migrates in the quickly frozen strawberries, and consequently, less polyphenols as well [93].

Literature on the effects of freezing/cooling on dietary polyphenol bioavailability is scarce. One study reported that freezing by immersion in liquid nitrogen and freeze-drying at −50 °C decreased the levels of total polyphenols and antioxidant activity in apples, both before and during in vitro gastric digestion. Raw apples, which served as control samples, retained the highest amount of polyphenols and exhibited small decreases in total polyphenol concentrations and antioxidant activity during in vitro gastric digestion [95]. As mentioned above, freezing can damage the food matrix due to ice crystal formation, especially in slow freezing. Consequently, polyphenols have been proposed to undergo higher extraction during digestion, which would enhance their bioavailability. At the same time, they are also more prone to oxidation and degradation, especially when food undergoes thermal treatment after freezing. Accordingly, it could be expected that freezing would have significant effects on polyphenol bioavailability; however, there are no data to address this question [45].

5.3. Biochemical Processing
Fermentation

Fermentation is a non-thermal process based on the activity of specific microorganisms and their enzymes that induce chemical alterations in food components, leading to a significantly transformed food product. Examples of such food products are fermented milk products (yogurt or cheese), bread, vegetal probiotic beverages, vinegar and alcoholic beverages. Today, these processes are well controlled and can yield products with desired characteristics by selecting an appropriate bacteria or yeast [96].

Fermentation is an affordable technique that transforms grains into edible foods by increasing their nutrient bioaccessibility and by positively affecting their antioxidant profile and activity in the end-products. Adebo et al. found higher levels of catechin, gallic acid, and quercetin in samples of fermented whole grain sorghum, while the total flavonoid content, total tannin content, and total phenolic content decreased [97]. The authors proposed that these decreases can be explained by the degradation and hydrolysis of the phenolic compounds, while the increase might be the consequence of fermentation by Lactobacillus strains. Another study reported an increase in total phenolic content in whole grain millet-koji, which might result from the mobilization of phenolic compounds from their bound form into a free form by the activity of the fermentation-produced enzymes [98].

Legumes have also been investigated as food classes in several studies. Eight commonly consumed legume varieties (black cow gram, mottled cowpea, speckled kidney beans, lentils, small rice beans, small runner beans, and two soya beans) were subjected to fermentation by naturally present bacteria and lactic acid bacteria. All fermented legumes had a high total phenolic content, probably owing to the biotransformation between bound and soluble phenolics. Thus, fermentation in legumes increases the bioavailability of polyphenols [99]. In four underutilized legumes (pigeon pea, Bambara groundnut, African yam bean, and kidney bean), a 4-day fermentation period increased the free soluble phenol content, whereas the bound phenolics were decreased. Free soluble phenolic compounds from fermented samples had a significantly higher reducing power, free radical scavenging ability, and inhibition of lipid peroxidation than the unfermented samples, confirming that fermentation led to enhanced antioxidant activity in the legumes [100]. Thus, in both cases, fermentation led to products with better nutrient profiles and antioxidant characteristics.

As observed in the case of heat treatment, the variety determines how fermentation affects polyphenol compounds as well. Fermentation of five different varieties of apple juice led to variable changes in the phenolic profile. In the three varieties, the levels of total phenolics remained the same after the process; however, in two of them, they decreased [101].

However, studies assessing the role of fermentation in improving red grape polyphenol bioavailability have indicated that fermentation may play a minor role. In a trial involving nine volunteers ingesting equal amounts of red wine and red grape juice (resulting in almost equal concentrations of anthocyanins), the authors observed higher urinary excretion of total anthocyanins in the case of juice (0.23%) than in wine (0.18%). They also reported that urinary recovery of five individual anthocyanins was different between the two grape products, without reaching significance in both. Thus, they suggested that these results might be because of the presence of ethanol in red wine [102]. This was not confirmed by Bub et al. [103], who compared the absorption of malvidin-3-glucoside between red grape juice, red wine, and dealcoholized red wine. The bioavailability of this compound was similar when volunteers consumed regular wine or those without alcohol; however, it was two-fold higher in the case of juice consumption. According to these results, it cannot be concluded that the ethanol produced by fermentation affects the accessibility of these red grape polyphenols.

Black tea is another fermented polyphenol-rich beverage widely consumed in the human diet. Both green and black teas are a great source of monomeric flavanols (catechins). The difference between these two types of tea is in the production process. Green tea is a product obtained by drying leaves of Camellia sinensis, while the production of black tea involves an additional fermentation step, resulting in the synthesis of oligomeric polyphenolic compounds from catechins. Thus, black tea contains lower levels of these flavanols than green tea [104]. In a trial comparing the absorption rate of catechin derived from black and green teas, the authors concluded that the tea variety did not determine the bioavailability of these flavonols. Plasma kaempferol and quercetin levels were similar in both cases, implying that fermentation did not affect the availability of polyphenols from the matrix [105].

5.4. Mechanical Processing

5.4.1. Peeling

Peeling is one of the necessary preparation steps for both industrial and domestic food processing. Peels of many fruits and vegetables contain higher concentrations of bioactive compounds than the rest of the fruit. Some of them are discarded as agro-waste and can be utilized as such for extracting these valuable compounds. For example, citrus peels are abundant in phenolic compounds, such as flavanones, flavones, flavonols, and anthocyanins [106]. Peels of some common fruits (apple, banana, mandarin, and nectarine) are sources of non-extractable polyphenols [107].

The effects of peeling on polyphenol content have been scarcely addressed in literature. In some cases, this preparation step does not considerably affect the food item's antioxidant capacity, as it is consumed without the peel, as in the case of bananas and citruses. However, it should be noted that, for example, the white layer in citruses is abundant in polyphenols; thus, a higher degree of peeling and removal of this layer would also lead to a lower polyphenol content in the consumed fruit. In addition, some fruits and vegetables can be consumed either with or without peels; thus, the difference in the polyphenol levels can be significant.

Studies have mainly focused on determining the phenolic composition and antioxidant activity of peels. However, few studies have addressed the effect of peeling on dietary polyphenols. For example, a study investigating how different heat-treatment regimes influenced onion flavonoids (quercetin and kaempferol) showed that the preprocessing step (peeling and trimming) caused the greatest loss in flavonoid content in onions (up to 39%) [108]. As onions contain multiple layers, the authors peeled only one layer in some cases and peeled several layers in other cases, resulting in a significant decrease in flavonoid content. This decrease in the flavonoid content could be because 90% of quercetin can be found in the first and second layers in onions [109].

Peeling of fruits and vegetables prior to processing was also observed to diminish phenolic bioactives. For example, peach puree containing peel tissues that underwent blanching and pasteurization had 7–11% higher antioxidant activity (measured by the β-carotene/linoleic acid assay) compared with the puree without the peel [110]. In another study, peeling caused a 13–48% loss in total phenolics in peaches, ranging between 316 and 397 mg kg^{-1} in peeled samples and between 376 and 609 mg kg^{-1} in unpeeled samples [111].

In the case of wine fermentation, there is also a big difference in whether the process is obtained with or without grape skin. Two white wine varieties were subjected to maceration at 5 °C for 24 h and further fermented with Saccharomyces bayanus BC commercial yeast. The authors reported that the total polyphenol index (representing the level of total polyphenols) and total flavonoids increased with an increase in alcohol content and the degree of fermentation. Higher increases were observed in the samples that contained skins, probably owing to a higher degree of polyphenol extraction [112].

5.4.2. Grinding

Grinding is a processing technique to reduce the size of solid particles, using mechanical forces [113]. It has been applied in the preparation of fruit and vegetable powders, spices, tea, and coffee, as well as flour production. Most studies that assessed how grinding affected polyphenol content in the raw food material showed that the extraction of these antioxidants was mostly enhanced. However, this largely depends on the particle size of the powder end-product.

Grinding of *Hieracium pilosella* L. (an invasive weed famous for its antiseptic, antibacterial, and anti-inflammatory properties) yielded powders with enhanced antioxidant capacity, which was followed by an increase in the content of identified flavonoids and phenolic acids. However, this was observed only in the case of two fractions, which implies that the granulometric class needs to be optimal to obtain the highest degree of extraction of bioactive compounds and their corresponding activity [114]. Another study explored the difference in phenolic content between three types of coffee: Turkish, Espresso, and American coffee. In the case of American and Espresso coffee, fine–coarse powder exhibited the highest total polyphenol content and corresponding antioxidant activity, while in the case of Turkish coffee, fine–coarse and coarse powders were similar. When comparing these three coffees, which differ according to the brewing method, Espresso exhibited the highest antioxidant content and capacity, followed by Turkish and American coffee [115]. In tea, the reduction in the particle size of green tea leaves led to a higher decrease in almost all catechins measured [116].

However, in some cases, the granulometric characteristics do not influence the degree of bioactive extraction caused by grinding. For example, superfine grinding of green propolis enhanced the extraction of bioactive compounds, resulting in increased total phenolic content and antioxidant activity, regardless of the particle size [117].

An overview of studies investigating the effects of the main food-processing techniques (type, procedure, food matrix, and investigated polyphenol), and their effects on polyphenols content and bioavailability/bioaccessibility were presented in Appendix A (Tables A1 and A2) respectively.

5.5. Emerging Food-Processing Technologies

Other emerging food-processing technologies, such as pulsed electric field, ultrasound treatments, high-pressure, and pulsed-light processing, have been developed in order to enhance the nutritive value, sensory properties, safety and preservation of several food components, including the improvement of polyphenol bioavailability in fruits and vegetables [45,118]. Through several physical and biochemicals changes of food components, these technologies contribute in reducing some food-related factors that impede polyphenols digestion, improving therefore their bioaccessibility and bioavailability [119]. The magnitude of these changes of the physicochemical and functional properties of food bioactive ingredients depends on the processing technology, the process parameters/conditions, and the food matrix [119,120]. Since we focused primarily on conventional food processing used at both domestic and industrial settings, these emerging technologies are beyond the scope of this review. However, it is important to investigate further their potential beneficial effects on dietary phytophenols in future studies and reviews to optimize their processing conditions according to each food matrix in order to maximize their bioaccessibility, bioavailability and health benefits.

6. Conclusions

As a large body of research evidence strongly supports the use of polyphenol-rich foods in the primary prevention and management of various chronic diseases, estimating their bioavailability is of great importance to draw straightforward conclusions regarding their actual efficacy. Since many fruits and vegetables are required to undergo food preparation prior to consumption, the summarized data regarding its influence on polyphenol content and bioavailability provide valuable insights into the actual benefits that could be obtained after consumption. Among the reviewed treatments that apply thermal processing, boiling is frequently reported to cause the most severe degradation in polyphenol content and bioavailability, mainly owing to their extensive leaching from the food matrix into the surrounding polar medium. Other treatments that utilize heat (such as canning and drying) have reported variable results. In canning, the presence of the surrounding medium plays an important role, while the intensity of the temperature regime and the duration of the process influence the end polyphenol content both when canning and drying are applied. Fermentation is reported to mainly lead to desirable changes in polyphenol content in food; however, bioavailability studies do not support the importance of fermentation in wine and black tea. Pickling can also yield products with an improved polyphenol profile, and studies have highlighted that this effect was mostly observed after an adequate fermentation period. Freezing and chilling are preservation techniques that are generally considered to produce minimal alterations in dietary polyphenols. Grinding is applied to facilitate the extraction of bioactive compounds, and this was mainly observed in polyphenols, with the particle size influencing their content. Data on the polyphenol-related effects of peeling are scarce; however, the existing evidence suggests that removing external layers can reduce the levels of polyphenols (and supposedly their bioavailability) in fruits and vegetables that contain polyphenol-rich peels (such as in the case of citruses). Although the bioavailability of polyphenols has gained popularity in the research community during the last decade, few studies have addressed this issue with regard to their bioavailability as influenced by food processing.

Funding: This research received no external funding.

Institutional Review Board Statement: Not applicable.

Informed Consent Statement: Not applicable.

Data Availability Statement: Data sharing not applicable.

Conflicts of Interest: The author declares no conflict of interest.

Appendix A

Table A1. Overview of studies investigating the food-processing effects on polyphenols content and antioxidant activity.

Food Processing	Procedure	Food Matrix	Investigated Polyphenols	Effects on Polyphenols Content and/or Antioxidant Activity	Reference
			Thermal Processing		
Heat treatment	Boiling for 60 min	Onions and asparagus	Flavonols	Flavonols decreased by 20.6% in onions and by 43.9% in asparagus. Antioxidant activity decreased by 10.65%.	[64]
	Cooking in smaller and larger amounts of water	Zucchini, beans, carrots, potatoes	Rutin (zucchini), rutin and quercitrin (beans), chlorogenic acid (carrots), caffeic acid (potatoes)	Cooking in small water volumes caused a decrease by 11.1% in rutin (zucchini), by 1.8% in rutin (beans), by 0.9% in quercetin (beans), by 25.4% in chlorogenic acid (carrots), and by 38.6% in caffeic acid (potatoes). Cooking in larger water volumes caused a decrease by 30.6% in rutin (zucchini), by 29.7% in rutin (beans), by 26.7% in quercetin (beans), by 62.8% in chlorogenic acid (carrots) and by 42.3% in caffeic acid (potatoes).	[66]
	Cooking 15 min at 100 °C	Cherry tomato	Naringenin and chlorogenic acid	NS difference in meals containing raw and cooked tomatoes, however, the content of analyzed polyphenols was higher in those with raw tomatoes.	[72]
	Microwave (900 W) cooking for 12 or 20 min	Purple carrots	Acylated and non-acylated anthocyanin content	Decrease in both acylated (by 22.93%) and non-acylated (by 22.52%) anthocyanin content.	[75]
	Pasteurization (HTST—90 °C for 30 s and PEF 4 μs bipolar pulse with an electric field strength of 35 kV/cm and a frequency of 1200 pulses per second)	Apple juice	TPC	TPC after HTST pasteurization decreased by 32.3%. TPC after PEF pasteurization decreased by 14.49%.	[71]
	Oven-roasting (180 °C/15 min and 200 °C/30 min); frying (180 °C/4 min and 180 °C/8 min); microwaving (450 W/4 min and 750 W/4 min); boiling (for 30 and 60 min)	Onions	Flavonols and anthocyanins	Quercetin diglucoside decreased after all treatments. Quercetin monoglucoside decreased after microwaving and boiling and increased after frying and oven-roasting. All anthocyanins (cyanidin 3-glucoside, cyanidin 3-laminaribioside, cyanidin 3-(6″-malonylglucoside), cyanidin 3-(6″-malonyl-laminaribioside) decreased after all treatments.	[65]

Table A1. Cont.

Food Processing	Procedure	Food Matrix	Investigated Polyphenols	Effects on Polyphenols Content and/or Antioxidant Activity	Reference
	Blanching 2.5 min at 96–98 °C and cooking 10 min at 100 °C	Kale leaves	Quercetin, kaempferol, caffeic acid, p-cumaric acid, sinapic acid, ferulic acid, total polyphenols	All analyzed compounds decreased, with more severe decrease observed in the case of cooking. Antioxidant activity decreased by 32.6% in steamed, and by 45.45% in cooked kale leaves.	[68]
	Boiling, steaming, and microwaving (700 W) for 5, 10, and 15 min	Eggplants (4 varieties)	TPC	TPC increased in all samples. Antioxidant activity increased in all samples.	[69]
	Baking (the baked product used 34 g of frozen blueberries as a polyphenol source; the comparison was carried out with a drink made by dissolving the same amount of frozen blueberries in water)	Blueberries	Total polyphenols, total anthocyanins, total procyanidins, quercetin, chlorogenic acid, caffeic acid, ferulic acid	Total polyphenols decreased but n.s. Total anthocyanins decreased significantly by 42.2% Total procyanidins increased but n.s. Quercetin increased but n.s. Chlorogenic acid increased significantly by 23.46% Caffeic acid increased but n.s. Ferulic acid increased but n.s.	[76]
	Tomato-sauce production (cooking for 60 min at 99 °C and crushing)	Tomato	Phenolic acids, flavanones and flavonols	Phenolic acids decreased by 43.18% Flavanones increased by 245.03% Flavonols increased by 17.21%	[73]
	Boiling, steaming, and microwaving	Cassava	Total extractable polyphenols	Total extractable polyphenols: increased by 152%, 236% and 164% after boiling, steaming and microwaving, respectively. Antioxidant activity: increased by 151.56%, 208.60% and 173.44% after boiling, steaming and microwaving, respectively.	[74]
	Sterilization until the temperature reached 123 °C	Runner bean	TPC	TPC decreased by 29.63% and 45.68% after 4 months and 12 months of storage, respectively. Antioxidant activity decreased by 87.89% and 89.47% after 4 months and 12 months of storage, respectively.	[70]

Table A1. Cont.

Food Processing	Procedure	Food Matrix	Investigated Polyphenols	Effects on Polyphenols Content and/or Antioxidant Activity	Reference
	Cooking in water (10 min), steaming (15 min, 97 ± 2 °C), microwaving (5 min, 800 W), and baking (15 min, 200 °C)	Sweet potatoes (2 varieties grown in Slovakia and Croatia)	TPC, TAC and phenolic acids (chlorogenic, neochlorogenic, and trans-ferulic)	TPC increased after almost all treatments and all varieties except in Beauregard from Croatia. chlorogenic acid decreased except after steaming in Beauregard from Slovakia. TAC increased in all samples. Neochlorogenic acid decreased in all samples. Trans-ferulic acid decreased in almost all samples except in boiled 414-purple from Croatia. Antioxidant activities increased in all samples.	[67]
	Canning in syrup with thermal treatment	Cherries	TAC	TAC decreased by 44.89% Antioxidant capacity decreased by 33.03% measured by FRAP assay.	[78]
	Canning in 5% brine	Peanuts	Trans-resveratrol and three conjugates, caffeic acid, luteolin, genistein, quercetin and catechin	All measured compounds (except genistein) decreased in all samples.	[80]
Canning	Canning—industrial vs. domestic thermal processing	Apricots	TPC, procyanidins, phenolic acids	TPC decreased by 13–47% in industrial setting and decrease by 2–33% in domestic setting Procyanidins decreased by 44% in industrial setting, and decreased by 2.4% in domestic setting Phenolic acids: higher decrease was observed in industrial vs. domestic cooking	[79]
	Canning of apricot pulps, followed by exhaustion under steam, and finally processed in an autoclave at 121 °C for 30 min	Apricots	Chlorogenic, neochlorogenic acid, catechin, kaempferol, quercetin, procyanidin B2	Chlorogenic acid increased by 31.31%, Neochlorogenic acid increased by 19.06%, Catechin increased by 37.19%, Kaempferol increased by 35.58%, Quercetin increased by 26.08%, Procyanidin B2 increased by 26.16% *The presented changes refer to only one variety, while two more varieties were used in the study.	[121]

Table A1. *Cont.*

Food Processing	Procedure	Food Matrix	Investigated Polyphenols	Effects on Polyphenols Content and/or Antioxidant Activity	Reference
	Canning vs. freezing (−18 °C) vs. drying (65 °C)	Apricots	Ellagic acid, gallic acid, ferulic acid, epicatechin, epigallocatechin, rutin	Ellagic acid, gallic acid, ferulic acid, epicatechin and epigallocatechin were all affected by the treatments in the following order: canning yielded the highest content, followed by freezing and drying (in all three varieties). Canning yielded the highest content in rutin, followed by freezing and drying in one variety, while in other two varieties the rutin content was the highest in the case of canning, followed by drying then freezing.	[122]
	Drying at 55 and 75 °C	Apricots (two cultivars)	Neochlorogenic, chlorogenic acid, catechin, epicatechin, rutin, quercetin-3-O-glucoside	Neochlorogenic and chlorogenic acid and catechin—decreased (higher decrease after 55 °C). Epicatechin, rutin and quercetin-3-0-glucoside—decreased (higher decrease after 75 °C). Antioxidant activity increased in one variety with higher increase after 75 °C drying.	[84]
	Drying (31–34 °C) for 8 days	Figs (2 varieties)	Total proanthocyanidin content	Total proanthocyanidin content increased in yellow figs And decreased in purple figs. Antioxidant activity (ABTS, DPPH, and FRAP assays) decreased in both varieties.	[88]
Drying	Convection-oven-drying, freeze-drying (FD), microwave-drying, and air-drying with the sun exposure and without the sun exposure	Spearmint	TPC, hydroxycinammic acid derivatives	TPC—FD gave the highest TPC, followed by air with sun exposure, without sun exposure, microwave-drying and finally convection-drying. Caffeic acid—FD gave the highest content, followed by air-drying with and then without sun, convection-oven-drying and microwave-drying. Antioxidant activity: FRAP—the highest value in FD sample, followed by air-drying with sun, without sun, convection-drying, and microwave-drying; DPPH—the highest value in FD sample, followed by air-drying with sun, without sun, while microwave-and oven-drying gave similar values.	[123]

Table A1. *Cont.*

Food Processing	Procedure	Food Matrix	Investigated Polyphenols	Effects on Polyphenols Content and/or Antioxidant Activity	Reference
	Convective hot-air-drying at 65 and 80 °C vs. freeze-drying (FD)	Murtilla fruit	TPC, TAC, gallic acid, catechin, quercetin-3-glucoside, myricetin, kaempferol, quercetin	TPC—decreased by 37.33% after 65 °C, increased by 27.24% and 90.77% after 80 °C and FD, respectively. TAC—decreased by 38.46% and 66.67%, respectively, after 65 °C and 80 °C, and increased by 71.79% after FD. Gallic acid increased in all samples Catechin increased in 80 °C and FD, decreased in 65 °C Quercetin 3-β-D-glucoside, myricetin, kaempferol—decreased in all samples Quercetin—increased in 65 °C and 80 °C, decreased in FD Antioxidant activity—increase in all samples	[124]
	Drying (70 °C, 36 h)	Tomatoes	TPC, TFC	Rutin apioside, rutin, naringenin chalcone, chlorogenic acid—decrease Naringenin—was not identified in raw, but it was in dried tomato Antioxidant activity—increase in antioxidant capacity (ABTS, DPPH, CUPRAC assays)	[87]
	Hot-air-oven-drying or freeze-drying (FD)	Pumpkin flower	Free, bound, total phenols	Free phenols—similar values in case of oven-drying and FD, bound and total phenols—higher values after oven-drying. Antioxidant activity—hot-air-oven-dried pumpkin flours had slightly higher antioxidant activities than FD pumpkin flour samples.	[89]
	Drying at 60, 70, and 80 °C, respectively, at relative humidity level of 50% for heating time ranging from 0 to 40 h	Cocoa beans	TPC	Maximum TPC at 70 °C, and it decreased with the increased drying time.	[85]
	Drying at 40, 50, and 60 °C	Cocoa beans	TPC	TPC decreased by 45% after drying at 40 °C. Higher decrease with higher temperature.	[83]

Table A1. *Cont.*

Food Processing	Procedure	Food Matrix	Investigated Polyphenols	Effects on Polyphenols Content and/or Antioxidant Activity	Reference
	Freeze-drying (FD), drying at 50 °C for 48 h, 65 °C for 20 h, or 130 °C for 2 h until a moisture 89 content below 15% was obtained	Berries	Anthocyanins (individual), TPC	Anthocyanins—FD preserved them the best, 130 °C drying degraded them. TPC—highest values obtained after 65 °C drying, followed by FD, 50 °C and 130 °C drying. Antioxidant activity: ABTS•+ radical scavenging activity and ferric-reducing power varied depending on the berry type—raspberry and boysenberry showed the highest ABTS in the case of 65°C drying and redcurrant and blackcurrant in the case of FD, the same was observed for ferric-reducing power	[86]
	Vacuum/microwave-drying (480, 120 W), hot-air-drying (70, 60, 50 °C), and combined methods, such as pre-drying and finish-drying (60 °C + 480/120 W)	Jujube fruits (3 varieties)	TPC	TPC decreased in all samples; the lowest decrease was observed in the lowest temperature regime and in the combined process. Antioxidant activity decreased in ORAC values after drying, higher decrease in the case of higher temperature; lower decrease in the case of microwave-drying. Combined treatment gave lower decrease than hot-air-drying.	[82]
	Drying at 65 °C	Apricots	Chlorogenic, neochlorogenic acid, catechin, kaempferol, quercetin, procyanidin B2	Chlorogenic acid decreased by 16.02% Neochlorogenic acid decreased by 2.52% Catechin decreased by 3.66% Kaempferol decreased by 9.20% Quercetin decreased by 11.80% Procyanidin B2 decreased by 14.57% *The presented changes refer to only one variety, while two more varieties were used in the study.	[121]
Cold Processing					
Freezing/ Chilling	Freezing at −30 °C	Red Raspberries	Total phenolics, anthocyanins, lambertianin C, sanguiin H-6, ellagic acid	There was n.s. change in all analyzed compounds.	[91]
	Individual quick-freezing process	Berries	TPC, total monomeric anthocyanins	There was n.s. change in all analyzed compounds.	[94]

Table A1. *Cont.*

Food Processing	Procedure	Food Matrix	Investigated Polyphenols	Effects on Polyphenols Content and/or Antioxidant Activity	Reference
	Freezing	Blanched/cooked kale leaves	TPC	TPC decreased by 3%. Antioxidant activity decreased by 7%	[68]
	Cooling at 5 °C in the refrigerator, or freezing at −20 °C	Maqui fruits	Polyphenol and anthocyanin concentration	Polyphenol and anthocyanin increased in both cases, with higher increase in the case of frozen samples.	[92]
	Freezing by immersion at liquid nitrogen and freeze-drying at −50 °C	Apples	TPC	TPC decreased before digestion in both freezing methods. Antioxidant activity decreased before and after digestion (ABTS, CUPRAC, and FRAP assays).	[95]
	Slow vs. quick freezing	Strawberries	TPC and total monomeric anthocyanin content	TPC and total monomeric anthocyanin content increased in the case of quick-frozen samples compared with slow frozen samples.	[93]
	Deep-freezing to −18 °C	Apricots	Chlorogenic, neochlorogenic acid, catechin, kaempferol, quercetin, procyanidin B2	Chlorogenic acid increased by 6.55% Neochlorogenic acid increased by 1.08% Catechin increased by 17.69% Kaempferol increased by 15.95% Quercetin increased by 4.35% Procyanidin B2 increased by 7.95% *The presented changes refer to only one variety, while two more varieties were used in the study.	[121]
	Freeze-drying vs. hot-air-drying vs. infrared-drying vs. pasteurization of apple puree)	Red-fleshed apples	Phenolic acids, flavan-3-ols, flavonols, anthocyanins, flavanones, dihydrochalcones	Compared with the freeze-dried snack: Infrared-drying caused important losses in most of the apple (poly)phenolics Purée pasteurization maintained 65% the (poly)phenols Hot-air-drying maintained 83% the (poly)phenols Anthocyanins were degraded to a higher extend after all thermal processing technologies.	[125]
Biochemical Processing					
	Fermentation of red grape	Red wine, dealcoholized red wine, and red grape juice	Malvidin-3-glucoside (M-3-G)	M-3-G—red wine (68 mg), dealcoholized red wine (58 mg) and red grape juice 117 mg	[103]

Table A1. Cont.

Food Processing	Procedure	Food Matrix	Investigated Polyphenols	Effects on Polyphenols Content and/or Antioxidant Activity	Reference
Fermentation	Black-tea fermentation	Black vs. green tea	Quercetin, kaempferol	Eight cups of black tea (4 g tea solids) provided 108 µmol of quercetin glycosides (equivalent to 32.5 mg as free quercetin) and 72 µmol of kaempferol glycosides. The green tea (4 g tea solids) provided 104 µmol of quercetin glycosides and 58 µmol of kaempferol glycosides per day.	[105]
	Fermentation (red-wine production)—comparison between red wine and red grape juice	Red grape	Anthocyanins	Total anthocyanin content was almost equal in both red grape juice and red wine.	[102]
	Fermentation to apple cider	Apple (5 varieties)	TPC, catechin, caffeic acid	TPC decreased only in two varieties. Catechin increased in all varieties Caffeic acid increased in two varieties	[101]
	Natural fermentation	Legumes—pigeon pea, bambara groundnut, African yam bean, and kidney bean	Free and bound soluble phenol content	Free soluble phenol content increased, Bound phenol content decreased Antioxidant activity: free soluble phenolic compounds of fermented legumes had increased reducing power, free radical scavenging ability, and inhibition of lipid peroxidation compared with unfermented legumes.	[100]
	Fermentation with naturally present bacteria and with lactic acid bacteria	Eight legumes: black cow gram, mottled cowpea, speckled kidney bean, lentil, small rice bean, small runner bean and two soya beans	TPC	TPC increased in almost all samples Antioxidant activity increased in mottled cowpea, speckled kidney bean and small rice bean, and n.s. changes in all other samples.	[99]
	Fermentation with *Aspergillus awamori*	Millet	TPC	TPC—increase (more than 2-fold) Antioxidant activity (measured both by DPPH and ABTS assays)—slight increase by 3.75% and by 2.12%	[98]
	Ting fermentation (at different time and temperature regimes)	Sorghum	TPC, total flavonoid and total tannin content	All analyzed compounds—optimal values at 27 °C for 72 h Antioxidant activity—the best one was obtained in a sample fermented at 27 °C for 24 h	[97]

Table A1. Cont.

Food Processing	Procedure	Food Matrix	Investigated Polyphenols	Effects on Polyphenols Content and/or Antioxidant Activity	Reference
	Lactic acid fermentation (milk enriched with dates)	Two types of yoghurt enriched with dates	TPC and antioxidant activity	TPC: 34 and 37 mg of GAE 100 g^{-1} for, respectively, yogurt made with dates blended with milk and yogurt produced using small pieces of dates that were added to milk. Antioxidant activity (measured by DDPH) was 51% and 57% for yogurt made with dates blended with milk and yogurt produced using small pieces of dates that were added to milk, respectively.	[126]
	Pickling (with variable salinity and the addition of *Lactobacillus plantarum*)	Potherb mustard	The total free phenolic acids, the total phenolic acids, total phenolics	Total free phenolic acids increased. Total phenolics and total phenolic acids decreased. Antioxidant activity decreased by 35%.	[127]
	Pickling	Papaya	TPC, TFC	TPC decreased by 68.40% TFC decreased by 65.90% Antioxidant activity (DDPH assay) decreased.	[128]
Pickling	Pickling	Green beans, green pepper, chili pepper, white cabbage, cauliflower, cucumber, sneak melon, tomato, carrot, garlic	TPC	TPC—after 15 days—decreased in all vegetable; after 30 and 60 days increased in all vegetables. Antioxidant activity: the Trolox equivalent antioxidant capacity decreased after 15 days, then increased after 30 and 60 days for green beans, green pepper, chili pepper, cauliflower, white cabbage, cucumber and sneak melon. For tomato, carrot and garlic it increased during all time points. DPPH assay: RSA decreased followed by increase in all except green pepper, cauliflower, cucumber and sneak melon which decreased during all time points.	[129]
	Pickling	Soybeans	TPC, TPA content, TFC, naringenin, and vanillin	TPC and TFC increased by 47% and 42%, respectively. TPA decreased by 35% Naringenin and vanillin increased (24 and 2.5-fold, respectively).	[130]

Table A1. *Cont.*

Food Processing	Procedure	Food Matrix	Investigated Polyphenols	Effects on Polyphenols Content and/or Antioxidant Activity	Reference
Mechanical Processing					
	Peeling, trimming and chopping	Onions	Flavonoids (quercetin and kaempferol)	Flavonoids decreased by 39%.	[108]
Peeling	Removal of periderm material in purée processing	Peaches	TPC, chlorogenic, neochlorogenic acid, catechin, caffeic acid	TPC—minor differences between the samples with and without the peel. Chlorogenic and neochlorogenic acid decreased in puree with peel (vs. puree without peels) Catechin increased in samples with peels (vs. puree without peels). Caffeic acid—slight decreased slightly in puree with peels (vs. puree without peels). Antioxidant activity: Peach puree with periderm tissue that underwent blanching and pasteurization had 7–11% higher antioxidant activity (measured by beta-carotene/linoleic acid assay).	[110]
	Peeling	Clingstone peaches	TPC	TPC decreased by 13–48%	[111]
	Fermentation with *Saccharomyces bayanus* BC (with and without skins)	White grape	Total polyphenol index, total flavonoids	Total polyphenol index increased especially in grapes with skins. Total flavonoids decreased in samples without skins, while they increased in samples with skins.	[112]
	Superfine grinding (included sieving through a 180 µm sieve once, or for 20–120 min)	Green tea	Catechins	Catechins decreased in all analyzed catechins Antioxidant activity increased in OH scavenging rate between the sample that was once sieved through a 180 µm sieve and those that underwent sieving for 20–120 min.	[116]
Grinding	Grinding and sieving	*Hieracium pilosella* L.	Flavonoids and phenolic acids	Increase in luteolin-7-glucoside, umbelliferone, luteolin, 3,5-dicaffeoylquinic acid, and chlorogenic acid (the maximum values in the case of 180–315 and 315–500 µm). Antioxidant activity increased in sieved samples (the maximum activity obtained at 180–315 and 315–500 µm).	[114]

Table A1. Cont.

Food Processing	Procedure	Food Matrix	Investigated Polyphenols	Effects on Polyphenols Content and/or Antioxidant Activity	Reference
	Grinding to produce American, Turkish, and Espresso coffees	Coffee beans	TPC	TPC—the highest observed in the case of fine–coarse powder. Further grinding decreased TPC. Antioxidant activity—the highest observed in the case of fine–coarse powder. Further grinding decreased the antioxidant activity (DPPH assay).	[115]
	Superfine grinding method	Brazilian green propolis	TPC	TPC increased (regardless of the particle size) Antioxidant activity increased (measured by ABTS and DPPH, regardless of the particle size)	[117]

Abbreviations: TPC—total phenolic content; TAC—total anthocyanin content; TPA—total phenolic acid content; TFC—total flavonoid content; sig—significant; n.s.—non significant; DPPH—2,2-diphenyl-1-picrylhydrazyl; ABTS—2,2′-azino-bis(3-ethylbenzothiazoline-6-sulfonic acid; HSTS—high-temperature short-time; PEF—pulsed electric field; FRAP—ferric reducing antioxidant power; CUPRAC—cupric-reducing antioxidant capacity; GAE—gallic acid equivalent; RSA—radical scavenging activity.

Table A2. Overview of studies investigating the food-processing effects on polyphenols bioavailability/bioaccessibility.

Food Processing	Procedure	Food Matrix	Investigated Polyphenols	Type of Study	Effects on Polyphenols on Bioavailability/Bioaccessibility	Reference
Heat treatment	Cooking 15 min at 100 °C	Cherry tomato	Naringenin and chlorogenic acid	In vivo crossover human study on 5 subjects	Plasma naringenin increased 2 h after consumption Plasma chlorogenic acid increased 2 and 6 h after consumption	[72]
	Microwave (900 W) cooking for 12 or 20 min	Purple carrots	Acylated and non-acylated anthocyanin content	In vivo crossover human study, 12 subjects	Acylation of anthocyanins: 11–14-fold decreased in anthocyanin recovery in urine and an 8–10-fold decreased in anthocyanin recovery in plasma. Cooking increased the recovery of non-acylated anthocyanins but not acylated anthocyanins.	[75]
	Baking by using 34 g of frozen blueberries as a polyphenol source and comparison with blueberry drink.	Blueberries	Total polyphenols, total anthocyanins, total procyanidins, quercetin, chlorogenic acid, caffeic acid, ferulic acid	In vivo crossover human RCT, 10 subjects	AUC of phenolic metabolites were compared between baked product and blueberry drink—increase in m-hydroxyphenylacetic, ferulic, isoferulic, and hydroxyhippuric acids and decrease in hippuric, benzoic, salicylic, and sinapic acids.	[76]

Table A2. Cont.

Food Processing	Procedure	Food Matrix	Investigated Polyphenols	Type of Study	Effects on Polyphenols on Bioavailability/Bioaccessibility	Reference
	Tomato sauce production (boiling for 60 min at 99 °C and crushing)	Tomato	Phenolic acids, flavanones and flavonols	In vivo crossover human RCT with 8 subjects	Increase of plasma concentration and urinary excretion of naringenin glucuronide.	[73]
	Thermal treatment at 90 °C for 60 s	Orange, kiwi, pineapple and mango juices	Total phenolic acids, total flavonoids, TPC	In vitro gastrointestinal digestion model	Bioaccessability of total phenolic acids decreased by 12.70% compared with the control sample Bioaccessability of total flavonoids increased by 2.65% compared with the control sample Bioaccessability of TPC decreased by 4.17% compared with the control sample	[131]
	Heating at 80 and 90 °C for 30 s	Apple, orange and grape juice	Total Polyphenols	In vitro gastrointestinal digestion model	Bioaccessibility of total polyphenols in heated apple juices did not change compared to the control juice. Bioaccessibility of total polyphenols in grape juice increased by 33.9% and 27.3% for those treated at 80 and 90 °C, respectively. Bioaccessibility of total polyphenols in orange juice increased by 19% and 29.2% for samples heated at 80 and 80 °C, respectively.	[132]
	Boiling, steaming, microwaving	Cassava	Total extractable polyphenols	In vitro gastrointestinal digestion model	Bioaccessibility for total extractable polyphenols was 72.94% after boiling, 74.54% after steaming, and 72.67% after microwaving Bioaccessibility for antioxidative activity was 34.78% after boiling, 36.71% after steaming and 36.85% after microwaving	[74]
	Drying (31–34 °C) for 8 days	Figs (2 varieties)	Total proanthocyanidin content	In vitro simulated gastrointestinal digestion model	Increase in bioaccessibility of total proanthocyanidins and chlorogenic acid content and decrease in anthocyanin bioaccessibility.	[88]
Drying	Drying (70 °C, 36 h)	Tomatoes	TPC, TFC	In vitro gastrointestinal digestion model	Compared with raw tomatoes, dried tomatoes had higher TPC and TFC values during digestion.	[87]
	Hot-air-oven-drying or Freeze-drying	Pumpkin flower	Free, bound, total phenols	In vitro digestion enzymatic extraction method	Phenolic bioaccessibility for oven-dried sample was 30.76% and for freeze-drying it was 29.19%.	[89]

Table A2. *Cont.*

Food Processing	Procedure	Food Matrix	Investigated Polyphenols	Type of Study	Effects on Polyphenols on Bioavailability/Bioaccessibility	Reference
	Freeze-drying vs. hot-air-drying vs. infrared-drying (35, 40, 50, and 60 °C) vs. pasteurization of apple puree	Apples puree	Total polyphenols	In vivo human crossover study, 3 subjects	Percentage of urine excretion of total polyphenols was the highest in the case of pasteurized puree, followed by hot-air-dried and then freeze-dried samples.	[125]
Freezing	Freezing by immersion at liquid nitrogen and freeze-drying at −50 °C	Apples	TPC	In vitro gastric digestion model	Decrease in TPC during and after digestion with both freezing methods.	[95]
	Individual quick freezing (IQF) and conventional freezing (CF)	Strawberries	TPC, TFC, TAC, TMAC	In vitro gastric digestion model	Overall, after the completion of in vitro digestion, bioaccessibility values for TPC, TFC, TMAC, and TAC were found to be 94–105%, 64–91%, 47–83%, and 55–84%, respectively. TMAC from frozen strawberries was significantly more bioaccessible than that of fresh strawberries ($P < 0.05$).	[133]
	Fermentation of red grape	Red wine, dealcoholized red wine and red grape juice	Malvidin-3-glucoside (M-3-G)	In vivo, crossover human RCT, 6 subjects	The plasma levels of M-3-G was similar between all three arms.	[103]
	Black tea fermentation	Black vs. green tea	Quercetin, kaempferol	In vivo human study, 18 subjects	Quercetin and kaempferol plasma levels showed no difference between the two tea types.	[105]
Fermentation	Fermentation of red wine and red grape juice	Wine vs. red grape juice	Anthocyanins	Acute in vivo human study, 9 subjects	Total dietary anthocyanins—higher bioavailability of those from red grape juice compared to those in red wine. Low urinary excretion of dietary anthocyanins with values below 1%. Only 0.25% and 0.18% of the administered dose of total anthocyanins was excreted within 7 h after red grape juice and red wine ingestion, respectively.	[102]

Table A2. *Cont.*

Food Processing	Procedure	Food Matrix	Investigated Polyphenols	Type of Study	Effects on Polyphenols on Bioavailability/Bioaccessibility	Reference
	Controlled alcoholic fermentation	Orange juice	A total of 24 (poly)phenol metabolites including both flavanone and phenolic acid derivatives	In vivo human crossover study, 9 subjects	Bioavailability of phenolic metabolites in urine in comparison with total intake of polyphenols was lower in fermented orange juice (around 46%) than in orange juice (59%).	[134]

Abbreviations: TPC—total phenolic content, TAC—total anthocyanin content, TPA—total phenolic acid content; TFC—total flavonoid content, RCT—randomized controlled trial, AUC—area under the ROC curve, M-3-G—malvidin-3-glucoside, FD—freeze-drying, TMAC—total monomeric anthocyanin content.

References

1. Duncan, M.J.; Kline, C.E.; Vandelanotte, C.; Sargent, C.; Rogers, N.L.; Di Milia, L. Cross-sectional associations between multiple lifestyle behaviors and health-related quality of life in the 10,000 Steps cohort. *PLoS ONE* **2014**, *9*, e94184. [CrossRef]
2. Tomás-Barberán, F.A.; Andrés-Lacueva, C. Polyphenols and health: Current state and progress. *J. Agric. Food Chem.* **2012**, *60*, 8773–8775. [CrossRef]
3. Afanas'ev, I.B.; Dcrozhko, A.I.; Brodskii, A.V.; Kostyuk, V.A.; Potapovitch, A.I. Chelating and free radical scavenging mechanisms of inhibitory action of rutin and quercetin in lipid peroxidation. *Biochem. Pharmacol.* **1989**, *38*, 1763–1769. [CrossRef]
4. Cory, H.; Passarelli, S.; Szeto, J.; Tamez, M.; Mattei, J. The Role of Polyphenols in Human Health and Food Systems: A Mini-Review. *Front. Nutr.* **2018**, *5*, 87. [CrossRef]
5. Caballero, B.; Allen, L.; Prentice, A. *Encyclopedia of Human Nutrition*, 2nd ed.; Academic Press: Cambridge, MA, USA, 2005; pp. 150–300.
6. Koli, R.; Erlund, I.; Jula, A.; Marniemi, J.; Mattila, P.; Alfthan, G. Bioavailability of Various Polyphenols from a Diet Containing Moderate Amounts of Berries. *J. Agric. Food Chem.* **2010**, *58*, 3927–3932. [CrossRef]
7. Ifie, I.; Marshall, L.J.; Yildiz, F. Food processing and its impact on phenolic constituents in food. *Cogent Food Agric.* **2018**, *4*, 1507782. [CrossRef]
8. Jiménez-Monreal, A.M.; García-Diz, L.; Martínez-Tomé, M.; Mariscal, M.; Murcia, M.A. Influence of cooking methods on antioxidant activity of vegetables. *J. Food Sci.* **2009**, *74*, H97–H103. [CrossRef] [PubMed]
9. Nayak, B.; Liu, R.H.; Tang, J. Effect of Processing on Phenolic Antioxidants of Fruits, Vegetables, and Grains—A Review. *Crit. Rev. Food Sci. Nutr.* **2015**, *55*, 887–918. [CrossRef] [PubMed]
10. D'Archivio, M.; Filesi, C.; Varì, R.; Scazzocchio, B.; Masella, R. Bioavailability of the polyphenols: Status and controversies. *Int. J. Mol. Sci.* **2010**, *11*, 1321–1342. [CrossRef] [PubMed]
11. Tsao, R. Chemistry and biochemistry of dietary polyphenols. *Nutrients* **2010**, *2*, 1231–1246. [CrossRef] [PubMed]
12. Haminiuk, C.W.I.; Maciel, G.M.; Plata-Oviedo, M.S.V.; Peralta, R.M. Phenolic compounds in fruits—An overview. *Int. J. Food Sci. Technol.* **2012**, *47*, 2023–2044. [CrossRef]
13. Amarowicz, R.; Carle, R.; Dongowski, G.; Durazzo, A.; Galensa, R.; Kammerer, D.; Maiani, G.; Piskula, M.K. Influence of postharvest processing and storage on the content of phenolic acids and flavonoids in foods. *Mol. Nutr Food Res.* **2009**, *53*, S151–S183. [CrossRef] [PubMed]
14. Crozier, A.; Del Rio, D.; Clifford, M.N. Bioavailability of dietary flavonoids and phenolic compounds. *Mol. Aspects Med.* **2010**, *31*, 446–467. [CrossRef] [PubMed]
15. Williams, C.A. Flavone and flavonol O-glycosides. In *Flavonoids: Chemistry, Biochemistry and Applications*; Andersen, O.M., Markham, K.R., Eds.; CRC Press: Boca Raton, FL, USA, 2006; pp. 749–856.
16. Quideau, S. *Flavonoids. Chemistry, Biochemistry and Applications*; Andersen, Ø.M., Markham, K.R., Eds.; Wiley Online Library: Hoboken, NJ, USA, 2006. [CrossRef]
17. Cardozo, L.F.; Pedruzzi, L.M.; Stenvinkel, P.; Stockler-Pinto, M.B.; Daleprane, J.B.; Leite, M., Jr.; Mafra, D. Nutritional strategies to modulate inflammation and oxidative stress pathways via activation of the master antioxidant switch Nrf2. *Biochimie* **2013**, *95*, 1525–1533. [CrossRef]
18. Siriwardhana, N.; Kalupahana, N.S.; Cekanova, M.; LeMieux, M.; Greer, B.; Moustaid-Moussa, N. Modulation of adipose tissue inflammation by bioactive food compounds. *J. Nutr. Biochem.* **2013**, *24*, 613–623. [CrossRef]
19. Wang, S.; Moustaid-Moussa, N.; Chen, L.; Mo, H.; Shastri, A.; Su, R.; Bapat, P.; Kwun, I.S.; Shen, C.L. Novel insights of dietary polyphenols and obesity. *J. Nutr. Biochem.* **2014**, *25*, 1–18. [CrossRef]
20. Bose, M.; Lambert, J.D.; Ju, J.; Reuhl, K.R.; Shapses, S.A.; Yang, C.S. The major green tea polyphenol, (-)-epigallocatechin-3-gallate, inhibits obesity, metabolic syndrome, and fatty liver disease in high-fat-fed mice. *J. Nutr.* **2008**, *138*, 1677–1683. [CrossRef]
21. Isaak, C.K.; Petkau, J.C.; Blewett, H.; Karmin, O.; Siow, Y.L. Lingonberry anthocyanins protect cardiac cells from oxidative-stress-induced apoptosis. *Can. J. Physiol. Pharmacol.* **2017**, *95*, 904–910. [CrossRef] [PubMed]
22. Rossi, A.; Serraino, I.; Dugo, P.; Di Paola, R.; Mondello, L.; Genovese, T.; Morabito, D.; Dugo, G.; Sautebin, L.; Caputi, A.P.; et al. Protective effects of anthocyanins from blackberry in a rat model of acute lung inflammation. *Free Radic. Res.* **2003**, *37*, 891–900. [CrossRef]
23. Lee, M.; Sorn, S.R.; Park, Y.; Park, H.K. Anthocyanin rich-black soybean testa improved visceral fat and plasma lipid profiles in overweight/obese Korean adults: A randomized controlled trial. *J. Med. Food* **2016**, *19*, 995–1003. [CrossRef]
24. Silveira, J.Q.; Dourado, G.K.Z.S.; Cesar, T.B. Red-fleshed sweet orange juice improves the risk factors for metabolic syndrome. *Int. J. Food Sci. Nutr.* **2015**, *66*, 830–836. [CrossRef]
25. Fisher, N.D.L.; Hughes, M.; Gerhard-Herman, M.; Hollenberg, N.K. Flavanol-rich cocoa induces nitric-oxide-dependent vasodilation in healthy humans. *J. Hypertens.* **2003**, *21*, 2281–2286. [CrossRef]
26. Argani, H.; Ghorbanihaghjo, A.; Vatankhahan, H.; Rashtchizadeh, N.; Raeisi, S.; Ilghami, H. The effect of red grape seed extract on serum paraoxonase activity in patients with mild to moderate hyperlipidemia. *Sao Paulo Med. J.* **2016**, *134*, 234–239. [CrossRef] [PubMed]

27. Brüll, V.; Burak, C.; Stoffel-Wagner, B.; Wolffram, S.; Nickenig, G.; Müller, C.; Langguth, P.; Alteheld, B.; Fimmers, R.; Naaf, S.; et al. Effects of a quercetin-rich onion skin extract on 24 h ambulatory blood pressure and endothelial function in overweight-to-obese patients with (pre-)hypertension: A randomised double-blinded placebo-controlled cross-over trial. *Br. J. Nutr.* **2015**, *114*, 1263–1277. [CrossRef]
28. Choi, E.Y.; Lee, H.; Woo, J.S.; Jang, H.H.; Hwang, S.J.; Kim, H.S.; Kim, W.S.; Kim, Y.S.; Choue, R.; Cha, Y.J.; et al. Effect of onion peel extract on endothelial function and endothelial progenitor cells in overweight and obese individuals. *Nutrition* **2015**, *31*, 1131–1135. [CrossRef] [PubMed]
29. Potì, F.; Santi, D.; Spaggiari, G.; Zimetti, F.; Zanotti, I. Polyphenol health effects on cardiovascular and neurodegenerative disorders: A review and meta-analysis. *Int. J. Mol. Sci.* **2019**, *20*, 351. [CrossRef] [PubMed]
30. Hanhineva, K.; Törrönen, R.; Bondia-Pons, I.; Pekkinen, J.; Kolehmainen, M.; Mykkänen, H.; Poutanen, K. Impact of dietary polyphenols on carbohydrate metabolism. *Int. J. Mol. Sci.* **2010**, *11*, 1365–1402. [CrossRef]
31. Rienks, J.; Barbaresko, J.; Oluwagbemigun, K.; Schmid, M.; Nöthlings, U. Polyphenol exposure and risk of type 2 diabetes: Dose-response meta-analyses and systematic review of prospective cohort studies. *Am. J. Clin. Nutr.* **2018**, *108*, 49–61. [CrossRef] [PubMed]
32. Yang, W.S.; Wang, W.Y.; Fan, W.Y.; Deng, Q.; Wang, X. Tea consumption and risk of type 2 diabetes: A dose-response meta-analysis of cohort studies. *Br. J. Nutr.* **2014**, *111*, 1329–1339. [CrossRef] [PubMed]
33. Wang, P.Y.; Fang, J.C.; Gao, Z.H.; Zhang, C.; Xie, S.Y. Higher intake of fruits, vegetables or their fiber reduces the risk of type 2 diabetes: A meta-analysis. *J. Diabetes Investig.* **2016**, *7*, 56–69. [CrossRef]
34. Gowd, V.; Xie, L.; Sun, C.; Chen, W. Phenolic profile of bayberry followed by simulated gastrointestinal digestion and gut microbiota fermentation and its antioxidant potential in HepG2 cells. *J. Funct. Foods* **2020**, *70*, 103987. [CrossRef]
35. Briguglio, G.; Costa, C.; Pollicino, M.; Giambò, F.; Catania, S.; Fenga, C. Polyphenols in cancer prevention: New insights (Review). *Int. J. Funct. Nutr.* **2020**, *1*, 9. [CrossRef]
36. Christensen, K.Y.; Naidu, A.; Parent, M.É.; Pintos, J.; Abrahamowicz, M.; Siemiatycki, J.; Koushik, A. The risk of lung cancer related to dietary intake of flavonoids. *Nutr. Cancer* **2012**, *64*, 964–974. [CrossRef] [PubMed]
37. Woo, H.D.; Lee, J.; Choi, I.J.; Kim, C.G.; Lee, J.Y.; Kwon, O.; Kim, J. Dietary flavonoids and gastric cancer risk in a Korean population. *Nutrients* **2014**, *6*, 4961–4973. [CrossRef] [PubMed]
38. Hoensch, H.; Groh, B.; Edler, L.; Kirch, W. Prospective cohort comparison of flavonoid treatment in patients with resected colorectal cancer to prevent recurrence. *World J. Gastroenterol.* **2008**, *14*, 2187–2193. [CrossRef] [PubMed]
39. Zhang, G.; Wang, Y.; Zhang, Y.; Wan, X.; Li, J.; Liu, K.; Wang, F.; Liu, Q.; Yang, C.; Yu, P.; et al. Anti-Cancer Activities of Tea Epigallocatechin-3-Gallate in Breast Cancer Patients under Radiotherapy. *Curr. Mol. Med.* **2012**, *12*, 163–176. [CrossRef] [PubMed]
40. Grosso, G.; Micek, A.; Marranzano, M.; Mistretta, A.; Giovannucci, E.L. Dietary polyphenols and cancer incidence: A comprehensive meta-analysis. *Eur. J. Public Health* **2015**, *25*, ckv175.177. [CrossRef]
41. Flanagan, E.; Müller, M.; Hornberger, M.; Vauzour, D. Impact of Flavonoids on Cellular and Molecular Mechanisms Underlying Age-Related Cognitive Decline and Neurodegeneration. *Curr. Nutr. Rep.* **2018**, *7*, 49–57. [CrossRef] [PubMed]
42. Bell, L.; Lamport, D.J.; Butler, L.T.; Williams, C.M. A review of the cognitive effects observed in humans following acute supplementation with flavonoids, and their associated mechanisms of action. *Nutrients* **2015**, *7*, 10290–10306. [CrossRef]
43. Evans, H.M.; Howe, P.R.C.; Wong, R.H.X. Effects of resveratrol on cognitive performance, mood and cerebrovascular function in post-menopausal women; A 14-week randomised placebo-controlled intervention trial. *Nutrients* **2017**, *9*, 27. [CrossRef] [PubMed]
44. Heaney, R.P. Factors influencing the measurement of bioavailability, taking calcium as a model. *J. Nutr.* **2001**, *131*, 1344S–1348S. [CrossRef]
45. Ribas-Agustí, A.; Martín-Belloso, O.; Soliva-Fortuny, R.; Elez-Martínez, P. Food processing strategies to enhance phenolic compounds bioaccessibility and bioavailability in plant-based foods. *Crit. Rev. Food Sci. Nutr.* **2018**, *58*, 2531–2548. [CrossRef] [PubMed]
46. Holst, B.; Williamson, G. Nutrients and phytochemicals: From bioavailability to bioefficacy beyond antioxidants. *Curr. Opin. Biotechnol.* **2008**, *19*, 73–82. [CrossRef] [PubMed]
47. Courraud, J.; Berger, J.; Cristol, J.P.; Avallone, S. Stability and bioaccessibility of different forms of carotenoids and vitamin A during in vitro digestion. *Food Chem.* **2013**, *136*, 871–877. [CrossRef] [PubMed]
48. Rein, M.J.; Renouf, M.; Cruz-Hernandez, C.; Actis-Goretta, L.; Thakkar, S.K.; da Silva Pinto, M. Bioavailability of bioactive food compounds: A challenging journey to bioefficacy. *Br. J. Clin. Pharmacol.* **2013**, *75*, 588–602. [CrossRef]
49. Carbonell-Capella, J.M.; Buniowska, M.; Barba, F.J.; Esteve, M.J.; Frígola, A. Analytical methods for determining bioavailability and bioaccessibility of bioactive compounds from fruits and vegetables: A review. *Compr. Rev. Food Sci. Food Saf.* **2014**, *13*, 155–171. [CrossRef] [PubMed]
50. Manach, C.; Scalbert, A.; Morand, C.; Rémésy, C.; Jiménez, L. Polyphenols: Food sources and bioavailability. *Am. J. Clin. Nutr.* **2004**, *79*, 727–747. [CrossRef]
51. Aura, A.-M.; Martin-Lopez, P.; O'Leary, K.A.; Williamson, G.; Oksman-Caldentey, K.-M.; Poutanen, K.; Santos-Buelga, C. In vitro metabolism of anthocyanins by human gut microflora. *Eur. J. Nutr.* **2005**, *44*, 133–142. [CrossRef]
52. Day, A.J.; Bao, Y.; Morgan, M.R.; Williamson, G. Conjugation position of quercetin glucuronides and effect on biological activity. *Free Radic. Biol. Med.* **2000**, *29*, 1234–1243. [CrossRef]

53. Inada, K.O.P.; Silva, T.B.R.; Lobo, L.A.; Domingues, R.M.C.P.; Perrone, D.; Monteiro, M. Bioaccessibility of phenolic compounds of jaboticaba (Plinia jaboticaba) peel and seed after simulated gastrointestinal digestion and gut microbiota fermentation. *J. Funct. Foods* **2020**, *67*, 103851. [CrossRef]
54. Karakaya, S. Bioavailability of Phenolic Compounds. *Crit. Rev. Food Sci. Nutr.* **2004**, *44*, 453–464. [CrossRef]
55. Prior, R.L.; Wu, X. Anthocyanins: Structural characteristics that result in unique metabolic patterns and biological activities. *Free Radic. Res.* **2006**, *40*, 1014–1028. [CrossRef] [PubMed]
56. Hollands, W.; Brett, G.M.; Radreau, P.; Saha, S.; Teucher, B.; Bennett, R.N.; Kroon, P.A. Processing blackcurrants dramatically reduces the content and does not enhance the urinary yield of anthocyanins in human subjects. *Food Chem.* **2008**, *108*, 869–878. [CrossRef] [PubMed]
57. Kahle, K.; Huemmer, W.; Kempf, M.; Scheppach, W.; Erk, T.; Richling, E. Polyphenols are intensively metabolized in the human gastrointestinal tract after apple juice consumption. *J. Agric. Food Chem.* **2007**, *55*, 10605–10614. [CrossRef] [PubMed]
58. Serrano, J.; Puupponen-Pimiä, R.; Dauer, A.; Aura, A.M.; Saura-Calixto, F. Tannins: Current knowledge of food sources, intake, bioavailability and biological effects. *Mol. Nutr. Food Res.* **2009**, *53*, S310–S329. [CrossRef] [PubMed]
59. Pandey, K.B.; Rizvi, S.I. Plant polyphenols as dietary antioxidants in human health and disease. *Oxid. Med. Cell. Longev.* **2009**, *2*, 270–278. [CrossRef]
60. Rothwell, J.A.; Medina-Remón, A.; Pérez-Jiménez, J.; Neveu, V.; Knaze, V.; Slimani, N.; Scalbert, A. Effects of food processing on polyphenol contents: A systematic analysis using Phenol-Explorer data. *Mol. Nutr. Food Res.* **2015**, *59*, 160–170. [CrossRef] [PubMed]
61. Peleg, H.; Naim, M.; Rouseff, R.L.; Zehavi, U. Distribution of bound and free phenolic acids in oranges (*Citrus sinensis*) and Grapefruits (*Citrus paradisi*). *J. Sci. Food Agric.* **1991**, *57*, 417–426. [CrossRef]
62. Minatel, I.O.; Borges, C.V.; Ferreira, M.I.; Gomez, H.A.G.; Chen, C.-Y.O.; Lima, G.P.P. Phenolic Compounds: Functional Properties, Impact of Processing and Bioavailability. *Phenolic Compd. Biol. Act.* **2017**. [CrossRef]
63. Miglio, C.; Chiavaro, E.; Visconti, A.; Fogliano, V.; Pellegrini, N. Effects of different cooking methods on nutritional and physicochemical characteristics of selected vegetables. *J. Agric. Food Chem.* **2008**, *56*, 139–147. [CrossRef]
64. Makris, D.P.; Rossiter, J.T. Domestic processing of onion bulbs (*Allium cepa*) and asparagus spears (*Asparagus officinalis*): Effect on flavonol content and antioxidant status. *J. Agric. Food Chem.* **2001**, *49*, 3216–3222. [CrossRef] [PubMed]
65. Rodrigues, A.S.; Pérez-Gregorio, M.R.; García-Falcón, M.S.; Simal-Gándara, J. Effect of curing and cooking on flavonols and anthocyanins in traditional varieties of onion bulbs. *Food Res. Int.* **2009**, *42*, 1331–1336. [CrossRef]
66. Andlauer, W.; Stumpf, C.; Hubert, M.; Rings, A.; Fürst, P. Influence of cooking process on phenolic marker compounds of vegetables. *Int. J. Vitam. Nutr. Res.* **2003**, *73*, 152–159. [CrossRef]
67. Musilova, J.; Lidikova, J.; Vollmannova, A.; Frankova, H.; Urminska, D.; Bojnanska, T.; Toth, T. Influence of Heat Treatments on the Content of Bioactive Substances and Antioxidant Properties of Sweet Potato (*Ipomoea batatas* L.) Tubers. *J. Food Qual.* **2020**, *2020*, 8856260. [CrossRef]
68. Korus, A.; Lisiewska, Z. Effect of preliminary processing and method of preservation on the content of selected antioxidative compounds in kale (*Brassica oleracea* L. var. *acephala*) leaves. *Food Chem.* **2011**, *129*, 149–154. [CrossRef]
69. Chumyam, A.; Whangchai, K.; Jungklang, J.; Faiyue, B.; Saengnil, K. Effects of heat treatments on antioxidant capacity and total phenolic content of four cultivars of purple skin eggplants. *ScienceAsia* **2013**, *39*, 246–251. [CrossRef]
70. Wołosiak, R.; Druzynska, B.; Piecyk, M.; Majewska, E.; Worobiej, E. Effect of sterilization process and storage on the antioxidative properties of runner bean. *Molecules* **2018**, *23*, 1409. [CrossRef] [PubMed]
71. Aguilar-Rosas, S.F.; Ballinas-Casarrubias, M.L.; Nevarez-Moorillon, G.V.; Martin-Belloso, O.; Ortega-Rivas, E. Thermal and pulsed electric fields pasteurization of apple juice: Effects on physicochemical properties and flavour compounds. *J. Food Eng.* **2007**, *83*, 41–46. [CrossRef]
72. Bugianesi, R.; Salucci, M.; Leonardi, C.; Ferracane, R.; Catasta, G.; Azzini, E.; Maiani, G. Effect of domestic cooking on human bioavailability of naringenin, chlorogenic acid, lycopene and β-carotene in cherry tomatoes. *Eur. J. Nutr.* **2004**, *43*, 360–366. [CrossRef]
73. Martínez-Huélamo, M.; Tulipani, S.; Estruch, R.; Escribano, E.; Illán, M.; Corella, D.; Lamuela-Raventós, R.M. The tomato sauce making process affects the bioaccessibility and bioavailability of tomato phenolics: A pharmacokinetic study. *Food Chem.* **2015**, *173*, 864–872. [CrossRef]
74. De Lima, A.C.S.; da Rocha Viana, J.D.; de Sousa Sabino, L.B.; da Silva, L.M.R.; da Silva, N.K.V.; de Sousa, P.H.M. Processing of three different cooking methods of cassava: Effects on in vitro bioaccessibility of phenolic compounds and antioxidant activity. *LWT Food Sci. Technol.* **2017**, *76*, 253–258. [CrossRef]
75. Kurilich, A.C.; Clevidence, B.A.; Britz, S.J.; Simon, P.W.; Novotny, J.A. Plasma and urine responses are lower for acylated vs nonacylated anthocyanins from raw and cooked purple carrots. *J. Agric. Food Chem.* **2005**, *53*, 6537–6542. [CrossRef]
76. Rodriguez-Mateos, A.; del Pino-García, R.; George, T.W.; Vidal-Diez, A.; Heiss, C.; Spencer, J.P.E. Impact of processing on the bioavailability and vascular effects of blueberry (poly)phenols. *Mol. Nutr. Food Res.* **2014**, *58*, 1952–1961. [CrossRef] [PubMed]
77. Vergara-Balderas, F.T. Canning: Process of Canning. In *Encyclopedia of Food and Health*; Caballero, B., Finglas, P.M., Toldra, F., Eds.; Elsevier Inc.: Amsterdam, The Netherlands, 2016; pp. 628–632.
78. Chaovanalikit, A.; Wrolstad, R.E. Anthocyanin and Polyphenolic Composition of Fresh and Processed Cherries. *J. Food Sci.* **2004**, *69*, FCT73–FCT83. [CrossRef]

79. Le Bourvellec, C.; Gouble, B.; Bureau, S.; Reling, P.; Bott, R.; Ribas-Agusti, A.; Audergon, J.M.; Renard, C.M.G.C. Impact of canning and storage on apricot carotenoids and polyphenols. *Food Chem.* **2018**, *240*, 615–625. [CrossRef] [PubMed]
80. Chukwumah, Y.; Walker, L.; Ogutu, S.; Wambura, P.; Verghese, M. Effect of canning and storage on the phenolic composition of peanuts. *J. Food Process. Preserv.* **2013**, *37*, 582–588. [CrossRef]
81. Sontakke, M.S.; Salve, S.P. Solar Drying Technologies: A Review. *Int. Refereed J. Eng. Sci.* **2015**, *4*, 29–35.
82. Wojdyło, A.; Lech, K.; Nowicka, P.; Hernandez, F.; Figiel, A.; Carbonell-Barrachina, A.A. Influence of different drying techniques on phenolic compounds, antioxidant capacity and colour of ziziphus jujube mill. Fruits. *Molecules* **2019**, *24*, 2361. [CrossRef] [PubMed]
83. Alean, J.; Chejne, F.; Rojano, B. Degradation of polyphenols during the cocoa drying process. *J. Food Eng.* **2016**, *189*, 99–105. [CrossRef]
84. Madrau, M.A.; Piscopo, A.; Sanguinetti, A.M.; Del Caro, A.; Poiana, M.; Romeo, F.V.; Piga, A. Effect of drying temperature on polyphenolic content and antioxidant activity of apricots. *Eur. Food Res. Technol.* **2009**, *228*, 441–448. [CrossRef]
85. Abhay, S.; Hii, C.; Law, C.; Suzannah, S.; Djaeni, M. Effect of hot-air drying temperature on the polyphenol content and the sensory properties of cocoa beans. *Int. Food Res. J.* **2016**, *23*, 1479–1484.
86. Bustos, M.C.; Rocha-Parra, D.; Sampedro, I.; De Pascual-Teresa, S.; León, A.E. The Influence of Different Air-Drying Conditions on Bioactive Compounds and Antioxidant Activity of Berries. *J. Agric. Food Chem.* **2018**, *66*, 2714–2723. [CrossRef]
87. Kamiloglu, S.; Demirci, M.; Selen, S.; Toydemir, G.; Boyacioglu, D.; Capanoglu, E. Home processing of tomatoes (*Solanum lycopersicum*): Effects on in vitro bioaccessibility of total lycopene, phenolics, flavonoids, and antioxidant capacity. *J. Sci. Food Agric.* **2014**, *94*, 2225–2233. [CrossRef]
88. Kamiloglu, S.; Capanoglu, E. Investigating the in vitro bioaccessibility of polyphenols in fresh and sun-dried figs (*Ficus carica* L.). *Int. J. Food Sci. Technol.* **2013**, *48*, 2621–2629. [CrossRef]
89. Aydin, E.; Gocmen, D. The influences of drying method and metabisulfite pre-treatment onthe color, functional properties and phenolic acids contents and bioaccessibility of pumpkin flour. *LWT Food Sci. Technol.* **2015**, *60*, 385–392. [CrossRef]
90. Tucker, G.S. *Food Biodeterioration and Preservation*; Blackwell Publishing: Hoboken, NJ, USA, 2008; pp. 81–135.
91. Mullen, W.; Stewart, A.J.; Lean, M.E.J.; Gardner, P.; Duthie, G.G.; Crozier, A. Effect of freezing and storage on the phenolics, ellagitannins, flavonoids, and antioxidant capacity of red raspberries. *J. Agric. Food Chem.* **2002**, *50*, 5197–5201. [CrossRef] [PubMed]
92. González, B.; Vogel, H.; Razmilic, I.; Wolfram, E. Polyphenol, anthocyanin and antioxidant content in different parts of maqui fruits (Aristotelia chilensis) during ripening and conservation treatments after harvest. *Ind. Crop. Prod.* **2015**, *76*, 158–165. [CrossRef]
93. Yanat, M.; Baysal, T. Effect of freezing rate and storage time on quality parameters of strawberry frozen in modified and home type freezer. *Hrvat. Čas. Prehrambenu Tehnol. Biotehnol. Nutr.* **2018**, *13*, 154–158. [CrossRef]
94. Poiana, M.A.; Moigradean, D.; Raba, D.; Aida, L.M.; Popa, M. The effect of long-term frozen storage on the nutraceutical compounds, antioxidant properties and color indices of different kinds of berries. *J. Food Agric. Environ.* **2010**, *1*, 54–58.
95. Dalmau, M.E.; Bornhorst, G.M.; Eim, V.; Rosselló, C.; Simal, S. Effects of freezing, freeze drying and convective drying on in vitro gastric digestion of apples. *Food Chem.* **2017**, *215*, 7–16. [CrossRef]
96. Van Boekel, M.; Fogliano, V.; Pellegrini, N.; Stanton, C.; Scholz, G.; Lalljie, S.; Somoza, V.; Knorr, D.; Jasti, P.R.; Eisenbrand, G. A review on the beneficial aspects of food processing. *Mol. Nutr. Food Res.* **2010**, *54*, 1215–1247. [CrossRef]
97. Adebo, O.A.; Njobeh, P.B.; Adebiyi, J.A.; Kayitesi, E. Co-influence of fermentation time and temperature on physicochemical properties, bioactive components and microstructure of ting (a Southern African food) from whole grain sorghum. *Food Biosci.* **2018**, *25*, 118–127. [CrossRef]
98. Salar, R.K.; Purewal, S.S.; Bhatti, M.S. Optimization of extraction conditions and enhancement of phenolic content and antioxidant activity of pearl millet fermented with Aspergillus awamori MTCC-548. *Resour. Effic. Technol.* **2016**, *2*, 148–157. [CrossRef]
99. Gan, R.-Y.; Shah, N.P.; Wang, M.-F.; Lui, W.-Y.; Corke, H. Fermentation alters antioxidant capacity and polyphenol distribution in selected edible legumes. *Int. J. Food Sci. Technol.* **2016**, *51*, 875–884. [CrossRef]
100. Oboh, G.; Ademiluyi, A.O.; Akindahunsi, A.A. Changes in Polyphenols Distribution and Antioxidant Activity during Fermentation of Some Underutilized Legumes. *Food Sci. Technol. Int.* **2009**, *15*, 41–46. [CrossRef]
101. Nogueira, A.; Guyot, S.; Marnet, N.; Lequéré, J.M.; Drilleau, J.F.; Wosiacki, G. Effect of alcoholic fermentation in the content of phenolic compounds in cider processing. *Braz. Arch. Biol. Technol.* **2008**, *51*, 1025–1032. [CrossRef]
102. Frank, T.; Netzel, M.; Strass, G.; Bitsch, R.; Bitsch, I. Bioavailability of anthocyanidin-3-glucosides following consumption of red wine and red grape juice. *Can. J. Physiol. Pharmacol.* **2003**, *81*, 423–435. [CrossRef]
103. Bub, A.; Watzl, B.; Heeb, D.; Rechkemmer, G.; Briviba, K. Malvidin-3-glucoside bioavailability in humans after ingestion of red wine, dealcoholized red wine and red grape juice. *Eur. J. Nutr.* **2001**, *40*, 113–120. [CrossRef]
104. Balentine, D.A.; Wiseman, S.A.; Bouwens, L.C.M. The chemistry of tea flavonoids. *Crit. Rev. Food Sci. Nutr.* **1997**, *37*, 693–704. [CrossRef] [PubMed]
105. Hollman, P.C.H.; Hof, K.H.V.H.; Tijburg, L.B.M.; Katan, M.B. Addition of milk does not affect the absorption of flavonols from tea in man. *Free Radic. Res.* **2001**, *34*, 297–300. [CrossRef]
106. Rafiq, S.; Kaul, R.; Sofi, S.A.; Bashir, N.; Nazir, F.; Ahmad Nayik, G. Citrus peel as a source of functional ingredient: A review. *J. Saudi Soc. Agric. Sci.* **2018**, *17*, 351–358. [CrossRef]

107. Pérez-Jiménez, J.; Saura-Calixto, F. Fruit peels as sources of non-extractable polyphenols or macromolecular antioxidants: Analysis and nutritional implications. *Food Res. Int.* **2018**, *111*, 148–152. [CrossRef] [PubMed]
108. Ewald, C.; Fjelkner-Modig, S.; Johansson, K.; Sjöholm, I.; Åkesson, B. Effect of processing on major flavonoids in processed onions, green beans, and peas. *Food Chem.* **1999**, *64*, 231–235. [CrossRef]
109. Kwak, J.H.; Seo, J.M.; Kim, N.H.; Arasu, M.V.; Kim, S.; Yoon, M.K.; Kim, S.J. Variation of quercetin glycoside derivatives in three onion (*Allium cepa* L.) varieties. *Saudi J. Biol. Sci.* **2017**, *24*, 1387–1391. [CrossRef]
110. Talcott, S.T.; Howard, L.R.; Brenes, C.H. Contribution of periderm material and blanching time to the quality of pasteurized peach puree. *J. Agric. Food Chem.* **2000**, *48*, 4590–4596. [CrossRef]
111. Asami, D.K.; Hong, Y.-J.; Barrett, D.M.; Mitchell, A.E. Processing-induced changes in total phenolics and procyanidins in clingstone peaches. *J. Sci. Food Agric.* **2003**, *83*, 56–63. [CrossRef]
112. Lamçe, F.; Gozhdari, K.; Kongoli, R.; Meta, B.; Kyçyk, O. Evaluation of the content of polyphenols and flavonoids during the fermentation of white wines (cv. Pulëz and Shesh i bardhë) with and without skins. *Albanian J. Agric. Sci.* **2018**, 568–571.
113. Murthy, C.T.; Rani, M.; Rao, P.N.S. Optimal grinding characteristics of black pepper for essential oil yield. *J. Food Process. Eng.* **1999**, *22*, 161–173. [CrossRef]
114. Becker, L.; Zaiter, A.; Petit, J.; Karam, M.-C.; Sudol, M.; Baudelaire, E.; Scher, J.; Dicko, A. How do grinding and sieving impact on physicochemical properties, polyphenol content, and antioxidant activity of *Hieracium pilosella* L. powders? *J. Funct. Foods* **2017**, *35*, 666–672. [CrossRef]
115. Derossi, A.; Ricci, I.; Caporizzi, R.; Fiore, A.; Severini, C. How grinding level and brewing method (Espresso, American, Turkish) could affect the antioxidant activity and bioactive compounds in a coffee cup. *J. Sci. Food Agric.* **2018**, *98*, 3198–3207. [CrossRef]
116. Hu, J.; Chen, Y.; Ni, D. Effect of superfine grinding on quality and antioxidant property of fine green tea powders. *LWT Food Sci. Technol.* **2012**, *45*, 8–12. [CrossRef]
117. Augusto-Obara, T.R.; de Oliveira, J.; da Gloria, E.M.; Spoto, M.H.F.; Godoy, K.; de Souza Vieira, T.M.F.; Scheuermann, E. Benefits of superfine grinding method on antioxidant and antifungal characteristic of Brazilian green propolis extract. *Sci. Agric.* **2019**, *76*, 398–404. [CrossRef]
118. Calugar, P.C.; Coldea, T.E.; Salanță, L.C.; Pop, C.R.; Pasqualone, A.; Burja-Udrea, C.; Zhao, H.; Mudura, E. An Overview of the Factors Influencing Apple Cider Sensory and Microbial Quality from Raw Materials to Emerging Processing Technologies. *Processes* **2021**, *9*, 502. [CrossRef]
119. Li, S.; Zhang, R.; Lei, D.; Huang, Y.; Cheng, S.; Zhu, Z.; Wu, Z.; Cravotto, G. Impact of ultrasound, microwaves and high-pressure processing on food components and their interactions. *Trends Food Sci. Technol.* **2021**, *109*, 1–15. [CrossRef]
120. Klepacka, J.; Najda, A. Effect of commercial processing on polyphenols and antioxidant activity of buckwheat seeds. *Int. J. Food Sci. Technol.* **2021**, *56*, 661–670. [CrossRef]
121. Wani, S.M.; Masoodi, F.; Haq, E.; Ahmad, M.; Ganai, S. Influence of processing methods and storage on phenolic compounds and carotenoids of apricots. *LWT* **2020**, *132*, 109846. [CrossRef]
122. Wani, S.M.; Masoodi, F.; Yousuf, S.; Dar, B.; Rather, S. Phenolic compounds and antiproliferative activity of apricots: Influence of canning, freezing, and drying. *J. Food Process. Preserv.* **2020**, *44*, e14887. [CrossRef]
123. Orphanides, A.; Goulas, V.; Gekas, V. Effect of Drying Method on the Phenolic Content and Antioxidant Capacity of Spearmint. *Czech. J. Food Sci* **2013**, *31*, 509–513. [CrossRef]
124. Alfaro, S.; Mutis, A.; Quiroz, A.; Seguel, I.; Scheuermann, E. Effects of Drying Techniques on Murtilla Fruit Polyphenols and Antioxidant Activity. *J. Food Res.* **2014**, *3*, 73. [CrossRef]
125. Yuste, S.; Macià, A.; Motilva, M.-J.; Prieto-Diez, N.; Romero, M.-P.; Pedret, A.; Solà, R.; Ludwig, I.A.; Rubió, L. Thermal and non-thermal processing of red-fleshed apple: How are (poly) phenol composition and bioavailability affected? *Food Funct.* **2020**, *11*, 10436–10447. [CrossRef]
126. Arfaoui, L. Total polyphenol content and radical scavenging activity of functional yogurt enriched with dates. *Czech. J. Food Sci.* **2020**, *38*, 287–292. [CrossRef]
127. Fang, Z.; Hu, Y.; Liu, D.; Chen, J.; Ye, X. Changes of phenolic acids and antioxidant activities during potherb mustard (Brassica juncea, Coss.) pickling. *Food Chem.* **2008**, *108*, 811–817. [CrossRef] [PubMed]
128. Nurul, S.; Asmah, R. Evaluation of antioxidant properties in fresh and pickled papaya. *Int. Food Res. J.* **2012**, *19*, 1117.
129. Sayin, K.F.; Alkan, S.B. The effect of pickling on total phenolic contents and antioxidant activity of 10 vegetables. *J. Food Health Sci.* **2015**, *1*, 135–141. [CrossRef]
130. Chung, I.-M.; Oh, J.-Y.; Kim, S.-H. Comparative study of phenolic compounds, vitamin E, and fatty acids compositional profiles in black seed-coated soybeans (*Glycine Max* (L.) Merrill) depending on pickling period in brewed vinegar. *Chem. Cent. J.* **2017**, *11*, 64. [CrossRef]
131. Rodríguez-Roque, M.J.; de Ancos, B.; Sánchez-Moreno, C.; Cano, M.P.; Elez-Martínez, P.; Martín-Belloso, O. Impact of food matrix and processing on the in vitro bioaccessibility of vitamin C, phenolic compounds, and hydrophilic antioxidant activity from fruit juice-based beverages. *J. Funct. Foods* **2015**, *14*, 33–43. [CrossRef]
132. He, Z.; Tao, Y.; Zeng, M.; Zhang, S.; Tao, G.; Qin, F.; Chen, J. High pressure homogenization processing, thermal treatment and milk matrix affect in vitro bioaccessibility of phenolics in apple, grape and orange juice to different extents. *Food Chem.* **2016**, *200*, 107–116. [CrossRef]

133. Kamiloglu, S. Effect of different freezing methods on the bioaccessibility of strawberry polyphenols. *Int. J. Food Sci. Technol.* **2019**, *54*, 2652–2660. [CrossRef]
134. Castello, F.; Fernández-Pachón, M.-S.; Cerrillo, I.; Escudero-López, B.; Ortega, Á.; Rosi, A.; Bresciani, L.; Del Rio, D.; Mena, P. Absorption, metabolism, and excretion of orange juice (poly) phenols in humans: The effect of a controlled alcoholic fermentation. *Arch. Biochem. Biophys.* **2020**, *695*, 108627. [CrossRef]

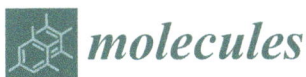

Article

Evaluation of Innovative Dried Purée from Jerusalem Artichoke—In Vitro Studies of Its Physicochemical and Health-Promoting Properties

Jan Oszmiański [1], Sabina Lachowicz [2,*], Paulina Nowicka [1], Paweł Rubiński [3] and Tomasz Cebulak [4]

[1] Department of Fruit, Vegetables and Nutraceutical Technology, Wrocław University of Environmental and Life Science, Chełmońskiego 37, 51-630 Wrocław, Poland; jan.oszmianski@upwr.edu.pl (J.O.); paulina.nowicka@upwr.edu.pl (P.N.)
[2] Department of Fermentation and Cereals Technology, Wrocław University of Environmental and Life Science, Chełmońskiego 37, 51-630 Wrocław, Poland
[3] Calisia University, Nowy Świat 4, 62-800 Kalisz, Poland; pawel.rubinski@interia.pl
[4] Department of Food Technology and Human Nutrition, University of Rzeszow, Zelwerowicza 4, 35-601 Rzeszów, Poland; tomcebulak@gmail.com
* Correspondence: sabina.lachowicz@upwr.edu.pl

Abstract: The present study aimed to evaluate the effect of Jerusalem artichoke processing methods and drying methods (freeze drying, sublimation drying, vacuum drying) on the basic physicochemical parameters, profiles and contents of sugars and polyphenolic compounds, and health-promoting properties (antioxidant activity, inhibition of the activities of α-amylase, α-glucosidase, and pancreatic lipase) of the produced purée. A total of 25 polyphenolic compounds belonging to hydroxycinnamic phenolic acids (LC-PDA-MS-QTof) were detected in Jerusalem artichoke purée. Their average content in the raw material was at 820 mg/100 g dm (UPLC-PDA-FL) and was 2.7 times higher than in the cooked material. The chemical composition and the health-promoting value of the purées were affected by the drying method, with the most beneficial values of the evaluated parameters obtained upon freeze drying. Vacuum drying could offer an alternative to freeze drying, as both methods ensured relatively comparable values of the assessed parameters.

Keywords: functional food; innovative food; drying; natural food; *Helianthus tuberosus*; pro-healthy properties

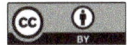

1. Introduction

The Jerusalem artichoke (*Helianthus tuberosus*; (JA)) is a species of sunflower from the genus Helianthus, belonging to the family Asteraceae, and derived from the North America. In Europe, it has been cultivated since the 17th century [1,2]. It is characterized by a fast growth rate, is tolerant to droughts, salinity, and frost, and is resistant to diseases and pests [2,3]. Due to its valuable chemical composition and scientifically proven health-promoting properties, JA has spurred a growing interest as an edible plant [4]. Its tubers contain ca. 80% of water, 2% of protein, and ca. 20% of carbohydrates, ca. 90% of which are represented by inulin [2]. JA is also valuable considering its bioactive compounds, such as, e.g., polyphenolic compounds, including phenolic acids, which exhibit strong antioxidant properties, and has also been confirmed to elicit antiviral, antibacterial, anti-inflammatory, and anti-carcinogenic effects [1,5]. In turn, as a prebiotic and soluble dietary fiber, inulin contained in JA tubers and stalks (considered to be its richest sources) ensures a hypoglycemic effect in diabetes treatment. In the gastrointestinal tract, inulin undergoes fermentation by the gut microbiota, affecting the state of eubiosis. In addition, it contributes to the increased availability of such minerals as Fe, Mg, and Ca, and influences lipid metabolism [1,6,7]. Furthermore, JA improves immunity and concentration, alleviates stress, and eliminates toxic metabolites from the body [8]. Its main applications include the production of inulin [9], feedstuff, fructose syrup, flour, French fries, biochemical materials, and bioethanol [10–12]. JA tubers processed with various cooking methods were evaluated for their sensory profiles [12]. Thus, taking into account their beneficial effects of providing valuable substances, it is necessary to develop a product with the lowest possible losses of these valuable substances and high storage stability.

Considering the above, we proposed JA purée preserved with a properly selected drying method. The use of the drying process will enable the preservation of the product, making it available all year round, and not only in the maturity period. The most common drying method is convective drying due to its low cost and relatively high efficiency [13]. In turn, sublimation drying (SD) requires high temperatures, is relatively long, which in turn leads to large losses of compounds valuable to the human body, resulting from the high access of oxygen [13]. On the other hand, freeze drying (FD) is the best method to obtain products with the lowest thermal degradation of bioactive compounds during water removal; however, it is relatively costly. Hence, vacuum drying (VD) can be an alternative to SD because it offers a shorter drying time, due to the reduced pressure, and heat supply by conduction [14]. In addition, it allows temperature control, which can reduce the thermal degradation of thermolabile compounds, such as polyphenolic compounds, and is relatively economical. However, different drying processes can affect the quality and induce different positive or negative changes in the finished product. Therefore, it is important to monitor these changes depending on the product being dried. Furthermore, the impact of the technological treatment and changes induced by drying on the content of inulin and polyphenols, and health-promoting values in the innovative dried purée from JA (raw and cooked tubers) has not been studied so far. Considering the above, the present study aimed to evaluate the effect of Jerusalem artichoke processing and drying methods (freeze drying, sublimation drying, vacuum drying) based on the analysis of physicochemical parameters, profiles and contents of sugars and polyphenolic compounds, and health-promoting properties (antioxidant, anti-diabetic, and anti-obesity activity) of the produced purée.

2. Results
2.1. Chemical Parameters
2.1.1. Basic Chemical Parameters

The results of analyses of six variants of dry purées obtained from fresh and cooked JA are presented in Table 1. Both the drying methods and the purée preparation technology statistically significantly affected the ash and pectin contents, while they had no significant effect on the dry matter content, total acidity, and pH ($p < 0.05$). The FD products showed a higher content of dry matter, ash, and pectins. In turn, the lowest contents of pectin, ash, and dry matter were obtained in the products after SD. Therefore, this method was proved the most advantageous for the preparation of the innovative dried JA purée; however, due to its high costs, the VD can be used as an alternative. Taking into account the JA preparation technology, the greatest differences were noted in SD products, where the contents of dry matter and ash were 5% and 9% higher in the purée prepared from cooked JA, while pectin content was 41% higher in the purée made of fresh material. In the case of pectins, after VD and FD, their content was 12% and 28% lower in the purée made from the cooked material than from the raw one. This is because cooking causes plant tissues to break down into individual cells and pectins to leach out. This phenomenon is also characteristic of potatoes and JA, but it is not observed when cooking root vegetables due to their thicker and harder cell membranes [15]. In addition, pectin is a form of soluble fiber that helps prevent cardiovascular diseases, diabetes, and obesity [16]. Therefore, a purée prepared from raw JA will be a more desirable product, especially when designing products dedicated to obese and diabetic patients.

Table 1. The results of analyzes of purées and dried JA.

Type of Analysis	FDC	FDR	SDC	SDR	VDC	VDR
Dry matter (g/100 g)	98.88 ± 0.20 a[a]	98.88 ± 0.20 a	97.14 ± 0.19 b	92.66 ± 0.19 e	95.90 ± 0.19 c	95.60 ± 0.19 d
Water activity (a_w)	0.01 ± 0.00 c	0.02 ± 0.00 c	0.15 ± 0.00 c	0.36 ± 0.00 a	0.19 ± 0.00 ab	0.11 ± 0.00 c
Ash (g/100 g)	4.28 ± 0.01 a	4.18 ± 0.01 a	4.10 ± 0.01 b	3.74 ± 0.01 c	3.88 ± 0.01 c	4.16 ± 0.01 b
pH	5.86 ± 0.01 ab	5.83 ± 0.01 ab	5.77 ± 0.01 ab	5.68 ± 0.01 b	5.80 ± 0.01 ab	5.90 ± 0.01 a
Total acidity (g/100 g)	1.08 ± 0.00 a	1.09 ± 0.00 a	1.07 ± 0.00 a	1.06 ± 0.00 a	1.09 ± 0.00 a	1.04 ± 0.00 a
Pectins (g/100 g)	3.10 ± 0.01 d	4.33 ± 0.01 a	1.44 ± 0.00 f	2.46 ± 0.01 e	3.60 ± 0.01 c	4.09 ± 0.01 b
Inulin (g/100 g)	40.08 ± 0.08 e	43.32 ± 0.09 a	43.06 ± 0.09 b	41.22 ± 0.08 c	40.94 ± 0.08 d	38.94 ± 0.08 f
Fructose (g/100 g)	0.10 ± 0.00 b	0.14 ± 0.00 b	0.12 ± 0.00 b	0.40 ± 0.00 a	0.09 ± 0.00 b	0.40 ± 0.00 a
Sucrose (g/100 g)	1.33 ± 0.00 d	1.84 ± 0.00 b	1.23 ± 0.00 d	1.61 ± 0.00 c	1.55 ± 0.00 c	2.06 ± 0.00 a

[a] Values are means ± standard deviation, n = 3. Mean values within a row with different letters as a, b, c, d, e, f are significantly different at $p < 0.05$. Abbreviations: FDC, freeze drying of cooked material; FDR, freeze drying of raw material; SDC, sublimation drying of cooked material; SDR, freeze drying of raw material; VDC, vacuum drying of cooked material; VDR, vacuum drying of raw material.

2.1.2. Determination of Sugar Changes

Table 1 presents the results of sugar content determination by ultra-efficient liquid chromatography coupled with an ELSD detector. The assessed material contained three types of sugars, i.e., inulin (accounting for 95.8% of total sugars on average from all analyzed sample) > sucrose (3.7%) > fructose in trace amounts (0.5%). The highest amount of total sugar was ranged from 41.4 g/100 g in sample made of raw material after the VD drying method to 45.3 g/100 g in sample made of raw material after the FD drying method. In turn, the highest content of inulin was determined in the purée from raw JA after FD (43.3 g/100 g), and the lowest one in the purée from raw JA after VD (38.9 g/100 g). Similar results concerning inulin content in the material subjected to FD were obtained by Michalska-Ciechanowska et al. [17] and Cieslik et al. [18]. In the case of fructose, it has been noted that the higher the inulin content was, the lower was the fructose content. This means that inulin has not been hydrolyzed to fructose, which usually occurs by an acid or by inulinase [19]. The authors state that JA contains the highest amounts of inulin during the harvest period from October to December, and that in the remaining months, inulin is hydrolyzed to a simple sugar [19]. However, it was noted that the purée made of raw JA contained from 29% to 78% more fructose after the FD and VD drying method, respectively, compared to the purée made of cooked JA. Thus, this may be related to inulin hydrolysis. According to Böhm et al. [20] the 1 h heat treatment at 100 to 135 °C after the acid hydrolysis of chicory inulin did not affect its degradation, which may also explain the slight differences between the purées prepared from the cooked and raw JA.

2.1.3. Determination of Polyphenolic Compounds

The detailed identification of polyphenolic compounds in dried JA purée made of raw and cooked material dried with all drying methods using LC-PDA-MS-QTof and UPLC-PDA-FL showed the presence of 25 compounds, all of which belonged to the class of hydroxycinnamic phenolic acids (Table 2). Similar results were obtained by Kapusta et al. [21] and Michalska-Ciechanowska et al. [17]. The obtained results indicate that the drying method used had a significant ($p < 0.05$) effect on the content of polyphenolic compounds. The highest total content of polyphenols, reaching 923.5 mg/100 g d.m., was found in the purée made of raw JA after FD. It was about five times higher compared to the content of polyphenolic compounds determined by Kapusta et al. [21]. Depending on the drying method used, the result obtained after FD was 21% (made of cooked material) and 15% (made of raw material) higher compared to the results obtained after SD and VD drying, respectively. According to Michalska et al. [14], the drying method had a significant impact on the final content of bioactive compounds in the finished product; hence, it is essential to select the appropriate drying method that would allow the maintenance of a relatively high content of the tested compounds. In the present study, the content of polyphenols was also statistically significantly affected by the technological treatment of JA. The purée made of cooked JA tubers contained 62% for FD, 69% for SD, and 60% for VD less bioactive compounds than the purée obtained from the unprocessed raw material dried by FD, SD, and VD, respectively. Similar results were reported in the study by Laib and Barkat [22], in which the content of polyphenolic compounds was much lower in cooked potatoes than those that were not heat-treated. This is probably due to the fact that these compounds are thermolabile, thus were destroyed and leached out to the solution.

Table 2. Analysis results of phenolic compounds (mg/100 g dm) in dry JA samples.

Compounds	MS/MS	R.t. (min)	FDC	FDR	SDC	SDR	VDC	VDR
Hydroxyferulic acid hexoside [a]	371/353/209	3.01	2.07 ± 0.00 a [e]	1.76 ± 0.00 b	1.36 ± 0.01 c	1.47 ± 0.01 c	1.85 ± 0.00 b	1.68 ± 0.01 b
Caffeoylquinic acid [b] (isomer of chlorogenic acid)	353/191/179/135	3.31	33.25 ± 0.07 a	20.90 ± 0.04 c	20.46 ± 0.04 d	1.85 ± 0.00 f	28.39 ± 0.06 b	16.27 ± 0.03 e
Hydroxyferulic acid hexoside(isommer) [a]	371/353/209	3.50	2.75 ± 0.01 b	2.28 ± 0.00 c	2.31 ± 0.01 c	5.69 ± 0.01 a	2.74 ± 0.01 b	5.61 ± 0.01 a
Hydroxyferulic acid hexoside(isommer) [a]	371/353/209	3.66	0.40 ± 0.00 b	0.40 ± 0.00 b	0.27 ± 0.00 b	0.87 ± 0.00 a	0.35 ± 0.00 b	0.84 ± 0.00 a
Caffeoylquinic acid-quinon sulfite [b]	415/387/258//191/179/161	3.83	nd	87.36 ± 0.17 c	nd	99.81 ± 0.20 a	nd	98.14 ± 0.20 b
Caffeoylquinic acid [b]	353/191/135	3.87	2.52 ± 0.01 f	76.77 ± 0.15 c	3.47 ± 0.01 d	87.71 ± 0.18 a	2.85 ± 0.01 e	86.24 ± 0.17 b
caffeoyl-gucoside [c]	341/179/135	4.25	7.71 ± 0.02 f	8.63 ± 0.02 e	10.98 ± 0.02 b	10.19 ± 0.02 c	8.87 ± 0.02 d	11.37 ± 0.02 a
3-O-Caffeoylquinic acid [d]	353/191/135	4.36	83.20 ± 0.17 d	150.46 ± 0.30 a	51.46 ± 0.10 f	111.94 ± 0.22 c	72.38 ± 0.14 e	119.73 ± 0.24 b
Caffeoylquinic acid [b]	353/191/179/173/135	4.51	38.54 ± 0.08 a	11.73 ± 0.02 f	26.95 ± 0.05 c	14.21 ± 0.03 d	33.02 ± 0.07 b	13.34 ± 0.03 e
Caffeoylquinic acid [b]	353/191/179/173/135	4.79	14.19 ± 0.03 c	6.19 ± 0.01 d	14.26 ± 0.03 c	20.25 ± 0.04 b	14.31 ± 0.03 c	37.94 ± 0.08 a
Caffeoylquinic acid [b]	353/191/179/173/135	5.13	27.31 ± 0.05 e	91.61 ± 0.18 a	23.44 ± 0.05 f	71.29 ± 0.14 c	27.63 ± 0.06 d	75.10 ± 0.15 b
Caffeoyl glucopyranose [c]	341/179/135	5.33	4.42 ± 0.01 d	8.88 ± 0.02 c	3.02 ± 0.01 f	12.74 ± 0.03 a	3.50 ± 0.01 e	10.47 ± 0.02 b
Dicaffeoylquinic acid [b]	515/353/191/179/173/161	5.58	13.96 ± 0.03 b	53.89 ± 0.11 a	10.12 ± 0.02 e	11.38 ± 0.02 d	12.52 ± 0.03 c	7.90 ± 0.02 f
Dicaffeoylquinic acids- quinon sulfite [b]	577/415/387/258//191/179	5.75	nd	99.58 ± 0.20 a	nd	77.63 ± 0.16 c	nd	83.43 ± 0.17 b
Caffeoylquinic acid [b]	353/191/179/173/135	6.14	9.36 ± 0.02 d	17.15 ± 0.03 c	4.86 ± 0.01 f	21.25 ± 0.04 a	7.33 ± 0.01 e	17.84 ± 0.04 b
Caffeoylquinic acid-quinon sulfite [b]	415/387/258//191/179/161	6.25	nd	12.89 ± 0.03 a	nd	7.78 ± 0.02 b	Nd	6.04 ± 0.01 c
Hydroxyferulic acid hexoside (isomer 3) [a]	371/353/209	6.33	2.05 ± 0.01 d	4.47 ± 0.01 b	1.44 ± 0.01 f	4.88 ± 0.01 a	1.77 ± 0.01 e	3.36 ± 0.01 c
Hydroxyferulic acid hexoside(isomer 3) [a]	371/353/209	6.57	4.02 ± 0.01 b	4.70 ± 0.01 a	2.38 ± 0.01 e	2.84 ± 0.01 d	3.34 ± 0.01 c	1.80 ± 0.01 f
Hydroxyferulic acid hexoside (isomer 3) [a]	371/353/209	6.96	1.37 ± 0.00 d	26.36 ± 0.05 a	0.95 ± 0.00 e	24.90 ± 0.05 b	1.11 ± 0.00 e	19.28 ± 0.04 c
Dicaffeoylquinic acids- quinon sulfite [b]	577/415/387/258//191/179	7.04	nd	75.95 ± 0.15 a	nd	71.74 ± 0.14 b	Nd	55.55 ± 0.11 c
3,4-Di-O-caffeoylquinic acid [b]	515/353/191	7.51	36.42 ± 0.07 d	24.15 ± 0.05 c	20.28 ± 0.04 d	19.23 ± 0.04 e	31.14 ± 0.06 b	12.88 ± 0.03 f
3,5-Di-O-caffeoylquinic acid) [b]	515/353/191	7.77	34.89 ± 0.07 d	118.37 ± 0.24 a	17.69 ± 0.04 f	68.39 ± 0.14 c	28.66 ± 0.06 e	77.14 ± 0.15 b
Hydroxyferulic acid hexoside (isomer 3) [a]	371/353/209	7.94	1.38 ± 0.00 d	2.64 ± 0.01 a	0.77 ± 0.00 e	1.75 ± 0.00 c	0.90 ± 0.00 e	1.97 ± 0.00 b
1,5-Di-O-caffeoylquinic acid [b]	515/353/191	8.21	32.40 ± 0.06 a	14.80 ± 0.03 d	17.26 ± 0.03 c	11.24 ± 0.02 e	27.39 ± 0.05 b	9.37 ± 0.02 g
Hydroxyferulic acid hexoside (isomer 3) [a]	371/353/209	8.48	0.83 ± 0.00 d	1.58 ± 0.01 a	0.40 ± 0.00 f	1.14 ± 0.00 b	0.63 ± 0.00 e	0.99 ± 0.00 bc
Sum of phenolic acids			353.05 ± 19.87 d	923.53 ± 43.70 a	234.13 ± 12.35 f	762.16 ± 35.70 b	310.68 ± 17.23 e	774.28 ± 36.67 c

[a] The calibration curve of ferulic acid was used to quantify; [b] the calibration curve of 5-O-caffeoylquinic was used to quantify; [c] the calibration curve of caffeic acid was used to quantify; [d] the calibration curve of 3-O-caffeoylquinic acid was used to quantify; [e] values are means ± standard deviation, $n = 3$. Mean values within a row with different letters as a, b, c, d, e, f are significantly different at $p < 0.05$. Abbreviations: FDC, freeze drying of cooked material; FDR, freeze drying of raw material; SDC, sublimation drying of cooked material; SDR, freeze drying of raw material; VDC, vacuum drying of cooked material; VDR, vacuum drying of raw material; R.t., retention time; nd, not detected.

3-O-caffeoylquinic acid (with main ion at m/z 353) and 3,5-di-O-caffeoylquinic acid (with main ion at m/z 515) were the major compounds [17] and, on average, accounted for 18% (from 16% of FDR to 24% of FDC) and 11% (from 8% of SDC to 13% of FDR) of total phenolic hydroxycinnamic acids, respectively. Their contents were also significantly dependent on the drying method and technological treatment, with the highest ones determined in the purées prepared from raw JA after FD, while the lowest ones were in the purée made of cooked JA after SD. During the peeling of Jerusalem artichoke, sulfur dioxide was added to protect the color. The UPLC-PDA chromatograms (Supplementary Materials Figure S1) of purées made of raw JA tuber revealed additional peaks of compounds, which were identified as derivatives of quinones, i.e., phenolic acid oxidation products in combination with a sulfite molecule. Such a combination with quinone sulfite was noted in caffeoylquinic acid (with main ion at m/z 415), compounds, whose fragmentation ions were found at m/z 387, 258, 191, 179, and 161, and in dicaffeoylquinic acid compounds (with main ion at m/z 577) whose fragmentation ions were found at m/z 415, 387, 258, 191, 179, and 161. The contribution of derivatives of quinones on the total polyphenolic compound concentration ranged from 30% for FDR to 34% for SDR. In turn, these compounds were not identified in the purées made of cooked JA tubers. They were probably washed out from the root surface by the water solutions in which they were cooked. In addition, the high cooking temperature contributed to the inactivation of enzymes that could cause the oxidation of phenolic acids to quinones. The use of sulfur dioxide as a preservative had a significant impact on the protection of bioactive compounds in the purées made of raw rather than cooked material. Similar observations regarding the protection of polyphenolic compounds were noted upon the use of sulfur dioxide in white wines [23]. In addition, compounds such as caffeoylquinic acids (isomer of chlorogenic acid; with main ion at m/z 353) and 1,5-dicaffeoylquinic acid (with main ion at m/z 515) were significantly influenced by cooking, as their contents in the purées were on average 57% and 52% lower, respectively, compared to those determined in the purées made of raw tubers. Similar observations were made by Laib and Barkat [22], who investigated the effect of heat treatment, including cooking, on the content of compounds in potato tubers. The analyzed compounds were probably released during heat treatment because some polyphenols, including phenolic acids, may be associated with non-digestible components of the cellular structure and may be released and/or solubilized during this structure's damage [22,24]. Moreover, the loss of the analyzed compounds is also strongly affected by their chemical structure, because the cooking process may differently influence compounds classified into one subclass. These losses can be influenced by the hydroxylation pattern, particle size, solubility, polarity, and sugar bonding [25]. Therefore, it is important to monitor changes during the selection of the most advantageous drying technique. The best method to obtain the dried purées turned out to be the freeze drying; however, due to its costs, the vacuum drying seems a fine alternative. In turn, depending on the chemical composition of the finished product, the raw material processing method can be used appropriately when designing new products. Considering the content of bioactive compounds, it is more advisable to produce the dried purée from raw JA tubers, irrespective of the compounds released during processing.

2.2. Physical Parameters
Color Parameters and Water Activity

The dried purées were found to differ significantly in their color parameters as affected by both the technological treatment and drying method (Table 3). The best in terms of brightest turned out to be the dried purée prepared from raw JA after FD compared to that made of boiled JA. In contrast, the use of VD and SD for product preservation caused 5% and 9% darkening of the purée made of the raw tubers and 5% and 4% darkening of the purée made of the cooked tubers. The a * and b * color parameters of the tested material indicated that JA cooking intensified the green color and darkened the yellow color of the purées, while purées made of the raw material were more yellow with a slight hue of green. Similar dependencies were observed in the measurements of the a* and b* color parameters depending on the drying method used; the FD purées were characterized by a light hue of green and a dark hue of yellow. An opposite tendency was noted in SD products, revealing a darker hue of green and a lighter hue of yellow. The results obtained for the purée after FD were comparable with the color measurement results reported by Antal et al. [2] for JA subjected to FD drying only. Those authors demonstrated a similar dependency; namely that the color of the dried material depended on the drying method used, and thus the brightest products were also obtained after FD [2].

The evaluation of the dried purées in terms of water activity (aw) showed statistically significant differences caused by both the drying method and the method of purée preparation (Table 1). The lowest aw, reaching 0.012 for FDC and 0.015 for FDR, was determined for the FD purée, and this value was on average 18 and 11 times lower compared to SD and VD purées, respectively. On the other hand, the a_w value determined after VD was two times lower compared to the value determined after SD. According to the results reported by Antal et al. [2], the a_w value recorded for freeze-dried JA without technological treatment was seven times higher compared to our study. A lower a_w value of dried fruits of Saskatoon berry was also noted after FD, whereas there was a higher value after SD [26]. In turn, regardless of the drying method used, the purées made of raw material were characterized by an on average 40% higher a_w value. This can be explained by the slight evaporation of water during the cooking process of [12]. However, regardless of the drying method and preparation technology used, the aw of all dried purées was below the critical level (a_w = 0.60). This means that they meet the requirement of a product safe from microbiological spoilage, i.e., from contamination with bacteria and mold, because the a_w value above 0.60 may cause microbiological spoilage of the finished product [2].

Table 3. Color measurement results.

Type of Sample	L *	a *	b *
FDR	92.51 ± 0.19 a [a]	−1.22 ± 0.01 e	12.11 ± 0.02 c
FDC	90.22 ± 0.18 b	−1.45 ± 0.01 f	10.88 ± 0.02 e
SDR	88.32 ± 0.18 c	−0.40 ± 0.00 b	14.10 ± 0.03 b
SDC	85.76 ± 0.17 e	−0.94 ± 0.00 d	11.67 ± 0.02 d
VDR	84.63 ± 0.17 f	−0.79 ± 0.00 c	14.05 ± 0.03 b
VDC	86.99 ± 0.17 d	−0.26 ± 0.00 a	14.59 ± 0.03 a

[a] Values are means ± standard deviation, $n = 3$. Mean values within a row with different letters as a, b, c, d, e, f are significantly different at $p < 0.05$. Abbreviations: FDC, freeze drying of cooked material; FDR, freeze drying of raw material; SDC, sublimation drying of cooked material; SDR, freeze drying of raw material; VDC, vacuum drying of cooked material; VDR, vacuum drying of raw material.

2.3. Pro-Healthy Properties

The study also determined the health-promoting properties of JA preserved using various drying methods. The purées were analyzed in terms of their antioxidant, anti-diabetic (the ability to inhibit α-amylase and α-glucosidase), and anti-obesity properties (the ability to inhibit pancreatic lipase). Finding effective inhibitors of α-amylase and α-glucosidase would allow a delay in sugar absorption and a reduction in postprandial blood glucose. On the other hand, finding an effective inhibitor of pancreatic lipase activity by stimulating the cell membrane permeability would enable the apt functioning of the pancreas as a gland responsible for the proper insulin secretion. Additionally, pancreatic lipase is a key dietary fat-absorbing enzyme responsible for the hydrolysis of triglycerides to 2-monoacylglycerides and free fatty acids that can be absorbed by enterocytes. Its inhibition is used to reduce the rate of dietary fat absorption and, therefore, may offer an alternative approach to treating overweight and obesity [27].

The analysis of the antioxidant activity of the studied variants of JA purées showed that the greatest antioxidant effect was obtained in JA dried using the vacuum and sublimation methods (Table 4). It was proved that not only the drying method, but also the type of raw material used for drying, played a significant role in modeling the antioxidant properties of the tested material. Hence, a much better effect in developing the health-promoting properties was obtained by drying fresh than the previously cooked material.

A slightly different trend was observed in the JA ability to inhibit pancreatic lipase, α-amylase, and α-glucosidase (Table 4). A more effective inhibitor turned out to be SDC. An opposite effect was observed with the vacuum method. It was shown to be the most effective in modeling both anti-diabetic and anti-obesity properties. Moreover, as in the case of antioxidant properties, it appeared more effective to dry fresh raw material than the cooked one. In general, it can be concluded that the produced dried purées were characterized by a high anti-diabetic potential—similar results were obtained for both α-amylase (IC_{50} values from 130 µg/mL to 736 µg/mL) and α-glucosidase (IC_{50} values from 120 µg/mL to 898 µg/mL). A study by Wang et al. [28] has shown that the ability to inhibit α-glucosidase is stimulated by hydroxycinnamic acid derivatives. However, no such trend was observed in the present study. It has been shown that procyanidin polymers can also be involved in enzyme inhibition. This tendency was confirmed by Boath et al. [29], who suggested that fruit extracts rich in procyanidins were effective inhibitors of α-amylase because they had the ability to form tannin–enzyme complexes, which effectively inhibited the hydrolysis of polysaccharides to simple sugars. Other authors have shown that the effective blocking of diabetes-related enzymes may be due to high concentrations of inulin [30].

Table 4. The degree of metabolism and absorption of sugars derived from JA products.

Type of Sample	α-Glucosidase	α-Amylase	Pancreatic Lipase	ABTS	FRAP
	IC$_{50}$ (mL/mL)	IC$_{50}$ (ug/mL)	IC$_{50}$ (mL/mL)	(mmol TE/100 g dm)	(mmol TE/100 g dm)
FDR	166.70 ± 0.33 e [a]	177.98 ± 0.36 c	43.75 ± 0.09 c	3.73 ± 0.01 d	1.69 ± 0.01 e
FDC	193.29 ± 0.39 f	297.90 ± 0.60 f	45.86 ± 0.09 e	7.65 ± 0.02 a	2.67 ± 0.01 a
SDR	123.60 ± 0.25 b	136.98 ± 0.27 b	31.48 ± 0.06 a	2.78 ± 0.01 f	1.46 ± 0.00 f
SDC	135.52 ± 0.27 c	185.87 ± 0.37 d	58.34 ± 0.12 f	6.91 ± 0.01 c	2.60 ± 0.01 b
VDR	150.94 ± 0.30 d	221.19 ± 0.44 e	45.06 ± 0.09 d	2.85 ± 0.01 e	1.97 ± 0.01 d
VDC	120.31 ± 0.24 a	129.97 ± 0.26 a	33.08 ± 0.07 b	7.09 ± 0.01 b	2.14 ± 0.01 c

[a] Values are means ± standard deviation, $n = 3$. Mean values within a row with different letters as a, b, c, d, e, f, are significantly different at $p < 0.05$. Abbreviations: FDC, freeze drying of cooked material; FDR, freeze drying of raw material; SDC, sublimation drying of cooked material; SDR, freeze drying of raw material; VDC, vacuum drying of cooked material; VDR, vacuum drying of raw material.

It should be emphasized, however, that JA was the most effective pancreatic lipase inhibitor. The IC$_{50}$ values determined for this enzyme ranged from 31 µg/mL (air-dried Jerusalem artichoke, previously cooked) to 58 µg/mL (air-dried JA, fresh). The observed trend may again be due to the high concentration of inulin in this product. Recently, it has been proved that inulin effectively prevents the occurrence of obesity and diabetes, i.a., by lowering the blood levels of triglycerides, cholesterol, and glucose [31].

The conducted research has shown that JA is an interesting raw material with a wide spectrum of health-promoting properties that can be modulated in certain ranges by selecting appropriate processing and preservation methods.

3. Materials and Methods

3.1. Materials

Acetonitrile, formic acid, methanol, ABTS (2,2′-azinobis(3-ethylbenzothiazoline-6-sulfonic acid), 6-hydroxy-2,5,7,8-tetramethylchroman-2-carboxylic acid (Trolox), 2,4,6-tri(2-pyridyl)-s-triazine (TPTZ), 2,2-Di(4-tert-octylphenyl)-1-picrylhydrazyl (DPPH), methanol, acetic acid, 2,2′-azobis (2-amidino-propane) dihydrochloride (AAPH), fluorescein disodium (FL), potassium persulfate, TPTZ (2,4,6-tripyridyl-1,3,5-triazine), FeCl3, phloroglucinol, 3,5-dinitrosalicylic acid, potassium sodium tartrate tetrahydrate, sodium phosphate monobasic, starch from potato, α-amylase from porcine pancreas (type VI-8), dipotassium hydrogen orthophosphate dihydrogen, p-nitrophenyl-α-D-glucopyranoside, α-glucosidase from Saccharomyces cerevisiae (type I), sugar, and polyphenolic standards were purchased from Sigma-Aldrich (Steinheim, Germany). Acetonitrile for ultra-performance liquid chromatography (UPLC; gradient grade) and ascorbic acid were from Merck (Darmstadt, Germany).

Helianthus tuberosus was harvested at the organic cultivation Gospodarstwo Rolno-Ogrodnicze Marek Strojs in Kalisz (Poland). Jerusalem artichoke (around 10 kg) "Albik" cultivar was collected in August 2020.

3.2. Sample Preparation

The production process of dried Jerusalem artichoke purée included 3 main stages:

(a) Peeling: samples were peeled for 3 min at room temperature with the addition of 0.5% sodium metabisulfate dissolved in water (1:1) on a modified vegetable peeler (YATO YG-03087 firmy (TOYA S.A Wrocław Poland).

(b) Preparation of two variants of material for drying, i.e., from fresh and cooked raw material: (i) in the first variant, 1 kg of peeled fresh material was ground in a Thermomix Varoma with the addition of 0.5% sodium metabisulphate (5 min/20 °C); whereas (ii) in the second variant, 1 kg of peeled Jerusalem artichoke was cooked in a basket of the Thermomix in water with the addition of 0.5% sodium metabisulphate (30 min/98 °C); afterward, the water was drained and the cooked sample was ground (5 min/20 °C).

(c) Drying: both cooked and raw samples were dried using three methods: (i) freeze drying (FD)—carried out in a freeze dryer—(Christ Alpha 1–4 LSC; Osterode am

Harz, Germany) for 24 h, (ii) sublimation drying (SD)—carried out in a (KC 100/200 Wytwórnia Aparatury Elektronicznej i Medycznej Warszawa) for 8 h at 80 °C, (iii) vacuum drying (VD)—carried out in a VACUCELL 111 ECO LINE vacuum dryer (MMM Medcenter Einrichtungen GmbH, Planegg, Germany) for 8 h at 80 °C.

All drying experiments were performed in duplicate. The samples obtained were milled by a laboratory mill (IKA A.11, Wilmington, NC, USA), and vacuum sealed. The powders were kept in a freezer (-20 °C) until the extracts' preparation.

3.3. Chemical Parameters

3.3.1. Basic Parameters

The dry matter was determined by mixing the sample with diatomaceous earth, pre-drying, and final drying under reduced pressure. Total acidity was extracted by mixing with water in 100 mL flasks, cooking for 20 min, and cooling for 20 min. Total acidity (TA) was analyzed supernatant (8 mL) by the titration of products with 0.1N NaOH to pH 8.1 and the results were expressed as g malic acid/100 g. TA and pH were determined using an automatic pH titrator system (TitroLine 5000, Xylem Analytics GmbH, Weilheim in Oberbayern, Germany). The soluble solids content, dry matter, titratable acidity, and ash were taken according to European Standards, PN-EN 12143:2000, PN-EN 12145:2001, and PN-EN 12145:2000, PN-EN 450:1998, respectively. Pectin content (g/100 g) was measured according to the Morris method reported by Pijanowski et al. [32]. All measurements were taken three times.

3.3.2. Determination of Sugar by HPLC

An analysis of sugar by the HPLC-ELSD method was performed according to the protocol described by Oszmiański and Lachowicz [33]. Calibration curves ($R^2 = 0.9999$) were created for glucose, fructose, sorbitol, and sucrose. All data were obtained in triplicate. The results were expressed as g per 100 g dm.

3.3.3. Polyphenolic Compounds by UPLC

The extraction of the samples for phenolic compounds and their chromatographic analysis were performed exactly as described by Oszmiański and Lachowicz (2016). The samples were analyzed by an Ultra-Performance Liquid Chromatography Photodiode Array Detector (UPLC-PDA; Acquity UPLC System, Waters Corp., Milford, MA, USA). The study identified phenolic acids and their sums were calculated as chlorogenic acid, which is based on dominant compounds and compared with reference standards (Figure S1). All results were taken in triplicate and shown as mg/100 g dm (dry mass) of sample.

3.4. Physical Parameters

3.4.1. Color Parameters by CIE Lab System

The color properties (L *, a *, b *) of prepared products were determined by reflectance measurement with a Color Quest XE HunterLab colorimeter (Biosens, Warsaw, Poland). The samples were filled in a 1-cm cell, and L*, a*, b* values were determined using Illuminant D65 and 10° observer angle. Samples were measured against a white ceramic reference plate (L * = 93.92; a * = 1.03; b * = 0.52). The total change in color of powders (DE *) [34] and also EP, and Dom WL were measured. The data were the mean of three measurements.

3.4.2. Water Activity

Water activity (a_w) was measured in triplicate ($n = 3$) at 25 °C $\pm$ 2 using an AQUA LAB DewPoint water activity meter (Pullman, WA, USA) [26].

3.5. Pro-Helathy Properties

3.5.1. The Antioxidants Activity

The extraction procedure of the radical activity (ABTS), reducing potency (FRAP), and the oxygen radical absorbance capacity (ORAC) test was the same for all determinations and was carried out identically, as described by Lachowicz, Świeca, and Pejcz [35], and Nowicka, Wojdyło, Laskowski [36]. The FRAP, ABTS, and ORAC tests were prepared as previously described by Benzie and Strain [37], Re et al. [38], and Ou et al. [39], respectively. The antioxidant capacity was expressed as millimoles of Trolox per 100 g of sample. The ORAC assay was carried out on an RF-5301 PC spectrofluorometer (Shimadzu, Kyoto, Japan). Measurements by means of ABTS, and FRAP method involved a UV-2401 PC spectrophotometer (Shimadzu, Kyoto, Japan).

3.5.2. Activity of α-Amylase, α-Glucosidase, Pancreatic Lipase Inhibitors

The α-amylase and α-glucosidase inhibitory effect of the sample extracts was assayed according to the procedure described previously by Nowicka, Wojdyło, Samoticha [36] while the inhibition of lipase activity was determined according to Podsędek et al. [40], respectively. Acarbose was included in the case of α-amylase and α-glucosidase as a positive control, while the orlistat was used as a positive control for pancreatic lipase. The results were expressed as IC_{50} value.

3.6. Statistics Methods

Statistical analysis was conducted using Statistica version 13 (StatSoft, Krakow, Poland). Significant differences ($p \leq 0.05$) between means were evaluated by two-way ANOVA and Tuckey's multiple range test. All data included in this study are presented as the mean value ± standard deviation and were performed at least three times.

4. Conclusions

The analyses of the content of polyphenolic compounds and the health-promoting activity of selected purée variants showed that the best results were obtained in JA dried with FD. It has been proved that not only the drying method but also the type of raw material used for drying played a significant role in modulating the antioxidant, anti-diabetic, and anti-obesity properties of the tested material. Hence, much better effects regarding the contents of pectin and health-promoting compounds as well as modeling health-promoting properties were obtained by drying the raw rather than the previously cooked material. The best effects of preserving the natural light color after production were obtained in the freeze-dried samples; however, due to the high costs of this method, it can be replaced by vacuum drying.

Supplementary Materials: Supplementary Materials Figure S1: chromatograms registered at 280 nm of dried purée from Jerusalem artichoke: with derivatives of SO_2 (1), without derivatives of SO_2 (2).

Author Contributions: Conceptualization, J.O., P.R., S.L., P.N.; material, P.R. methodology, J.O., S.L., P.N.; formal analysis, J.O., S.L., P.N.; T.C.; writing—original draft preparation, J.O., S.L., P.N. All authors have read and agreed to the published version of the manuscript.

Funding: The research is financed under the Operational Program: Smart Growth: Priority Axis 2 Support for the environment and the potential of enterprises to conduct R & D & I activity, measure 2.3 Pro-innovative services for enterprises, sub-measure 2.3.2. The project is carried out by FNT Food and Technology Sp. z o.o.–Wrocław, Poland. Number of project: POIR.02.03.02-02-0027/18.

Institutional Review Board Statement: Not applicable.

Informed Consent Statement: Not applicable.

Data Availability Statement: The authors declare that the data is available.

Conflicts of Interest: The authors declare no conflict of interest.

Sample Availability: Samples of the compounds as JA are available from the authors.

References

1. Amarowicz, R.; Cwalina-Ambroziak, B.; Janiak, M.A.; Bogucka, B. Effect of N Fertilization on the Content of Phenolic Compounds in Jerusalem artichoke (*Helianthus tuberosus* L.) Tubers and Their Antioxidant Capacity. *Agronomy* **2020**, *10*, 1215. [CrossRef]
2. Antal, T.; Tarek, M.; Tarek-Tilistyák, J.; Kerekes, B. Comparative effects of three different drying methods on drying kinetics and quality of J.A. (*Helianthus tuberosus* L.). *J. Food Process. Preserv.* **2017**, *41*, e12971. [CrossRef]
3. Yang, L.; He, Q.S.; Corscadden, K.; Udenigwe, C.C. The prospects of Jerusalem artichoke in functional food ingredients and bioenergy production. *Biotechnol. Rep.* **2015**, *5*, 77–88. [CrossRef] [PubMed]
4. Cieslik, E.; Gebusia, A. Jerusalem artichoke (*Helianthus tuberosus* L.)—Tuber with pro-healthily nutritive properties. *Postępy Nauk. Rol.* **2010**, *62*, 91.
5. Koroleva, O.; Torkova, A.; Nikolaev, I.; Khrameeva, E.; Fedorova, T.; Tsentalovich, M.; Amarowicz, R. Evaluation of the antiradical properties of phenolic acids. *Int. J. Mol. Sci.* **2014**, *15*, 16351–16380. [CrossRef] [PubMed]
6. Fotschki, B.; Jurgonski, A.; Fotschki, J.; Majewski, M.; Ognik, K.; Juskiewicz, J. Dietary chicory inulin-rich meal exerts greater healing effects than fructooligosaccharide preparation in rats with trinitrobenzenesulfonic acid-induced necrotic colitis. *Pol. J. Food Nutr. Sci.* **2019**, *69*, 147–155. [CrossRef]
7. Kalyani Nair, K.; Kharb, S.; Thompkinson, D.K. Inulin dietary fiber with functional and health attributes—A review. *Food Rev. Int.* **2010**, *26*, 189–203. [CrossRef]
8. Lee, Y.J.; Lee, M.G.; Yu, S.Y.; Yoon, W.B.; Lee, O.H. Changes in physicochemical characteristics and antioxidant activities of Jerusalem artichoke tea infusions resulting from different production processes. *Food Sci. Biotechnol.* **2014**, *23*, 1885–1892. [CrossRef]
9. Rubel, I.A.; Iraporda, C.; Novosad, R.; Cabrera, F.A.; Genovese, D.B.; Manrique, G.D. Inulin rich carbohydrates extraction from Jerusalem artichoke (*Helianthus tuberosus* L.) tubers and application of different drying methods. *Food Res. Int.* **2018**, *103*, 226–233. [CrossRef]
10. Tchoné, M.; Barwald, G.; Annemuller, G.; Fleischer, L. Separation and identification of phenolic compounds in Jerusalem artichoke (Helianthus tuberosus L.). *Sci. Aliment.* **2006**, *26*, 394. [CrossRef]
11. Kim, M.J.; An, D.J.; Moon, K.B.; Cho, H.S.; Min, S.R.; Sohn, J.H.; Kim, H.S. Highly efficient plant regeneration and Agrobacterium-mediated transformation of *Helianthus tuberosus* L. *Ind. Crop. Prod.* **2016**, *83*, 670–679. [CrossRef]
12. De Santis, D.; Frangipane, M.T. Evaluation of chemical composition and sensory profile in Jerusalem artichoke (*Helianthus tuberosus* L.) tubers: The effect of clones and cooking conditions. *Int. J. Gastron. Food Sci.* **2018**, *11*, 25–30. [CrossRef]
13. Figiel, A. Drying kinetics and quality of beetroots dehydrated by combination of convective and vacuum-microwave methods. *J. Food Eng.* **2010**, *98*, 461–470. [CrossRef]
14. Michalska, A.; Wojdyło, A.; Lech, K.; Łysiak, G.P.; Figiel, A. Physicochemical properties of whole fruit plum powders obtained using different drying technologies. *Food Chem.* **2016**, *207*, 223–232. [CrossRef]
15. Komolka, P.; Górecka, D. Wpływ obróbki cieplnej na strukturę wybranych warzyw i owoców®. *Postępy Tech. Przetwórstwa Spożywczego* **2017**, *2*, 67–73.
16. Mudgil, D.; Barak, S. Composition, properties and health benefits of indigestible carbohydrate polymers as dietary fiber: A review. *Int. J. Biol. Macromol.* **2013**, *61*, 1–6. [CrossRef]
17. Michalska-Ciechanowska, A.; Wojdyło, A.; Bogucka, B.; Dubis, B. Moderation of inulin and polyphenolics contents in three cultivars of *Helianthus tuberosus* L. by potassium fertilization. *Agronomy* **2019**, *9*, 884. [CrossRef]
18. Cieslik, E.; Florkiewicz, A.; Filipiak-Florkiewicz, A. Wplyw terminu zbioru na zawartosc weglowodanow w bulwach topinamburu (*Helianthus tuberosus* L.). *Zyw. Człowieka Metab.* **2003**, *3*, 1076–1080.
19. Chekroun, M.B.; Amzile, J.; Yachioui, M.E.; Haloui, N.E.; Prevost, J. Qualitative and quantitative development of carbohydrate reserves during the biological cycle of Jerusalem artichoke (*Helianthus tuberosus* L.) tubers. *N. Z. J. Crop. Hortic. Sci.* **1994**, *22*, 31–37. [CrossRef]
20. Böhm, A.; Kaiser, I.; Trebstein, A.; Henle, T. Heat-induced degradation of inulin. *Eur. Food Res. Technol.* **2005**, *220*, 466–471. [CrossRef]
21. Kapusta, I.; Krok, E.S.; Jamro, D.B.; Cebulak, T.; Kaszuba, J.; Salach, R.T. Identification and quantification of phenolic compounds from Jerusalem artichoke (*Helianthus tuberosus* L.) tubers. *J. Food Agric. Environ.* **2013**, *11*, 601–606.
22. Laib, I.; Barkat, M. Optimization of conditions for extraction of polyphenols and the determination of the impact of cooking on total polyphenolic, antioxidant, and anticholinesterase activities of potato. *Foods* **2018**, *7*, 36. [CrossRef] [PubMed]
23. Santos, C.V.A.; da Silva, M.G.; Cabrita, M.J. Impact of SO2 and bentonite addition during fermentation on volatile profile of two varietal white wines. *LWT Food Sci. Technol.* **2020**, *133*, 109893. [CrossRef]
24. Acosta-Estrada, B.A.; Gutiérrez-Uribe, J.A.; Serna-Saldívar, S.O. Bound phenolics in foods, a review. *Food Chem.* **2014**, *152*, 46–55. [CrossRef]
25. Rothwell, J.A.; Medina-Remón, A.; Pérez-Jiménez, J.; Neveu, V.; Knaze, V.; Slimani, N.; Scalbert, A. Effects of food processing on polyphenol contents: A systematic analysis using Phenol-Explorer data. *Mol. Nutr. Food Res.* **2015**, *59*, 160–170. [CrossRef]
26. Lachowicz, S.; Michalska, A.; Lech, K.; Majerska, J.; Oszmiański, J.; Figiel, A. Comparison of the effect of four drying methods on polyphenols in saskatoon berry. *LWT Food Sci. Technol.* **2019**, *111*, 727–736. [CrossRef]
27. Sergent, T.; Vanderstraeten, J.; Winand, J.; Beguin, P.; Schneider, Y.J. Phenolic compounds and plant extracts as potential natural anti-obesity substances. *Food Chem.* **2012**, *135*, 68–73. [CrossRef]

28. Wang, Y.C.; Hu, H.F.; Ma, J.W.; Yan, Q.J.; Liu, H.J.; Jiang, Z.Q. A novel high maltose-forming α-amylase from *Rhizomucor miehei* and its application in the food industry. *Food Chem.* **2020**, *305*, 125447. [CrossRef]
29. Boath, A.S.; Stewart, D.; MSDougall, G.J. Berry components inhibit α-glucosidase in vitro: Synergies between acarbose and polyphenols from black currant and rowanberry. *Food Chem.* **2012**, *135*, 929–936. [CrossRef]
30. Gao, L.; Chi, Z.; Sheng, J.; Wang, L.; Li, J.; Gong, F. Inulinase-producing marine yeasts: Evaluation of their diversity and inulin hydrolysis by their crude enzymes. *Microb. Ecol.* **2007**, *54*, 722–729. [CrossRef]
31. Simsek, S.; Sánchez-Rivera, L.; El, S.N.; Karakaya, S.; Recio, I. Characterisation of *in vitro* gastrointestinal digests from low fat caprine kefir enriched with inulin. *Int. Dairy J.* **2017**, *75*, 68–74. [CrossRef]
32. Pijanowski, J.; New, R. Comparison of Various Methods for Computing the Axially Backscattered Field of a Prolate Spheroid. *J. Acoust. Soc. Am.* **1973**, *53*, 374. [CrossRef]
33. Oszmiański, J.; Lachowicz, S. Effect of the production of dried fruits and juice from chokeberry (*Aronia melanocarpa* L.) on the content and antioxidant activity of bioactive compounds. *Molecules* **2016**, *21*, 1098. [CrossRef]
34. Nowicka, P.; Wojdyło, A.; Teleszko, M.; Samoticha, J. Sensory attributes and changes of physicochemical properties during storage of smoothies prepared from selected fruit. *LWT Food Sci. Technol.* **2016**, *71*, 102–109. [CrossRef]
35. Lachowicz, S.; Świeca, M.; Pejcz, E. Biological activity, phytochemical parameters, and potential bioaccessibility of wheat bread enriched with powder and microcapsules made from Saskatoon berry. *Food Chem.* **2021**, *338*, 128026. [CrossRef]
36. Nowicka, P.; Wojdyło, A.; Samoticha, J. Evaluation of phytochemicals, antioxidant capacity, and antidiabetic activity of novel smoothies from selected Prunus fruits. *J. Funct. Foods* **2016**, *25*, 397–407. [CrossRef]
37. Benzie, I.F.; Strain, J.J. The ferric reducing ability of plasma (FRAP) as a measure of "antioxidant power": The FRAP assay. *Anal. Biochem.* **1996**, *239*, 70–76. [CrossRef]
38. Re, R.; Pellegrini, N.; Proteggente, A.; Pannala, A.; Yang, M.; Rice-Evans, C. Antioxidant activity applying an improved ABTS radical cation decolorization assay. *Free Radic. Biol. Med.* **1999**, *26*, 1231–1237. [CrossRef]
39. Ou, B.; Huang, D.; Hampsch-Woodill, M.; Flanagan, J.A.; Deemer, E.K. Analysis of antioxidant activities of common vegetables employing oxygen radical absorbance capacity (ORAC) and ferric reducing antioxidant power (FRAP) assays: A comparative study. *J. Agric. Food Chem.* **2002**, *50*, 3122–3128. [CrossRef]
40. Podsedek, A.; Majewska, I.; Redzynia, M.; Sosnowska, D.; Koziołkiewicz, M. In vitro inhibitory effect on digestive enzymes and antioxidant potential of commonly consumed fruits. *J. Agric. Food Chem.* **2014**, *62*, 4610–4617. [CrossRef]

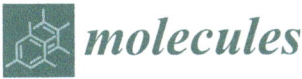

Communication

Antioxidant Activity of Polyphenols, from *Mauritia flexuosa* (Aguaje), Based on Controlled Dehydration

Hichem Bensaada [1], María Fernanda Soto-Garcia [2] and Juan Carlos Carmona-Hernandez [2,*]

1. Medical School, Ferhat Abbas University of Setif 1, Setif 19000, Algeria; dr.bensaada.h@gmx.com
2. Grupo de Investigación Médica, Línea Metabolismo-Nutrición-Polifenoles, Medical School, Universidad de Manizales, Manizales 17000, Colombia; mfsoto79169@umanizales.edu.co
* Correspondence: jucaca@umanizales.edu.co; Tel.: +57-300-586-8133

Abstract: Plant polyphenols offer several benefits for the prevention of diverse illnesses. Fruit's edible and inedible parts (pulp, seeds, peels, stems, flowers) are important sources of polyphenols. Different industrial processes for fruit treatment and commercialization affect the total polyphenol content (TPC), and probably the biological activity. The purpose of the present work was to determine the TPC and antioxidant activity (by DPPH) of polyphenols extracted from the pulp and seeds of *Mauritia flexuosa* (aguaje), in fresh and dehydrated forms, in order to determine the possible connection with the quantity of polyphenols and their specific antioxidant activity. The highest phenolic content for *M. flexuosa* seeds in fresh form (non-dehydrated) was 270.75 mg GAE/100 g with a 96-h extraction. With respect to the dehydrated samples, the best yield was quantified in the 96-h dehydrated seed sample. For all pulp and seeds, dehydrated for 24, 48, and 96 h, TPC showed a slightly decreasing pattern. The DPPH results were the highest in the 96-h dehydrated samples and the differences among all dehydrated pulp and seed samples were minimal. More studies testing the presence of other antioxidant components could help in understanding the detailed antioxidant activity, and related more to the specific action, rather than only total polyphenol content.

Keywords: polyphenols; antioxidant activity; *Mauritia flexuosa* (aguaje); controlled dehydration

Citation: Bensaada, H.; Soto-Garcia, M.F.; Carmona-Hernandez, J.C. Antioxidant Activity of Polyphenols, from *Mauritia flexuosa* (Aguaje), Based on Controlled Dehydration. *Molecules* **2022**, *27*, 3065. https://doi.org/10.3390/molecules27103065

Academic Editors: Jan Oszmianski and Sabina Lachowicz-Wiśniewska

Received: 3 March 2022
Accepted: 28 April 2022
Published: 10 May 2022

Publisher's Note: MDPI stays neutral with regard to jurisdictional claims in published maps and institutional affiliations.

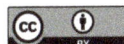

Copyright: © 2022 by the authors. Licensee MDPI, Basel, Switzerland. This article is an open access article distributed under the terms and conditions of the Creative Commons Attribution (CC BY) license (https://creativecommons.org/licenses/by/4.0/).

1. Introduction

The antioxidant benefit of fruit consumption is mainly connected to the polyphenol content; these types of phytochemicals display several other functions [1,2]. Multiple publications have reported improved lipid metabolism in overweight and obese humans due to a regular diet inclusion of plant polyphenols [3–5]. These phytochemicals offer a protective activity, leading to health benefits; several studies relate oxidative stress with the development of diseases such as cardiovascular diseases, neurodegenerative disorders, and cancer [6,7]. With respect to ovarian cancer, there is histological evidence of aortas showing promising anti-proliferative and anti-inflammatory effects and leading to a reduction of cancer cell viability [8,9]. Given the multiple health benefits of polyphenols, it is of general interest to know the phenolic content and major phenolic compounds, such as flavonoids, found in regularly harvested and consumed fruits [10–12].

The oxido-reducing activity of compounds containing phenolic rings is the most studied biological property in plant polyphenols. This type of chemical reaction is representative of a misbalance in oxidizing and reducing compounds; which at the cellular level can lead to molecular damage [13]. Plants and fruits can contribute to the reduction of negative side effects in different pathologies.

Commonly known as buriti plant, *Mauritia flexuosa* (Arecaceae) is a palm broadly cultivated in Colombia, Venezuela, the Guianas, Trinidad, Ecuador, Peru, Brazil, and Bolivia [2,14]. The fresh form of *M. flexuosa* fruits (Figure 1) has an orange, soft, water-soluble, and edible pulp and numerous small circular dark red and brown flat seeds. Several

South American aboriginal groups use this Amazonic fruit for medicinal purposes [15–19]. The mesocarp oil is used to treat respiratory symptoms, pneumonia, influenza, snake bites, and heart problems [20]. In Colombia, *M. flexuosa* is also named "aguaje" [2].

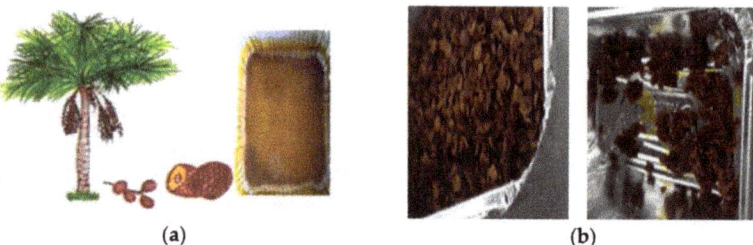

(a) (b)

Figure 1. (a) *Mauritia flexuosa* (aguaje) palm and fruit (seedless pulp) [2]. (b) Dehydrated aguaje samples, seeds and pulp.

Different variables can affect the total polyphenol content (TPC) and the antioxidant capacity of fruits, such as passing from a fresh to a dehydrated long-shelf-life state. This is still an area of active research, while conflicting results have been reported in the literature [21–23]. Information is lacking with respect to the specific activity and bio-accessibility of polyphenols, especially due to structural alterations, such as ring modifications, and polyphenol interaction with other food matrixes based on high or low water contents [24,25]. Multiple studies have focused on testing total phenolic content and antioxidant activity in *M. flexuosa*, but a comparison of the influence in dehydration states in pulp or seeds and its connection to antioxidant activity is still lacking in information and research [26–29]. The contradicting results show that some studies highlight decreasing TPC and higher antioxidant activity, while others report the opposite situations tested in a different food matrix, such as grapes, onions, rice, and other vegetables [30–33]. The goal of the present study was to determine a comparative approach to polyphenols from *M. flexuosa*, with high and low water content (fresh and de-hydrated samples), under active interconversion, and their relation to effective antioxidant activity.

2. Results and Discussion

2.1. Food Matrix Dehydration and Polyphenol Extraction

Samples of *M. flexuosa* pulp and seeds were treated by extraction and a controlled dehydration process at four different times (24, 48, 72, and 96 h). The biggest weight difference was recorded for the first 24 h of dehydration. The water content in pulp and seeds was approximately 85% and 44%, respectively. Dehydrated weights were stable at 96 h at 50 °C. Considering the high difference in water content for pulp and seeds, the dehydration pattern (Figure 2) yielded similar values.

Polyphenols from fresh pulp and seeds were extracted in ethanol (80% w/v) and more polyphenol extractions were done with seeds and pulp at three dehydration intervals (24, 48, and 96 h). The comparative extraction looked for differences in polyphenol content, based on conflicting studies that reported higher phenolics and antioxidant activity in fresh fruit, seeds, or peels [34,35]. Figure 3 shows the comparative values for total polyphenol content from pulp and seeds in fresh or dehydrated form.

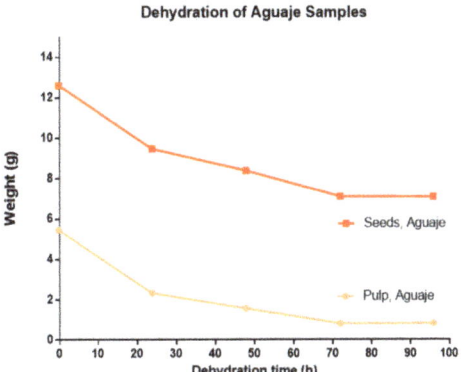

Figure 2. Dehydration curve for *M. flexuosa*, pulp and seeds at a constant 50 °C from 0 to 96 h.

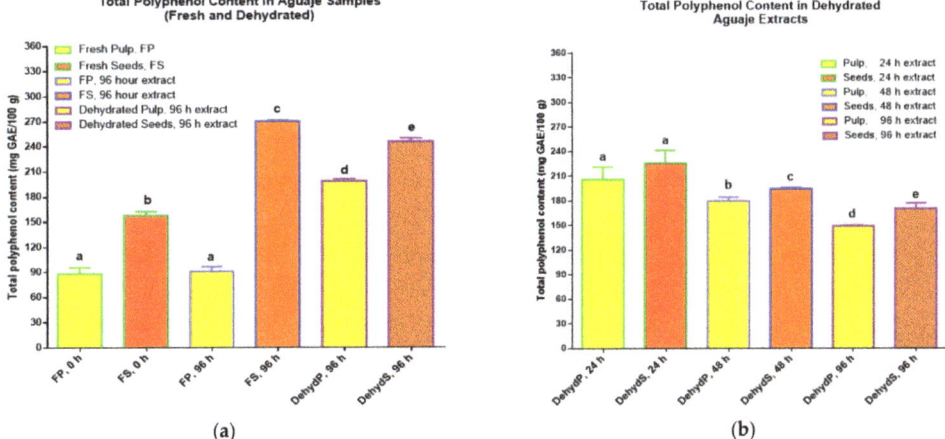

Figure 3. TPC (mg of gallic acid equivalents per 100 g) of fresh and dehydrated pulp and seeds of (**a**) *M. flexuosa* (aguaje) fresh and dehydrated pulp and seeds for the initial experimental assay and (**b**) TPC in *M. flexuosa* dehydrated pulp and seeds in a second assay. Data are means (±standard deviation), and lower-case letters represent significant differences, for total polyphenol content in mg GAE/100 g of initial sample, based on ANOVA followed by Tukey test ($p < 0.05$).

2.2. Total Polyphenol Content (TPC)

Polyphenols that were initially extracted from the fresh pulp of aguaje at 0 h of dehydration and the samples of fresh pulp that continued with the extraction process for another 96 h, in the dark without stirring, registered the lowest TPC with statistical significance, with respect to the phenolic content in fresh and dehydrated (96 h) seeds, registering approximately 90 mg GAE/100 g. The highest TPC was detected in fresh and dehydrated aguaje seeds (dehydration at 96 h) yielding more than 270 mg GAE/100 g in fresh seeds, as shown in Figure 3a that represents the results for the first experimental assays. The best aqueous conditions for polyphenol detection and reactions (fresh pulp matrix) did not favor higher TPC. These results suggest, coinciding with other researchers, that higher phenolic presence is more connected to the food matrix and the solvent affinity due to polyphenol polarity [35]. Nevertheless, in comparison with other fruits, we registered a high TPC; other studies reported *M. flexuosa*, with TPC values of 435.08 ± 6.97 and 362.90 ± 7.98 mg GAE/100 g of the whole pulp in fresh form [29,36]. The results here differed with studies where the TPC in fresh fruit, after food processing, was lowered or lost due to temperature or processing changes [31,32].

For the second experimental assay, concerning the TPC results for dehydrated *M. flexuosa* pulp and seeds, as shown in Figure 3b, a regular decreasing TPC pattern from 24 to 96 h of dehydration was registered. TPC values at the three different dehydration points were higher than the TPC in fresh pulp and seeds; the highest TPC was quantified at 24 h of dehydrating pulp and seeds at a constant 50 °C. The results at 48 and 96 h yielded slightly lower TPC values with statistical significance. The lowest phenolic content was measured in dehydrated pulp at 96 h (149.28 ± 0.81 mg GAE/100 g). This decreasing trend in phenolic concentration is consistent with research done with the purpose of evaluating TPC values in fruits processed with long effective storage time for exportation purposes [31].

2.3. Antioxidant Activity, DPPH (2,2-Diphenyl-1-picrylhydrazyl) Radical Scavenging Assays

The results for the antioxidant action of phenolic compounds, extracted in ethanol 80%, in a fresh and dehydrated matrix at different times for *M. flexuosa* (aguaje) samples are shown in Figure 4, showing the comparative results for two different experimental assays. The total inhibitory concentration, IC 50%, that yielded the best output was due to phenolics in dehydrated seeds at 96 h (78.28 ± 0.67 mg AAE/100 g of dehydrated sample). All DPPH results were higher in the extractions from fresh or dehydrated seeds. In both assays, Figure 4a,b, the antioxidant activity registered an increasing tendency. The best DPPH results, with statistical significance, were detected in *M. flexuosa* pulp and seeds dehydrated for 96 h.

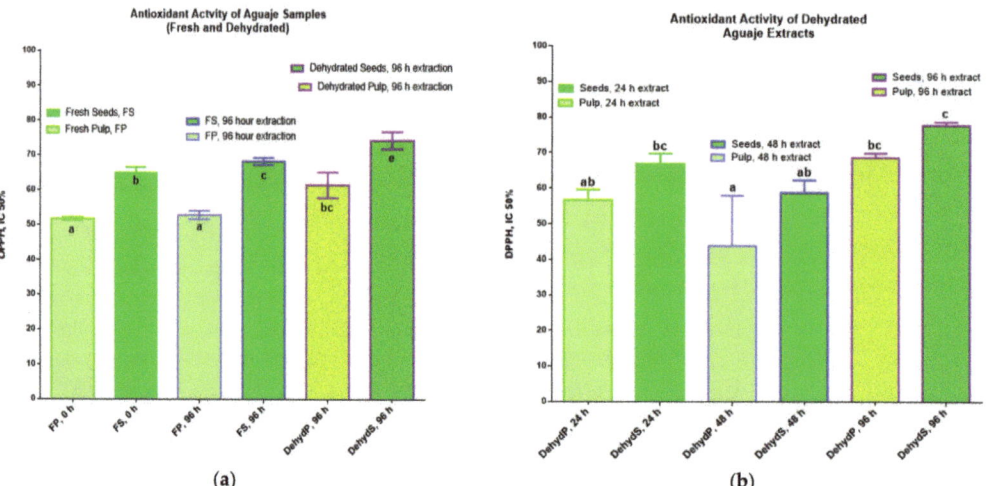

Figure 4. Antioxidant activity (mg AAE/100 g FP) of extracts in two different experimental assays. (**a**) fresh and dehydrated *M. flexuosa* and (**b**) dehydrated pulp and seeds at different times. Data are means (±standard deviation) and lower-case letters represent significant differences, for antioxidant activity of aguaje extracts according to DPPH (IC 50%), based on ANOVA followed by a Tukey test ($p < 0.05$).

These results for antioxidant activity coincide with the assays, in the same fruit, where other parts of the plant were evaluated [26,37]. The dehydration approaches in the present work led to improved DPPH values, with respect to the previously cited studies. The results are comparable and coincide with studies applying more complex dehydration processes [38,39]. Figure 5 represents a summary display of the dehydration process with respect to TPC and antioxidant activity seen in *M. flexuosa* pulp and seed extracts, as a comparative base for the various other studies.

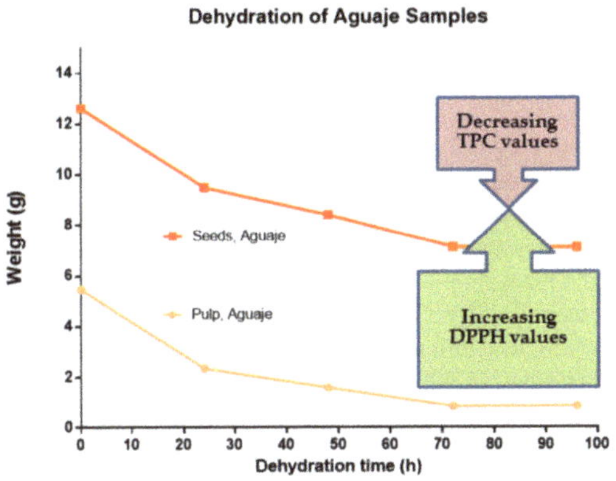

Figure 5. TPC (mg of gallic acid equivalents) and DPPH (mg ascorbic acid equivalents) in *M. flexuosa* (aguaje) pulp and seeds with respect to a constant dehydration pattern from 0 to 96 h. The stable flattening dehydration pattern is connected to lower TPC values and higher redox activity. From 72 to 96 h, the weight differences were stable, and statistical significance was registered at different points in the dehydration process.

Studies evaluating the biological activity of polyphenols in red raspberries showed that dehydration led to a lowering polyphenol content and less antioxidant activity, while the rate of this reduction was connected to the dehydration method, and this showed that a high dehydration temperature was linked to polyphenol content loss [40,41]. Increasing temperature promotes higher solubility and diffusion coefficient of polyphenolic compounds into the extracting solvents, and higher temperatures also enhance the penetration of solvents into the cell matrix; hence, increasing the TPC of the extracts [41].

Furthermore, the results confirmed a positive correlation between the total polyphenol content and the antioxidant activity for the aglycone compounds undergoing the drying process (74.7%). These lowering TPC values may be due to oxidative and thermal degradation of the phenolic compounds [42,43]. The major phenolic content drop, during fruit processing at high temperatures in enzymatic reactions, could be related to the action of oxidative enzymes such as polyphenol oxidases (PODs) and polyphenol peroxidases (PPOs) [43,44]. PODs can enhance the degradation of phenols when coexisting with PPOs; both the PPO and POD enzymatic activities play a key role in determining the phenolic profile of olive oil. In contrast, low temperatures during the dehydration process decrease the oxidation of volatile compounds [45].

When Cabernet Sauvignon and Merlot grapes were dried using a constant low temperature (7 °C) for several weeks, there was an increase in TPC and antioxidant activity [46]. This could be due to the effect of the concentration of the phenolic compounds as a result of water loss caused by the dehydration, even if the constant temperature (40 °C) was higher [47]. The results in these two previous studies partially coincide with the findings in the present work, with respect to the higher antioxidant activity of polyphenols in dehydrated aguaje fruit samples, but differ with respect to the decreasing phenolic content during d the dehydration process.

In a study evaluating the redox activity of phenolics from goldenberry, the levels of TPC and antioxidant activity (determined with the ferric reducing antioxidant power FRAP method) increased in dehydrated samples [20]. Furthermore, the highest TPC was registered in samples that were dried at 90 °C, coinciding with the results in this study, where samples were dehydrated at lower temperature (50 °C). The interconversion of phenolic compounds at high temperatures might be caused by the availability of phenolic precursor molecules through the non-enzymatic rearrangement between phenolic molecules [48]. This higher phenolic content may originate from the disruption of cell walls during processing or the breakdown of insoluble phenolic compounds. Therefore, this could lead to a better extractability for these particular types of phenolic compounds [49].

These comparative studies suggest that the antioxidant activity could be due to the combined reactions of total phenolics rather that certain individual components or the action of polyphenols as a whole group. The results in this study, using fresh and dehydrated aguaje seeds and pulp, coincide with the findings of Gupta et al. (2021), testing different parts of pomelo fruit (*Citrus grandis* (L.) Osbeck) in similar experiments for antioxidant activity. They found that TPC was highest in the membrane of the fruit, and DPPH registered the highest activity in the pomelo juice [50]. Considering the total polyphenols in the present study, the improvement in TPC could be a result of the destruction of the covering structure and the release of more phenolic compounds, facilitating and increasing the extraction yield [48]. Moreover, the dehydration process could induce metabolic pathways that can generate, and increase the number of, precursors for different categories of phenolic compounds [49].

3. Materials and Methods

3.1. Reagents and Chemicals

Ethanol, sodium carbonate, and Folin–Ciocalteu reagent were purchased from PanReac AppliChem, ITW Reagents, (Darmstadt, Germany), and methanol, from Sigma Aldrich (St. Louis, MO, USA). Ascorbic acid (Sebion) and DPPH (2,2-Diphenyl-1-picrylhydrazyl, Sigma-Aldrich) were purchased from Merck KGaA (Darmstadt, Germany).

3.2. Plant Material, Sample Preparation, and Polyphenol Extractions

M. flexuosa pulp with seeds was obtained in the Colombian city of Leticia. All samples were refrigerated before laboratory analyses. The extraction of total polyphenol compounds was performed following a previous method from this research group [2,51]. Different amounts of fresh and dehydrated pulp and seeds of *M. flexuosa* were placed in ethanol (80% w/v) at proportions of 1:5 per volume, stirred for 15 min at 500 rpm, homogenized, and stored at room temperature, in the dark, for 24 h without stirring. Two different extractions times (—*al fresco*—0 h and 96 h of extraction) for the first experimental assay, as an explorative comparison, and three different dehydration times (24, 48, and 96 h) at a constant of 50 °C, including only samples in dry state as a second assay, were considered in this experimental process. The extracts were centrifuged for 10 min at 3500 rpm, and the supernatant was recovered for polyphenol quantitation and antioxidant activity evaluation.

3.3. Total Polyphenol Content (TPC)

The total polyphenol content in *M. flexuosa* pulp and seeds (fresh and dehydrated matrix) was quantified following the Folin–Ciocalteu (F–C) assay [51]. Samples of 1 mL of each extract were mixed with 1 mL F–C reagent (10% w/v), allowed to react for 2 min, and mixed with 2 mL sodium carbonate, Na_2CO_3, (3.5% w/v). Reactants were kept in the dark at room temperature for 90 min. All runs were performed in triplicate. Absorbance was read at 655 nm in a UV-Vis spectrophotometer (Mecasys Optizen POP, Daejeon, Korea). All data were calculated based on a gallic acid standard calibration curve, with a range of 0–4.0 mg/L and r^2 of 0.9982). TPC is expressed as milligrams gallic acid equivalent (GAE) per 100 g of fresh or dehydrated sample (mg GAE/100 g).

3.4. DPPH Assay for Radical Scavenging Antioxidant Activity

The DPPH radical scavenging test is one of the most useful techniques to evaluate the antioxidant activity in polyphenols extracted from natural products. The DPPH compound is a stable free radical in methanol. The DPPH assay was performed following previous work from this research group [2]. Volumes of 1900 µL of DPPH (100 µM) prepared in pure methanol were mixed with 100 µL of each diluted (1:5) extract and left to react in the dark at room temperature for 30 min. The antioxidant activity from phenolics, in fresh and dehydrated pulp and seeds, of *M. flexuosa* was measured via spectrophotometry at

517 nm, comparing against a methanol blank. A positive control of ascorbic acid based on a calibration curve, and in triplicates for each colorimetric reaction, was applied in this methodology. The control curve was prepared with concentrations of comparable reference ascorbic acid (Merck KGaA, Darmstadt, Germany) in a concentration range from 50 to 600 µg/mL (r^2 of 0.9945). All dilutions followed the same DPPH reaction conditions for the antioxidant activity evaluated in fruit extracts. The slope taken from the calibration curve served as the calculation of the inhibition concentration (IC 50%), when 50% of the antioxidant component was reduced. The results for IC 50% were determined based on the equation:

$$\% \text{ scavenging DPPH free radical} = (ABS_{Control} - ABS_{Extracts} / ABS_{Control}) \times 100\%$$

The antioxidant activity of *M. flexuosa* extracted phenolics is expressed as mg of ascorbic acid equivalents per 100 g of fresh or dehydrated pulp or seeds (mg AAE/100 g).

3.5. Statistical Analysis

All analyses were carried out in triplicate, and TPC and DPPH values are expressed as mean ± standard deviation (SD). Means were tested for normality and homogeneity. Data were analyzed based on a ANOVA test followed by Tukey test ($p < 0.05$) with the IBM SPSS Statistics software version 20.0 (IBM Corp., Armonk, NY, USA).

4. Conclusions

The total polyphenol content and antioxidant activity of *M. flexuosa* pulp and seeds, in fresh and dehydrated form, were tested in this work. The water content in a food matrix allows for a specific polyphenol oriented chemical reaction, yielding better results in some cases where the water content is higher. A controlled dehydration process was considered in this experimental approach, with the purpose of evaluating the polyphenol availability and antioxidant action. TPC values were not directly proportional to antioxidant activity, suggesting that the polyphenol reactions for radical scavenging in pulp and seeds of *M. flexuosa* do not depend directly in the specific quantity of phenolic compounds, but rather on the specific chemical structure or on its re-accommodation or interconversion. More studies based on the specific polyphenol/flavonoid content and the presence of other antioxidants, such as C vitamin, in *M. flexuosa* could lead to understanding more of the specific antioxidant activity of this fruit with multiple processes of it edible parts.

Author Contributions: Conceptualization, formal analysis, data curation and writing—review and editing, H.B., M.F.S.-G. and J.C.C.-H.; methodology, H.B., M.F.S.-G. and J.C.C.-H.; supervision, J.C.C.-H.; project administration, H.B. and J.C.C.-H.; funding acquisition, J.C.C.-H. All authors have read and agreed to the published version of the manuscript.

Funding: This research received no external funding.

Institutional Review Board Statement: Not applicable.

Informed Consent Statement: Not applicable.

Data Availability Statement: The data presented in this study are available on request from the corresponding author.

Acknowledgments: The authors thank all laboratory members, especially Carmen Serna Hurtado, at Universidad de Manizales (Colombia) for their constant support and help.

Conflicts of Interest: The authors declare no conflict of interest.

Sample Availability: Samples of the compounds are not available from the authors.

References

1. Garzón, G.A.; Narváez, C.E.; Riedl, K.M.; Schwartz, S.J. Chemical composition, anthocyanins, non-anthocyanin phenolics and antioxidant activity of wild bilberry (*Vaccinium meridionale* Swartz) from Colombia. *Food Chem.* **2010**, *122*, 980–986. [CrossRef]
2. Carmona-Hernandez, J.C.; Le, M.; Idárraga-Mejía, A.M.; González-Correa, C.H. Flavonoid/Polyphenol Ratio in *Mauritia flexuosa* and *Theobroma grandiflorum* as an Indicator of Effective Antioxidant Action. *Molecules* **2021**, *26*, 6431. [CrossRef] [PubMed]
3. Solverson, P.M.; Rumpler, W.V.; Leger, J.L.; Redan, B.W.; Ferruzzi, M.G.; Baer, D.J.; Castonguay, T.W.; Novotny, J.A. Blackberry Feeding Increases Fat Oxidation and Improves Insulin Sensitivity in Overweight and Obese Males. *Nutrients* **2018**, *10*, 1048. [CrossRef] [PubMed]
4. Mir, S.A.; Shah, M.A.; Ganai, S.A.; Ahmad, T.; Gani, M. Understanding the role of active components from plant sources in obesity management. *J. Saudi. Soc. Agric. Sci.* **2019**, *18*, 168–176. [CrossRef]
5. Neri-Numa, I.A.; Cazarin, C.B.B.; Ruiz, A.L.T.G.; Paulino, B.N.; Molina, G.; Pastore, G.M. Targeting flavonoids on modulation of metabolic syndrome. *J. Funct. Foods* **2020**, *73*, 104132. [CrossRef]
6. Uttara, B.; Singh, A.V.; Zamboni, P.; Mahajan, R.T. Oxidative stress and neurodegenerative diseases: A review of upstream and downstream antioxidant therapeutic options. *Curr. Neuropharmacol.* **2009**, *7*, 65–74. [CrossRef]
7. Valko, M.; Rhodes, C.J.; Moncol, J.; Izakovic, M.; Mazur, M. Free radicals, metals and antioxidants in oxidative stress-induced cancer. *Chem. Biol. Interact.* **2006**, *160*, 1–40. [CrossRef] [PubMed]
8. Kleemann, R.; Verschuren, L.; Morrison, M.; Zadelaar, S.; van Erk, M.J.; Wielinga, P.Y.; Kooistra, T. Anti-inflammatory, antiproliferative and anti-atherosclerotic effects of quercetin in human in vitro and in vivo models. *Atherosclerosis* **2011**, *218*, 44–52. [CrossRef] [PubMed]
9. Luo, H.; Jiang, B.; Li, B.; Li, Z.; Jiang, B.-H.; Chen, Y.C. Kaempferol nanoparticles achieve strong and selective inhibition of ovarian cancer cell viability. *Int. J. Nanomed.* **2012**, *7*, 3951–3959.
10. Swallah, M.S.; Sun, H.; Affoh, R.; Fu, H.; Yu, H. Antioxidant Potential Overviews of Secondary Metabolites (Polyphenols) in Fruits. *Int. J. Food Sci.* **2020**, *2020*, 9081686. [CrossRef]
11. Kalinowska, M.; Gryko, K.; Wróblewska, A.M.; Jabłońska-Trypuć, A.; Karpowicz, D. Phenolic content, chemical composition and anti-/pro-oxidant activity of Gold Milenium and Papierowka apple peel extracts. *Sci. Rep.* **2020**, *10*, 14951. [CrossRef] [PubMed]
12. Dias, R.; Oliveira, H.; Fernandes, I.; Simal-Gandara, J.; Perez-Gregorio, R. Recent advances in extracting phenolic compounds from food and their use in disease prevention and as cosmetics. *Crit. Rev. Food Sci. Nutr.* **2021**, *61*, 1130–1151. [CrossRef] [PubMed]
13. Madamanchi, N.R.; Vendrov, A.; Runge, M.S. Oxidative stress and vascular disease. *Arter. Thromb. Vasc. Biol.* **2005**, *25*, 29–38. [CrossRef]
14. Virapongse, A.; Endress, B.A.; Gilmore, M.P.; Horn, C.; Romulo, C. Ecology, livelihoods, and management of the *Mauritia flexuosa* palm in South America. *Glob. Ecol. Conserv.* **2017**, *10*, 70–92. [CrossRef]
15. Trujillo-Gonzalez, J.M.; Torres-Mora, M.A.; Santana-Castañeda, E. The Moriche palm (*Mauritia flexuosa* L. f) represents astrategic ecosystem. *Orinoquía* **2011**, *15*, 62–70. [CrossRef]
16. Gragson, T.L. Pumé Exploitation of *Mauritia flexuosa* (Palmae) in the Llanos of Venezuela. *J. Ethnobiol.* **1995**, *15*, 177–188.
17. Case, C.; Lares, M.; Palma, A.; Brito, S.; Pérez, E.; Schroeder, M. Blood glucose and serum lipid levels in the Venezuelan Warao tribe: Possible relationship with moriche fruit (*Mauritia flexuosa* L.) intake. *Nut. Metabol. Cardiovasc. Dis.* **2007**, *17*, e1–e2. [CrossRef]
18. Martins, R.C.; Filgueiras, T.S.; de Albuquerque, U.P. Ethnobotany of *Mauritia flexuosa* (Arecaceae) in a Maroon Community in Central Brazil. *Econ. Bot.* **2011**, *66*, 91–98. [CrossRef]
19. Horn, C.M.; Gilmore, M.P.; Endress, B.A. Ecological and socio-economic factors influencing aguaje (*Mauritia flexuosa*) resource management in two indigenous communities in the Peruvian Amazon. *For. Ecol. Manag.* **2012**, *267*, 93–103. [CrossRef]
20. Lopez, J.; Vega-Gálvez, A.; Torres, M.J.; Lemus-Mondaca, R.; Quispe-Fuentes, I.; Di Scala, K. Effect of dehydration temperature on physico-chemical properties and antioxidant capacity of goldenberry (*Physalis peruviana* L.). *Chil. J. Agric. Res.* **2013**, *73*, 293–300. [CrossRef]
21. Tolić, M.-T.; Jurčević, I.L.; Krbavčić, I.P.; Marković, K.; Vahčić, N. Phenolic Content, Antioxidant Capacity and Quality of Chokeberry (*Aronia melanocarpa*) Products. *Food Technol. Biotechnol.* **2015**, *53*, 171–179. [CrossRef] [PubMed]
22. Chen, W.; Guo, Y.; Zhang, J.; Zhang, X.; Meng, Y. Effect of Different Drying Processes on the Physicochemical and Antioxidant Properties of Thinned Young Apple. *Int. J. Food Eng.* **2015**, *11*, 207–219. [CrossRef]
23. Eran Nagar, E.; Okun, Z.; Shpigelman, A. Digestive fate of polyphenols: Updated view of the influence of chemical structure and the presence of cell wall material. *Curr. Opin. Food Sci.* **2020**, *31*, 38–46. [CrossRef]
24. Starec, M.; Calabretti, A.; Berti, F.; Forzato, C. Oleocanthal Quantification Using ^{1}H-NMR Spectroscopy and Polyphenols HPLC Analysis of Olive Oil from the Bianchera/Belica Cultivar. *Molecules* **2021**, *26*, 242. [CrossRef] [PubMed]
25. Koolen, H.H.F.; da Silva, F.M.A.; Gozzo, F.C.; de Souza, A.Q.L.; de Souza, A.D.L. Antioxidant, antimicrobial activities and characterization of phenolic compounds from buriti (*Mauritia flexuosa* L. f.) by UPLC–ESI-MS/MS. *Food Res. Int.* **2013**, *51*, 467–473. [CrossRef]
26. de Oliveira, D.M.; Siqueira, E.P.; Nunes, Y.R.F.; Cota, B.B. Flavonoids from leaves of *Mauritia flexuosa*. *Rev. Bras. Farmacog.* **2013**, *23*, 614–620. [CrossRef]

27. Tauchen, J.; Bortl, L.; Huml, L.; Miksatkova, P.; Doskocil, I.; Marsik, P.; Villegas, P.P.P.; Flores, Y.B.; van Damme, P.; Lojka, B.; et al. Phenolic composition, antioxidant and anti-proliferative activities of edible and medicinal plants from the Peruvian Amazon. *Rev. Bras. Farmacog.* **2016**, *26*, 728–737. [CrossRef]
28. Abreu-Naranjo, R.; Paredes-Moreta, J.G.; Granda-Albuja, G.; Iturralde, G.; González-Paramás, A.M.; Alvarez-Suarez, J.M. Bioactive compounds, phenolic profile, antioxidant capacity and effectiveness against lipid peroxidation of cell membranes of *Mauritia flexuosa* L. fruit extracts from three biomes in the Ecuadorian Amazon. *Heliyon* **2020**, *6*, e05211. [CrossRef]
29. Mencarelli, F.; D'onofrio, C.; Bucci, S.; Baccelloni, S.; Cini, R.; Pica, G.; Bellincontro, A. Management of high-quality dehydrated grape in vinification to produce dry red wines. *Food Chem.* **2021**, *338*, 127623. [CrossRef]
30. Lund, M.N. Reactions of plant polyphenols in foods: Impact of molecular structure. *Trends Food Sci. Technol.* **2021**, *112*, 241–251. [CrossRef]
31. Nayeem, S.; Sundararajan, S.; Ashok, A.K.; Abusaliya, A.; Ramalingam, S. Effects of cooking on phytochemical and antioxidant properties of pigmented and non-pigmented rare Indian rice landraces. *Biocatal. Agric. Biotechnol.* **2021**, *32*, 101928. [CrossRef]
32. Aryal, S.; Baniya, M.K.; Danekhu, K.; Kunwar, P.; Gurung, R.; Koirala, N. Total Phenolic Content, Flavonoid Content and Antioxidant Potential of Wild Vegetables from Western Nepal. *Plants* **2019**, *8*, 96. [CrossRef] [PubMed]
33. Costanzo, G.; Vitale, E.; Iesce, M.R.; Naviglio, D.; Amoresano, A.; Fontanarosa, C.; Spinelli, M.; Ciaravolo, M.; Arena, C. Antioxidant Properties of Pulp, Peel and Seeds of Phlegrean Mandarin (*Citrus reticulata* Blanco) at Different Stages of Fruit Ripening. *Antioxidants* **2022**, *11*, 187. [CrossRef] [PubMed]
34. Wongnarat, C.; Srihanam, P. Phytochemical and Antioxidant Activity in Seeds and Pulp of Grape Cultivated in Thailand. *Orient. J. Chem.* **2017**, *33*, 113–121. [CrossRef]
35. Nakilcioğlu-Taş, E.; Ötleş, S. Influence of extraction solvents on the polyphenol contents, compositions, and antioxidant capacities of fig (*Ficus carica* L.) seeds. *Acad. Bras. Cienc.* **2021**, *93*, e20190526. [CrossRef]
36. Cândido, T.L.N.; Silva, M.R.; Agostini-Costa, T.S. Bioactive compounds and antioxidant capacity of buriti (*Mauritia flexuosa* L.f.) from the Cerrado and Amazon biomes. *Food Chem.* **2015**, *177*, 313–319. [CrossRef]
37. da Rocha Romero, A.B.; de Carvalho e Martins, M.; Moreira Nunes, P.H.; Trindale Ferreira, N.R.; de Lima, A.; de Assis, R.C.; Araújo, E.M. La actividad antioxidante in vitro e in vivo de la fruta buriti (*Mauritia flexuosa* L.f.). *Nutr. Hosp.* **2015**, *32*, 2153–2161.
38. Chong, C.H.; Law, C.L.; Figiel, A.; Wojdyło, A.; Oziembłowski, M. Colour, phenolic content and antioxidant capacity of some fruits dehydrated by a combination of different methods. *Food Chem.* **2013**, *141*, 3889–3896. [CrossRef]
39. Kidoń, M.; Grabowska, J. Bioactive compounds, antioxidant activity, and sensory qualities of red-fleshed apples dried by different methods. *LWT* **2021**, *136*, 110302. [CrossRef]
40. Mejia-Meza, E.I.; Yáñez, J.A.; Remsberg, C.M.; Takemoto, J.K.; Davies, N.M.; Rasco, B.; Clary, C. Effect of dehydration on raspberries: Polyphenol and anthocyanin retention, antioxidant capacity, and antiadipogenic activity. *J. Food Sci.* **2010**, *75*, 5–12. [CrossRef]
41. Taranto, F.; Pasqualone, A.; Mangini, G.; Tripodi, P.; Miazzi, M.M.; Pavan, S.; Montemurro, C. Polyphenol oxidases in crops: Biochemical, physiological and genetic aspects. *Int. J. Mol. Sci.* **2017**, *18*, 377. [CrossRef] [PubMed]
42. Zhang, W.; Liang, L.; Pan, X.; Lao, F.; Liao, X.; Wu, J. Alterations of phenolic compounds in red raspberry juice induced by high-hydrostatic-pressure and high-temperature short-time processing. *Innov. Food Sci. Emerg. Technol.* **2021**, *67*, 102569. [CrossRef]
43. Alfaro, S.; Mutis, A.; Quiroz, A.; Seguel, I.; Scheuermann, E. Effects of Drying Techniques on Murtilla Fruit Polyphenols and Antioxidant Activity. *J. Food Res.* **2014**, *3*, 73. [CrossRef]
44. Wan Mahmood, W.M.A.; Lorwirachsutee, A.; Theodoropoulos, C.; Gonzalez-Miquel, M. Polyol-Based Deep Eutectic Solvents for Extraction of Natural Polyphenolic Antioxidants from *Chlorella vulgaris*. *ACS Sustain. Chem. Eng.* **2019**, *7*, 5018–5026. [CrossRef]
45. Cirilli, M.; Bellincontro, A.; De Santis, D.; Botondi, R.; Colao, M.C.; Muleo, R.; Mencarelli, F. Temperature and water loss affect ADH activity and gene expression in grape berry during postharvest dehydration. *Food Chem.* **2012**, *132*, 447–454. [CrossRef] [PubMed]
46. Panceri, C.P.; Gomes, T.M.; De Gois, J.S.; Borges, D.L.G.; Bordignon-Luiz, M.T. Effect of dehydration process on mineral content, phenolic compounds and antioxidant activity of Cabernet Sauvignon and Merlot grapes. *Food Res. Int.* **2013**, *54*, 1343–1350. [CrossRef]
47. Marquez, A.; Serratosa, M.P.; Lopez-Toledano, A.; Merida, J. Colour and phenolic compounds in sweet red wines from Merlot and Tempranillo grapes chamber-dried under controlled conditions. *Food Chem.* **2012**, *130*, 111–120. [CrossRef]
48. Tepe, F.; Tepe, T.; Ekinci, A. Impact of air temperature on drying characteristics and some bioactive properties of kiwi fruit slices. *Chem. Ind. Chem. Eng.* **2021**, *7*, 26. [CrossRef]
49. Aguilera, Y.; Dueñas, M.; Estrella, I.; Hernández, T.; Benitez, V.; Esteban, R.M.; Martín-Cabrejas, M.A. Evaluation of phenolic profile and antioxidant properties of Pardina lentil as affected by industrial dehydration. *J. Agric. Food Chem.* **2010**, *58*, 10101–10108. [CrossRef]
50. Gupta, A.K.; Dhua, S.; Sahu, P.P.; Abate, G.; Mishra, P.; Mastinu, A. Variation in Phytochemical, Antioxidant and Volatile Composition of Pomelo Fruit (*Citrus grandis* (L.) Osbeck) during Seasonal Growth and Development. *Plants* **2021**, *10*, 1941. [CrossRef]
51. Carmona-Hernandez, J.C.; Taborda-Ocampo, G.; Gonzalez-Correa, C.H. Folin-Ciocalteu Reaction Alternatives for Higher Polyphenol Quantitation in Colombian Passion Fruits. *Int. J. Food Sci.* **2021**, *2021*, 8871301. [CrossRef] [PubMed]

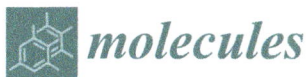

Article

Isoflavone Changes in Immature and Mature Soybeans by Thermal Processing

Shanshan Qu [1,†], Soon Jae Kwon [2,†], Shucheng Duan [1], You Jin Lim [1] and Seok Hyun Eom [1,*]

1. Department of Horticultural Biotechnology, College of Life Sciences, Kyung Hee University, Yongin 17104, Korea; qss1996@khu.ac.kr (S.Q.); dsc97@khu.ac.kr (S.D.); yujn0213@khu.ac.kr (Y.J.L.)
2. Advanced Radiation Technology Institute, Korea Atomic Energy Research Institute, Jeongeup 56212, Korea; soonjaekwon@kaeri.re.kr
* Correspondence: se43@khu.ac.kr
† These authors contributed equally to this work.

Abstract: The isoflavone changes occurring in mature soybeans during food processing have been well studied, but less information is available on the changes in immature soybeans during thermal processing. This study aimed to determine the effect of thermal processing by dry- or wet-heating on the changes in the isoflavone profiles of immature and mature soybeans. In the malonylglycoside forms of isoflavone, their deglycosylation was more severe after wet-heating than after dry-heating regardless of the soybean maturity. The malonyl forms of isoflavones in the immature seeds were drastically degraded after a short wet-heating process. In the acetylglycoside forms of isoflavone, dry-heating produced relatively low amounts of the acetyl types in the immature soybeans compared with those in the mature soybeans. These results were explained by the content of acetyldaidzin being relatively less changed after dry-heating immature soybeans but increasing four to five times in the mature soybeans. More of the other types of acetylglycoside were produced by dry-heating soybeans regardless of their maturity. Acetylgenistin in wet-heating was a key molecule because its content was unchanged in the immature soybeans during processing but increased in the mature soybeans. This determined the total acetylglycoside content after wet-heating. In contrast, most of the acetyl forms of isoflavone were produced after 90 to 120 min of dry-heating regardless of the seed maturity. It can be suggested that the pattern of isoflavone conversion was significantly affected by the innate water content of the seeds, with a lower water content in the mature soybeans leading to the greater production of acetyl isoflavones regardless of the processing method even if only applied for a relatively short time. The results suggested that the isoflavone conversion in the immature soybeans mainly follows the wet-heating process and can be promoted in the application of stronger processing.

Keywords: isoflavone conversion; thermal process; immature seeds; mature seeds; internal water content

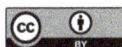

1. Introduction

Soybeans (*Glycine max* L.) are one of the most widely consumed legumes in the world. As well as their main role in providing protein, carbohydrates, and oil, soybeans are also a rich source of phytochemicals, particularly isoflavones [1,2]. The content of isoflavones, a type of flavonoid, is greater in soybeans than in other legumes [3]. The 12 major isoflavones in soybeans can be classified into four main forms: aglycones (daidzein, glycitein, and genistein); β-glycosides (daidzin, glycitin, and genistin); acetylglycosides (acetyldaidzin, acetylglycitin, and acetylgenistin); and malonylglycosides (malonyldaidzin, malonylglycosides, and malonylgenistin) [4,5]. Of these isoflavone groups, malonylglycosides are the predominant form in raw soybeans, followed by β-glycosides and acetylglycosides, with aglycones rarely observed [6]. Epidemiological studies have reported that the presence of different types of isoflavone in soybeans contributes to various biological activities, such as reducing the risk of cancer, cardiovascular disease, and osteoporosis, and relieving menopausal symptoms [7–12]. Among the four forms of isoflavones, the bioavailability of malonyl-conjugated isoflavones was lower than that of corresponding non-conjugated β-glycoside isoflavones [13], and that of isoflavone aglycons was highest because aglycones were more easily and quickly absorbed by the intestine [14]. Furthermore, some studies reported that non-conjugated glycoside isoflavones also possessed high-quality antioxidant activity similar to aglycones. Thus, soybeans with a high content of non-conjugated glycosides and aglycones had high-quality antioxidant activity [15].

Because of their grassy-beany flavor and bitter taste [16,17], raw mature soybeans are mainly consumed after thermal processing, such as boiling or roasting, which greatly improves the flavor of the soybeans and soy products [18–20]. It has also been reported that thermal processing causes the conversion or degradation of isoflavones [21–24]. The predominant isoflavone form (malonylglycosides) is usually converted into acetylglycosides and β-glycosides by thermal processing [25–30], with the patterns of conversion depending significantly on the severity of heating. In general, the increase in the contents of isoflavone acetylglycosides and β-glycosides occurs through the decarboxylation and deesterification of malonylglycosides, respectively [28,31]. The wet-heating method promotes deesterification more than dry-heating as it causes the rapid conversion of isoflavone malonylglycosides to β-glycosides rather than acetylglycosides [32,33]. Chien et al. [34] reported no changes in the glycosides and aglycones during dry-heating below 150 °C, but Huang and Chou [35] reported a decrease in the aglycones in soybeans steamed for 30 min at temperatures above 60 °C.

The changes in isoflavone content during thermal processing in mature soybeans have been widely reported, but those in immature soybeans have rarely been studied. Immature soybeans, also known as edamame or maodou, are harvested when the green seeds fill the pod and have a water content of 60 to 65% [36,37]. Immature soybeans are also rich in isoflavones. The difference in the isoflavone content between immature and mature soybeans is significantly affected by the cultivar. Simonne et al. [38] investigated the iso-flavone contents of immature and mature beans of five soybean cultivars and found that the immature beans contained twice the isoflavone content of the mature beans in four of the cultivars, whereas Kim et al. [39] reported that the mature soybeans of several cultivars contained more isoflavone than the immature soybeans. Immature soybeans also exhibit a beany off-flavor and unique taste compared with mature soybeans [40]. Traditionally, in East Asia, immature soybeans have also been consumed as vegetables and snacks after thermal processing, such as boiling [40]. Simonne et al. [38] studied the influence of processing methods, such as boiling and freeze-drying, on the distribution of isoflavones in immature soybeans, but the patterns of variation in isoflavone content in immature soybeans during thermal processing are still unclear, particularly compared with those in mature soybeans.

Therefore, the objectives of this study are: to compare the effects of thermal processing (dry- and wet-heating) on variations in the isoflavone profiles of immature and mature soybeans, and to determine the effect of the internal water content of soybeans on the isoflavone content during thermal processing by varying the soaking time of mature seeds before dry-heating. This study will provide basic information on utilizing isoflavones in soybeans with different levels of maturity.

2. Results and Discussion

2.1. Physiological Characteristics of Immature and Mature Soybeans

The physical characteristics of the raw immature and mature soybeans are shown in Table 1. The water contents of the immature and mature seeds were 66.87% and 13.04%, respectively. Takahashi et al. [37] reported that, in immature soybeans, the water contents of four different cultivars ranged from 61.5% to 76.8%, similar levels to those of the present study. It has also been reported that the moisture content of mature soybeans was 10–15%, a similar content to the present study [41,42]. The dry weight of 10 immature seeds

(0.66 g) was significantly lower than that of 10 mature seeds (0.88 g) (Table 1). As expected, a remarkable difference in the SSC of the immature (2.75 °Brix) and mature seeds (15.76 °Brix) was also observed (Table 1). Sale and Campbell [43] reported that a dramatic reduction in the water content of soybeans was accompanied by a steady accumulation of dry matter and SSC during seed maturation from the R6 (immature) to the R8 (mature) stages. Figure 1 shows the morphologies of the immature and mature soybeans before and after thermal processing. After dry-heating, the immature and mature soybeans had shrunk, particularly the immature soybeans, whereas they had both swelled after wet-heating, particularly the mature seeds. A significant variation in seed color (green to yellow) was also observed, particularly for the immature soybeans, possibly because of the Maillard reaction [44].

Table 1. Physical characteristics of immature and mature soybean seeds.

Seed Maturity	Water Content (%)	Dry Weight (g/10 ea)	SSC (°Brix)
Immature	66.87 ± 0.32 [a]	0.66 ± 0.02 [b]	2.75 ± 0.18 [b]
Mature	13.04 ± 0.22 [b]	0.88 ± 0.03 [a]	15.76 ± 0.31 [a]

SSC means soluble solids content. Different letters (a, b) in a column indicate significant differences at $p < 0.05$ by Tukey's studentized range (HSD) test. Results are given as mean ± SE ($n = 10$).

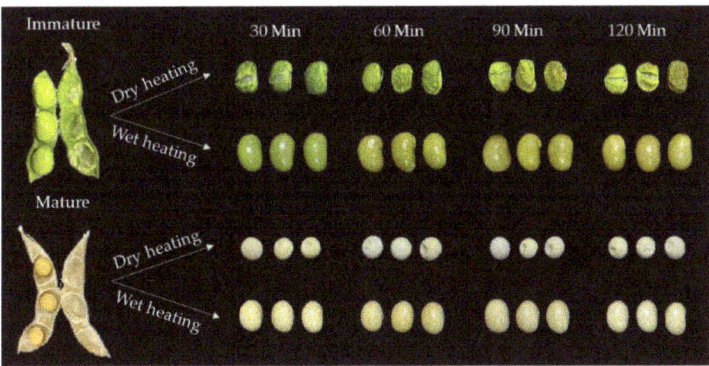

Figure 1. Morphologies of immature and mature soybeans after dry- and wet-heating for different times.

2.2. The Variation in the Total Isoflavone Content and Four Isoflavone Forms of Soybeans during Thermal Processing

Many studies have reported the effect of thermal processing on the isoflavone profiles of mature soybeans or soy products [25,28,30,32]. However, studies comparing the thermal transformation or degradation of isoflavones in soybeans at different maturity levels are still limited. The variations in the total isoflavone content (TI) and in the other four forms of isoflavone (total isoflavone malonylglycosides (TIMG); total isoflavone acetylglycosides (TIAG); total isoflavone β-glycosides (TIG); and total isoflavone aglycones (TIA)) in immature and mature soybeans during thermal processing are shown in Figure 2.

Before thermal treatment (freeze-dried, FD), the TI of the mature soybeans (304.51 mg/100 g DW) was 1.6 times higher than that of the immature soybeans. The isoflavone form with the highest content in both the immature and mature soybeans was TIMG, followed by TIG, with small amounts of TIAG and TIA (Figure 2). These results were consistent with those of Kim et al. [39], who reported that the TI of mature soybeans was higher than that of immature soybeans, with malonylglycoside isoflavones being the predominant form in both immature and mature soybeans, followed by the β-glycoside, acetylglycoside, and aglycone isoflavone forms.

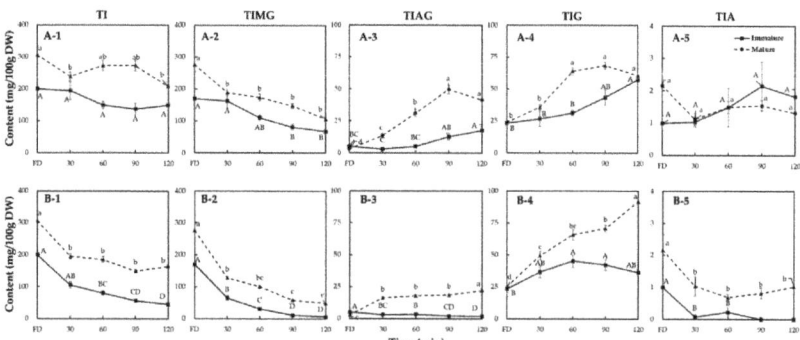

Figure 2. Changes in the total isoflavone (TI), total isoflavone malonylglycosides (TIMG), total isoflavone acetylglycosides (TIAG), total isoflavone β-glycosides (TIG), and total isoflavone aglycones (TIA) contents of immature and mature soybeans during dry-heating (**A**) and wet-heating (**B**). Data are shown as mean ± SE ($n = 3$). Different letters indicate significant differences at $p < 0.05$ by Tukey's studentized range (HSD) test.

After thermal processing, the TI content tended to decrease regardless of the seed maturity and processing method. The TI content decreased significantly after wet-heating: in mature soybeans from 304.51 to 163.49 mg/100 g DW; in immature soybeans from 199.34 to 44.63 mg/100 g DW; compared with dry-heating: in mature soybeans to 200.32 mg/100 g DW; and in immature soybeans to 147.15 mg/100 g DW). This may have been caused by the difference in humidity between wet- and dry-heating affecting the transfer of thermal energy [34,45], which accelerates the decrease in TI content. This decrease in the TI content of thermally treated soybeans or soy products has been widely reported [13,29,38]. However, the present study has been the first to compare changes in TI content in soybeans at different maturity levels and after different processing methods. The significant decrease in the TIMG content was considered to be the main reason for the reduction in the TI content (Figure 2). As mentioned previously, malonylglycoside isoflavones are the predominant form in soybeans. Similar to the TI content, the content of TIMG in both the immature and mature soybeans tended to decrease after thermal treatment, and soybeans with a higher internal water content under wet-heating conditions promoted this decreasing trend (Figure 2(A-2,B-2)). The relative thermal instability of malonyl-conjugated β-glycoside isoflavones has been reported previously [34]. Wet-heating degraded malonyl isoflavones more than dry-heating because of the higher moisture content in wet-heat process [32,45].

The decrease in the TIMG content, usually accompanied by an increase in the TIAG content in soybeans processed by thermal treatments, such as roasting [46] and baking [47], or in processed soy products, such as cooked soybeans [48] and soy milk [31], has been widely investigated. The increase in the TIAG content was caused by the decarboxylation of malonyl isoflavones during heat processing. Similarly, in mature soybeans, significant increases in the TIAG content after thermal processing were also observed (Figure 2(A-3,B-3)), with dry-heating increasing its content from 3.09 to 41.47 mg/100 g DW, thus being more effective than wet-heating, which increased its content from 3.09 to 22.23 mg/100 g DW. The difference in the effect of dry- and wet-heating on TIAG content can be explained by the maximum degradation rate of malonyl to acetyl isoflavones under the dry-heat condition, while a low conversion rate of malonyl to acetyl isoflavones was found under the wet-heat condition [34]. It indicated that wet-heating tended to convert or degrade malonylglycosides to other isoflavone derivatives instead of acetylglycosides, while the decarboxylation of malonyl isoflavones also occurred simultaneously. However, immature soybeans showed the reverse behavior in response to dry- and wet-heating: like the mature soybeans, dry-heating increased the TIAG content of immature beans from 5.20 to 19.36 mg/100 g DW, whereas wet-heating significantly decreased the TIAG content from 5.20 to 2.04 mg/100 g DW. As there has been no comparative study on the variation in the TIAG content in immature soybeans under dry- and wet-heating conditions, the present study is the first to report that the variation in the TIAG content of immature soybeans after thermal processing is different from that of mature beans. This may have been caused by the higher internal water content of immature soybeans significantly promoting the transfer of energy under wet-heating compared with dry-heating conditions. This led to the rapid conversion of acetylglycosides to β-glycosides, or the degradation of acetylglycosides [34], a speculation also supported by Huang and Chou [35], who reported that the acetyl isoflavones content of soaked black soybeans decreased after steaming at 100 °C for 30 min. Under dry-heat conditions, the TIAG content of the mature soybeans increased significantly compared with the immature soybeans (Figure 2(A-3)). This could be interpreted as the variation in the TIAG content of immature soybeans with their higher internal water content under dry-heating being similar to that of mature soybeans under wet-heating.

Thermal processing also increased the TIG content by deesterifying malonylglycoside and acetylglycoside isoflavones [46–50]. The patterns of variation in the TIG content were significantly affected by the processing methods and level of seed maturity (Figure 2(A-4,B-4)). In mature soybeans, the effect of wet-heating, increasing the TIG content from 25.16 to 91.64 mg/100 g DW, was better than that of dry-heating, where it increased from 25.16 to 59.00 mg/100 g DW. This can be partly explained by the deesterification of acetylglycoside isoflavones to form β-glycoside isoflavones under wet-heating (Figure 2(A-3,B-3)). Huang and Chou [35] have also reported that the TIG content of mature soybeans increased as the temperature of the thermal treatment increased. In contrast, the opposite patterns were observed for immature soybeans. The TIG content after dry-heating, ranging from 23.40 to 57.30 mg/100 g DW, was higher than that after wet-heating, which ranged from 23.40 to 45.26 mg/100 g DW. As mentioned earlier, the high internal moisture content of the soybeans under wet-heating may have led to excessive energy transfer, leading to the further conversion or degradation of the β-glycoside isoflavones. Thermal processes, such as oven drying [46], baking [47], frying [48], steaming [35], and autoclaving [50], have been reported as important methods for increasing the TIG content of mature soybeans. However, the effect of dry- and wet-heating on the variation in the TIG content of immature soybeans has not been studied. The results suggest that, unlike mature soybeans, dry-heating is more suitable for processing immature soybeans and leads to a higher TIG content than wet-heating.

As mentioned earlier, TIA accounts for only a small proportion of the TI in soybeans. Figure 2(A-5,B-5) shows the variation in the TIA content at different maturity levels of soybeans after thermal processing. The TIA content remained stable in the mature soybeans during dry-heating but decreased significantly during wet-heating. Similar results on mature soybeans have also been observed by Kao et al. [51] and Aguiar et al. [50] for dry- and wet-heating, respectively. The isoflavone deglycosylation from glycoside form to aglycone was observed only under high temperature, possibly because it was difficult to break down the glycoside groups to form aglycones at relatively low temperatures [52]. The present study has shown that the variation in the TIA content of the immature soybeans was similar to that of mature soybeans. In this study, because we used only one cultivar, further studies using numerous cultivars are required to understand the isoflavone deglycosylation patterns of soybeans regarding whether the isoflavone changes among immature soybean cultivars by thermal processing are presenting the same patterns or not.

2.3. Correlation Analysis between Isoflavone Form and Corresponding Individual Isoflavones in Immature and Mature Soybeans

To clarify the patterns of how isoflavones changed for different maturity levels of soybeans during thermal processing, the correlations between the contents of the isoflavone form and corresponding individual isoflavones were analyzed. Tables 2 and 3 show the variations in the content of 12 individual isoflavones (IMG (MDZI, MGLI, and MGNI), IAG (ADZI, AGLI, and AGNI), IG (DZI, GLI, and GNI), and IA (DZE, GLE, and GNE)) in immature and mature soybeans, respectively, after dry- and wet-heating. The profiles of 12 individual isoflavones detected by the reversed-phase high-performance liquid chromatography (HPLC) in immature and mature soybeans before treatment and after 120 min of thermal treatment are shown in Figure 3.

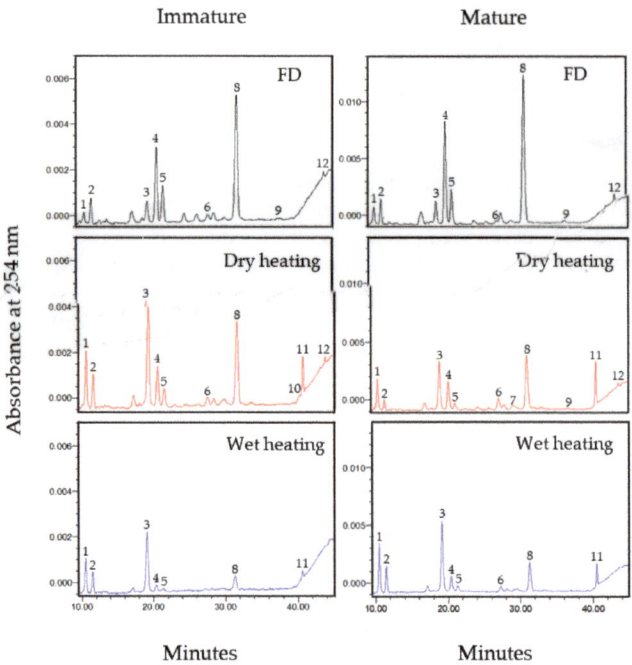

Figure 3. Twelve isoflavones of immature and mature soybean seeds after 120 min of dry- and wet-heat treatment determined by HPLC. 1, daidzin (DZI); 2, glycitin (GLI); 3, genistin (GNI); 4, malonyldaidzin (MDZI); 5, malonylglycitin (MGLI); 6, acetyldaidzin (ADZI); 7, acetylglycitin (AGLI); 8, malonylgenistin (MGNI); 9, daidzein (DZE); 10, glycitein (GNE); 11, acetylgenistin (AGNI); 12, genistein (GNE).

Of the three types of malonylglycoside isoflavones, MGNI (78.18 mg/100 g DW in immature soybeans; 141.25 mg/100 g DW in mature soybeans) and MDZI (62.32 mg/100 g DW in immature soybeans; 119.20 mg/100 g DW in mature soybeans) were the main isoflavones in the FD samples (Tables 2 and 3). The deglycosylation of MGNI, MDZI, and MGLI was more severe after wet-heating than after dry-heating regardless of the level of the seed maturity. Significantly positive correlations ($p < 0.001$) between the contents of MGNI, MDZI, and MGLI individually and of TIMG were observed in all the samples (Table 4). The contents of the three types of malonyl isoflavone in the immature soybeans did not change after 30 min of dry-heating but drastically decreased after 30 min of wet-heating. Similar results have also been observed by Chien et al. [34], where moist-heating at 100 °C reduced the MGNI (standard compound) content more than dry-heating at 100 °C.

Table 2. Isoflavone content (mg/100 g DW) in immature soybeans during thermal processing.

		FD (0 Min)	Dry-Heating				Wet-Heating			
			30 Min	60 Min	90 Min	120 Min	30 Min	60 Min	90 Min	120 Min
Malonyl glycosides	MDZI	62.32 ± 1.54 a	63.38 ± 9.37 a	34.81 ± 3.21 b	29.62 ± 3.55 b	23.01 ± 2.31 b,c	23.16 ± 2.64 b,c	9.39 ± 1.27 c,d	4.01 ± 0.08 d	2.03 ± 0.34 d
	MGLI	29.26 ± 2.47 a	26.09 ± 7.54 a	18.51 ± 3.35 a,b	10.51 ± 1.80 b,c	7.70 ± 0.63 c	5.73 ± 0.42 c	1.57 ± 0.44 c	0.62 ± 0.21 c	N.D.
	MGNI	78.18 ± 0.21 a	72.87 ± 9.58 a	57.24 ± 4.00 a,b	40.79 ± 4.76 b,c	37.21 ± 4.76 b,c	38.68 ± 2.06 b,c	20.07 ± 1.80 c,d	7.13 ± 0.83 d	4.23 ± 0.48 d
Acetyl glycosides	ADZI	5.20 ± 0.29 a	2.80 ± 0.62 b,c	2.64 ± 0.40 a,b	4.39 ± 0.70 a,b	5.66 ± 0.70 a	1.06 ± 0.20 c	0.68 ± 0.05 c	N.D.	N.D.
	AGLI	N.D.	Tr.	0.36 ± 0.19 a	2.56 ± 0.77 a	3.65 ± 1.23 a	N.D.	N.D.	N.D.	N.D.
	AGNI	Tr.	0.12 ± 0.12 c,d	2.20 ± 0.26 c,d	4.02 ± 1.83 b	9.94 ± 1.27 a	2.25 ± 0.25 c,d	2.86 ± 0.13 c	2.25 ± 0.17 c,d	2.04 ± 0.16 c,d
β-glycosides	DZI	3.71 ± 0.53 c	5.16 ± 1.17 b,c	6.23 ± 0.59 b,c	10.11 ± 2.81 a,b,c	15.45 ± 1.80 a	8.91 ± 1.47 a,b,c	11.72 ± 1.51 a,b	10.55 ± 1.02 a,b,c	9.11 ± 0.70 a,b,c
	GLI	11.62 ± 1.16 a	11.30 ± 3.98 a	10.82 ± 1.37 a	10.84 ± 2.27 a	11.70 ± 1.50 a	8.62 ± 1.08 a	7.42 ± 1.12 a	6.24 ± 0.80 a	7.31 ± 0.48 a
	GNI	8.08 ± 0.96 a	10.26 ± 1.90 d,e	14.30 ± 0.57 c,d,e	22.52 ± 2.20 a,b,c	30.16 ± 2.90 a	19.16 ± 1.80 b,c,d	26.12 ± 2.22 a,b	25.47 ± 2.30 a,b	19.9 ± 1.41 a,b
Aglycones	DZE	0.77 ± 0.12 a	0.33 ± 0.03 a	0.74 ± 0.42 a	0.61 ± 0.24 a	0.75 ± 0.32 a	N.D.	N.D.	N.D.	N.D.
	GLE	Tr.	0.28 ± 0.14 a	0.74 ± 0.17 a,b	1.13 ± 0.25 a	1.03 ± 0.42 a	N.D.	N.D.	N.D.	N.D.
	GNE	0.22 ± 0.11 a,b	0.70 ± 0.12 a,b	0.74 ± 0.17 a,b	0.87 ± 0.21 a	0.89 ± 0.14 a	0.07 ± 0.07 b	0.22 ± 0.14 a,b	N.D.	N.D.

Data are shown as mean with standard error ($n = 3$). Different letters (a–e) in a row indicate significant differences at $p < 0.05$ by Tukey's studentized range (HSD) test. N.D. indicates not detected; Tr. Indicates trace amount.

Table 3. Isoflavone content (mg/100 g DW) in mature soybeans during thermal processing.

		FD (0 Min)	Dry-Heating				Wet-Heating			
			30 Min	60 Min	90 Min	120 Min	30 Min	60 Min	90 Min	120 Min
Malonyl glycosides	MDZI	119.20 ± 11.24 a	68.96 ± 4.43 b	57.43 ± 3.54 b,c	47.09 ± 2.40 b,c,d	31.92 ± 1.20 d,e	48.00 ± 2.54 b,c,d	35.03 ± 1.36 c,d,e	20.91 ± 0.64 d,e	18.34 ± 1.20 e
	MGLI	24.18 ± 5.96 a	21.53 ± 1.52 a	22.27 ± 2.22 a,b	15.58 ± 2.61 b,c	14.15 ± 1.38 b,c	16.22 ± 2.80 b,c	12.87 ± 2.84 c	4.65 ± 0.28 c	4.09 ± 0.22 c
	MGNI	141.25 ± 7.92 a	89.11 ± 3.38 b	80.17 ± 3.10 b	68.91 ± 2.22 b,c,d	52.48 ± 3.44 d,e	63.58 ± 0.59 b,c	52.53 ± 0.48 c,d	32.76 ± 1.20 e	26.17 ± 0.76 e
Acetyl glycosides	ADZI	3.09 ± 0.35 d	5.74 ± 0.56 d	10.46 ± 0.61 b,c	15.83 ± 1.97 a	12.23 ± 0.98 a,b	5.96 ± 0.29 d	5.65 ± 0.30 d	6.32 ± 0.11 d	6.81 ± 0.35 c,d
	AGLI	N.D.	2.13 ± 0.83 c	6.12 ± 1.48 b,c	12.67 ± 1.04 a	8.67 ± 2.17 a,b	3.77 ± 0.66 b,c	3.22 ± 0.65 b,c	2.85 ± 0.25 c	3.57 ± 0.66 b,c
	AGNI	Tr.	5.62 ± 0.34 e	14.51 ± 0.78 b	21.10 ± 0.53 a	20.58 ± 1.61 a	6.57 ± 0.06 d,e	9.09 ± 0.19 c,d	9.42 ± 0.22 c,d	11.84 ± 0.35 b,c
β-glycosides	DZI	7.56 ± 0.80 e	11.22 ± 0.66 d,e	19.53 ± 1.11 b	19.92 ± 0.61 b	19.07 ± 0.88 b	13.62 ± 1.00 c,d	17.97 ± 2.20 b,c	20.03 ± 0.58 b	27.45 ± 0.38 a
	GLI	7.53 ± 1.96 a,b	7.71 ± 0.86 b	15.05 ± 0.43 a,b	14.47 ± 1.09 a,b	10.37 ± 0.98 a,b	14.82 ± 1.82 a,b	17.30 ± 2.20 a	13.97 ± 0.97 a,b	16.75 ± 0.57 a
	GNI	8.64 ± 1.99 e	16.83 ± 0.58 d	29.26 ± 1.04 c	33.99 ± 0.87 b	31.11 ± 2.08 b,c	21.07 ± 0.18 d	30.52 ± 0.71 b,c	36.74 ± 0.91 b	47.44 ± 1.62 a
Aglycones	DZE	1.21 ± 0.35 a	0.50 ± 0.10 a,b	0.78 ± 0.11 a,b	0.63 ± 0.05 a,b	0.59 ± 0.09 a,b	0.38 ± 0.03 b	0.29 ± 0.15 b	0.31 ± 0.16 b	0.57 ± 0.13 a,b
	GLE	Tr.	N.D.	N.D.	N.D.	N.D.	0.38 ± 0.02 a	N.D.	N.D.	N.D.
	GNE	0.94 ± 0.14 a	0.61 ± 0.08 a,b,c	0.70 ± 0.07 a,b,c	0.90 ± 0.12 a	0.72 ± 0.04 a,b	0.27 ± 0.06 c	0.30 ± 0.02 b,c	0.40 ± 0.10 a,b	0.45 ± 0.10 b,c

Data are shown as mean with standard error ($n = 3$). Different letters (a–e) next to data in a row indicate significant differences at $p < 0.05$ by Tukey's studentized range (HSD) test. N.D. indicates not detected; Tr. Indicates trace amount.

Table 4. Correlation coefficients between isoflavone forms and individual isoflavones in thermally treated soybeans.

Seed Maturation	Heating Methods		MDZI	MGLI	MGNI
Immature	D [z]	TIMG	0.983 ***	0.931 ***	0.970 ***
	W [y]	TIMG	0.999 ***	0.976 ***	0.944 ***
Mature	D	TIMG	0.996 ***	0.712 ***	0.987 ***
	W	TIMG	0.996 ***	0.889 ***	0.997 ***
			ADZI	**AGLI**	**AGNI**
Immature	D	TIAG	0.704 **	0.963 ***	0.967 ***
	W	TIAG	0.902 ***	-	−0.537 *
Mature	D	TIAG	0.961 ***	0.955 ***	0.980 ***
	W	TIAG	0.901 **	0.844 ***	0.983 ***
			DZI	**GLI**	**GNI**
Immature	D	TIG	0.939 ***	0.410 ns	0.946 ***
	W	TIG	0.972 ***	−0.314 ns	0.953 ***
Mature	D	TIG	0.943 ***	0.769 ***	0.956 ***
	W	TIG	0.983 ***	0.687 **	0.976 ***
			DZE	**GLE**	**GNE**
Immature	D	TIA	−0.053 ns	0.892 ***	0.420 ns
	W	TIA	1.000 ***	-	-
Mature	D	TIA	0.601 *	-	0.202 ns
	W	TIA	0.727 **	-	0.658 **

[z] and [y] indicate dry-heating and wet-heating, respectively. *, **, and *** indicate significances at $p < 0.05$, $p < 0.01$, and $p < 0.001$ in Tukey's HSD test. ns indicates no significance at the test. Data of 12 individual isoflavones, TIMG, TIAG, TIG, and TIA, for correlation analysis were calculated by the time-dependent dry-heating and wet-heating values, ranging from 0 to 120 min treatments.

Of the acetylglycoside isoflavones, ADZI (5.20 mg/100 g DW in immature soybeans; 3.09 mg/100 g DW in mature soybeans) was the main acetyl isoflavone in the FD samples (Tables 2 and 3). Only a trace amount of AGNI was detected in both the immature and mature soybeans, with no AGLI being detected. The three types of acetyl isoflavone in the soybeans of different maturity levels responded differently to thermal processing. The ADZI content changed relatively little in the dry-heated immature soybeans but increased by four to five times in the dry-heated mature soybeans. The ADZI content also decreased to undetectable levels in the wet-heated immature soybeans, but not in the wet-heated mature soybeans. More AGLI and AGNI were produced in the dry-heated soybeans regardless of the maturity level. The AGLI content of the immature soybeans did not change but increased slightly after wet-heating. The AGNI in wet-heating was a key molecule because its content was unchanged in the immature soybeans after processing but increased in the mature soybeans, thus determining the amount of total acetylglycosides after wet-heating. The increase in the AGNI content was greater than that in the contents of ADZI and AGLI, possibly because of the varying thermal stability of the three acetylglycoside isoflavones and the corresponding malonylglycoside isoflavones. In contrast, the content of most of the types of acetyl increased up to 90 to 120 min of dry-heating regardless of the seed maturity. Significant positive correlations were found between the contents of ADZI, AGLI, AGNI, and that of TIAG for all the treatment groups except for the wet-heated immature soybeans (Table 4). A high negative correlation between the contents of AGNI and TIAG was observed for wet-heated immature soybeans, unlike the significant positive correlations for the other samples. This indicated that the amount of total acetylglycosides depended mainly on the content of AGNI during thermal processing.

The β-glycosides, the non-conjugated form of isoflavones, are the second major group after malonylglycosides in raw soybeans [52,53]. Of the β-glycosides, the content of

GLI (11.62 mg/100 g DW) was higher than that of DZI (3.71 mg/100 g DW) and GNI (8.08 mg/100 g DW) in the FD immature soybeans (Table 2), similar to results from Simonne et al. [38]. The content of GLI (7.53 mg/100 g DW) was relatively lower than that of DZI (7.56 mg/100 g DW) and GNI (8.64 mg/100 g DW) in the FD mature soybeans (Table 3), results that are consistent with those of Kim et al. [54]. During thermal processing, different patterns of variation in the contents of GLI, GNI, and DZI arose. In the mature soybeans, the increase in the GLI content was small after heating compared with a significant increase in the DZI and GNI contents, similar to results reported by Toda et al. [48]. In the immature soybeans, no significant differences ($p > 0.05$) in GLI content were observed between FD and thermally treated soybeans. The contents of DZI and GNI both increased significantly after thermal treatment regardless of the seed maturity and processing method. Wet-heating was also more efficient in increasing β-glycoside isoflavones than dry-heating. The contents of GNI and DZI of all the treated samples were significantly positively correlated ($p < 0.001$) with the TIG content (Table 4). A good correlation ($p < 0.01$) between the GLI and TIG contents during thermal processing was found in the mature soybeans but not in the immature soybeans ($p > 0.05$). This indicated that the patterns of variation in the TIG content of soybeans were dominated more by the contents of DZI and GNI than the content of GLI during thermal processing even though the GLI content was relatively high in both FD samples.

In the FD soybeans, only small amounts of DZE (immature soybeans, 0.77 mg/100 g DW; mature soybeans, 1.21 mg/100 g DW) and GNE (immature soybeans, 0.22 mg/100 g DW; mature seeds, 0.94 mg/100 g DW) were detected, with a trace amount of GLE. The contents of the three aglycones in the immature soybeans were relatively stable under dry-heating but decreased to undetectable levels after 90 min of wet-heating. Both types of thermal processing decreased the contents of the three aglycones in the mature soybeans, particularly wet-heating. The variations in the contents of the three aglycones with the temperatures of thermal processing have been contradictory: Xu et al. [52] reported that aglycones in soybean flour extracts were generated with heat treatments above 135 °C, but Huang and Chou [35] reported that the contents of GNE, DZE, and GLE in black soybeans decreased at steaming temperatures of 60 °C or above for 30 min. A good correlation between the contents of DZE and TIA was found in all the treatments except for the dry-heated immature soybeans (Table 4). However, only the GLE content was well correlated with the TIA content in the immature soybeans under dry-heating with the content of GNE being well correlated with the TIA content in the mature soybeans under wet-heating.

The three isoflavone types (daidzein, glycitein, and genistein) showed different conversion patterns under heat processing. The MDZI and MGNI decreased more rapidly in the initial 30 min than the MGLI. Moreover, the production of AGNI and GNI by heat processing were higher than that of other isoflavone types. Glycitein conjugate types had relatively low thermal-change compared to daidzein and genistein types regardless of the seed maturity. Similar results have been reported by Stintzing et al. [55], where glycitein carrying a meth-oxy group at 6 position of A-ring has higher stability upon dry-heating. Moreover, Mathias et al. [56] reported that the heat-induced loss of daidzein glycosides was higher than that of genistein glycosides. These results indicate that different deglycosylation rates among isoflavone types occur during different thermal process methods.

2.4. Verification of the Relationship between Soybean Water Content and Changes in Patterns of Isoflavone Contents

It is important to note the different patterns of variation in the contents of acetylglycoside and β-glycoside isoflavones during the dry- and wet-heating of soybeans at two maturity levels. The internal moisture content of the soybeans affected the composition of isoflavones during thermal processing. To confirm this assumption, fully mature soybeans were soaked in distilled water for 0, 1, 2, 4, and 8 h to obtain different internal water contents, then dry-heated, followed by further observations of the patterns of variation in isoflavone content after heating for 1 h. Figure 4A shows the variations in the moisture content of the soybeans after soaking. The water content of the soybeans gradually increased from 6.34% to 57.04% as the soaking time increased. The contents of TI and of the four forms of isoflavone, TMIG, TAIG, TIG, and TIA, in the fully mature soybeans before and after the 1-h dry-heat treatment are shown in Figure 4B, C, D, E, and F, respectively.

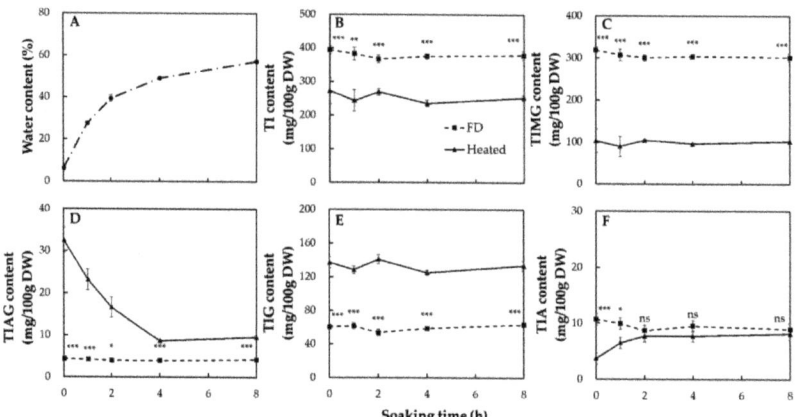

Figure 4. Water content of mature seeds during serial soaking (**A**), and isoflavone contents in soaked seeds after freeze-drying (FD) and dry-heating (**B**–**F**). (**A**), water content; (**B**), total isoflavone (TI); (**C**), total isoflavone malonylglycosides (TIMG); (**D**), total isoflavone acetylglycosides (TIAG); (**E**), total isoflavone β glycosides; (**F**), total isoflavone aglycones. Data are shown as mean with standard error ($n = 3$). Asterisks indicate statistically significant differences (*, $p < 0.05$; **, $p < 0.01$; ***, $p < 0.001$; ns indicates no significance).

Before heating, no significant differences in the TI content were observed between the unsoaked and soaked soybeans. Wang and Murphy [24] have also reported that soaking at room temperature for 10 to 12 h significantly increased the moisture content from 11.03% to 63.23% and retained the TI of the soaked soybeans. Heating significantly decreased the content of TI and TIMG and increased the content of TIAG and TIG of the soybeans compared with the FD samples (Figure 4B–E). The highest amount of TIAG generated was found in the unsoaked soybeans (0 h), and the lowest amount in soybeans soaked for a long time. There were no significant variations in the TIG content between the unsoaked and soaked soybeans after dry-heating for 1 h. These results were consistent with this report that the immature and mature beans had a similar TIG content after a long period of dry-heating, with even immature soybeans showing a lower TIAG content than mature soybeans (Figure 2). In contrast, the TIA content of the unsoaked soybeans was reduced by dry-heating, but, the longer the soaking time, the more TIA was generated after heating (Figure 4F). These results were different from the results we reported before, which may have been caused by differences between natural soybeans with a higher internal water content and artificially made soybeans with a higher water content. This also confirmed the assumption that the internal moisture content of soybeans was an important factor affecting the different patterns of variation in isoflavone content in soybeans of different maturity.

It is notable that, the longer the soaking time, the less TIAG was produced after heating. Lee and Lee [46] reported that the content of acetyl isoflavones in soybeans soaked for 12 h did not change during 120 min of oven drying but that, in unsoaked soybeans, it increased significantly after roasting at 200 °C. This indicated that soybeans with a higher internal water content produced a lower amount of acetyl isoflavones after heating, which confirmed the previous assumption that the water content of soybeans significantly affected the pattern of isoflavone conversion. Therefore, the differences between the content of acetyl isoflavones in mature and immature soybeans after heating were caused by the difference in the internal water content. The increase in the content of aglycone isoflavones was highly related to soaking and heating, results similar to those of Lima et al. [57], who found no significant difference in the content of aglycones in soybeans soaked at 25 °C but a significant increase after soaking for 1 h at 70 °C.

3. Materials and Methods

3.1. Chemical Reagents

The HPLC-grade acetonitrile and water (Daejung Chemical & Metals Co., Siheung, Korea) were used as mobile phases for isoflavones analysis. Standards of isoflavone aglycones (daidzein, glycitein, and genistein) and β-glycosides (daidzin, glycitin, and genistin) were purchased from LC Laboratories (Woburn, MA, USA). Isoflavone acetylglycosides (acetyldaidzin, acetylglycitin, and acetylgenistin) were obtained from Nacalai tesque (Kyoto, Japan), and malonylglycosides (malonyldaidzin, malonylglycitin, and malonylgenistin) were obtained from GenDEPOT (Katy, TX, USA).

3.2. Soybean Cultivation

Soybean seeds (*Glycine max* L. cv. *Pungwon*) used in this study were provided by the Pulmuone Food Co. (Chungbuk, Korea). The cultivar 'Pungwon' was registered to the Korea Seed & Variety Service (Gimcheon, Korea) in 2007 and had earlier matu-ration period and high content of isoflavones (more information described in Oh et al. [58]). The soybeans were germinated for 24 h at room temperature in a dark culture room after soaking with distilled water for 4 h. The germinated soybeans were planted in a horticultural soil (Baroker, Seoulbio Co., Eumseong, Korea) in pots (Plastic pot, 24 × 27 × 18 cm) in early June 2020 and then grown in the greenhouse of Kyung Hee University (Yongin, Korea) under natural sunlight. The average of temperature during the soybean growing season was 18–22 °C in June; 22–30 °C in July and August; 19–26 °C in September; 12–23 °C in October (based on Korean meteorological administration data). The average solar radiation period was 14 h/day in June to August and 12.5 h/day in September and October (based on Korean meteorological administration data). The average of relative humidity was 45–55% from June to October. The potted soybeans were maintained with several irrigations per week in the early stage of soybean plants and with daily irrigation in the period of seed formation. The soybean seeds were harvested at the immature stage on September 10 when the pods of soybeans contained green seeds that filled the pod cavity and harvested at the mature stage on October 10 when 95% of the pods exhibited the light brown color with dehydrating, as shown in Figure 1 in a previous report [36].

3.3. Physical Characteristics of Immature and Mature Seeds

The harvested soybean samples were weighed before and after freeze-drying. The dry weight of the immature and mature soybeans was expressed as the weight (g) of 10 raw seeds based on the mean value of ten replicates. The water content (%) was calculated as follows: $100 \times$ [fresh weight (g) − dry weight (g)]/[fresh weight (g)]. Fresh soybeans (0.3 g) were ground with a pestle and a mortar and added 0.6 mL of distilled water to measure the soluble solid content (SSC). After stirring the mixture, the sample was centrifuged at $14,240 \times g$ for 15 min. The SSC of the supernatant was evaluated using a hand refractometer (Atago Co., Tokyo, Japan) and expressed as degree of Brix (°Brix).

3.4. Thermal Treatment

The immature and mature soybean seeds were processed using three thermal processing methods: (1) freeze-drying (FD) at −80 °C for 72 h in a vacuum freeze-dryer (IlshinBioBase. Co. Ltd., Dongducheon, Korea) and stored in a −20 °C refrigerator; (2) dry-heating at 100 ± 3 °C for 30, 60, 90, and 120 min with a convective dryer (Koencon Co., Ltd., Hanam, Korea); and (3) wet-heating (steaming) at 100 ± 3 °C for 30, 60, 90, and 120 min with a steam cooker. All experiments were carried out in triplicate. The thermally treated samples were freeze-dried and stored in a −20 °C refrigerator before isoflavone analysis.

3.5. Extraction of Isoflavones

All samples were finely ground using a commercial grinder (JL-1000, Hibell, Hwaseong, Korea). The isoflavones extraction was performed by previously described method [59]. Briefly, 20 mg of ground sample mixed with 58% aqueous acetonitrile (1 mL, v/v) in a shaking incubator for 24 h at 25 °C and 120 rpm after sonication for 30 min. The supernatant was obtained after centrifuging at 14,240× g for 5 min. Then, two-fold volume of distilled water was added to dilute the supernatant. The diluted supernatant was filtered through a 0.45 μm hydrophilic PTFE membrane syringe filter (Futecs Co., Ltd., Daejeon, Korea) and used for isoflavones analysis.

3.6. Determination of Isoflavones

Extracts were analyzed using HPLC (Waters 2695 Alliance HPLC; Waters Inc., Milford, MA, USA) with the octadecylsilane column (Prontosil 120–5-C18-SH-EPS 5.0 μm (200 × 4.6 mm; Bischoff, Leonberg, Germany). According to the previously published method [59], the solvent A (0.1% formic acid in water) and solvent B (0.1% formic acid in acetonitrile) were used as mobile phase with the flow rate of 0.8 mL/min. The mobile phase B gradient was as follows: 16–25%, 0 to 35 min; 25–50%, 35 to 40 min; 50–65%, 40 to 47 min; 65–16%, 47 to 50 min. The injection volume was 5 μL. The peaks of 12 standard isoflavones were detected at 254 nm (Water 996 photodiode array detector (Waters Inc.)).

3.7. Statistical Analysis

All experiments were carried out in triplicate with the data expressed as the mean with standard error (n = 3). Analysis of variance was performed using SAS software (Enterprise guide 7.1 version, SAS Institute Inc., Cary, NC, USA). Significant differences between experimental treatments were evaluated using Tukey's student range test, with a significance level defined at $p < 0.05$.

4. Conclusions

This is the first study to compare the patterns of isoflavone changes between soybeans at two maturity levels after thermal processing. Overall, the patterns of the isoflavone changes in the soybeans depended significantly on the soybean maturity and the processing method, which affected the decarboxylation of malonylglycoside or the deesterification of acetylglycoside isoflavones. The decreases in the TI in all the samples were mainly caused by the decrease in the TIMG during thermal processing. The deglycosylation of the three types of malonyl isoflavones was more severe in wet- than in dry-heating regardless of the seed maturity. In the acetylglycoside isoflavones, dry-heating produced a relatively low amount of acetyl isoflavones in the immature seeds compared with that in the mature seeds. The ADZI was relatively less changed in the dry-heated immature seeds but increased significantly in the processed mature seeds. AGLI and AGNI were produced in greater amounts in the dry-heated samples regardless of the seed maturity. The AGNI in wet-heating was the key molecule because its content remained unchanged in the immature soybeans during processing but increased in the mature soybeans, which determined the total amount of acetylglycoside in wet-heating. Wet-heating increased the amount of β-glycoside isoflavones in the mature soybeans more than in dry-heating, while, interestingly, the immature soybeans exhibited the opposite behavior. The aglycone isoflavones were stable under dry-heating, but their contents decreased significantly after wet-heating. The internal moisture content of the soybeans was an important factor affecting the deglycosylation of isoflavones during thermal processing, also confirmed by the verification experiment (Section 2.4). This is the first study to highlight the importance of the internal water content of soybeans on the distribution of isoflavones during thermal processing. The results of the present study will provide basic information on the different uses of immature and mature soybeans after thermal processing.

Author Contributions: Conceptualization, S.H.E.; methodology, S.Q., S.J.K. and S.H.E.; software, S.Q.; validation, S.H.E.; formal analysis, S.Q. and S.D.; investigation, S.Q.; resources, S.H.E.; data curation, S.Q. and Y.J.L.; writing—original draft preparation, S.Q.; writing—review and editing, S.J.K. and S.H.E.; visualization, S.Q. and S.D.; supervision, S.H.E.; funding acquisition, S.H.E. All authors have read and agreed to the published version of the manuscript.

Funding: This work was supported by Radiation Technology R&D program (NRF-2017M2A2A6A050-18538) through the National Research Foundation of Korea funded by the Ministry of Science and ICT. This work was also supported by the National Research Foundation of Korea (NRF) grant funded by the Korean government (MSIT) (NO. NRF-2019R1A2C1009623).

Institutional Review Board Statement: Not applicable.

Informed Consent Statement: Not applicable.

Data Availability Statement: The data presented in this study are available on request from the corresponding author.

Conflicts of Interest: The authors declare no conflict of interest.

Sample Availability: Samples of the compounds are not available from the authors.

References

1. O'Keefe, S.; Bianchi, L.; Sharman, J. Soybean nutrition. *J. Nutr. Metab.* **2015**, *1*, 1006.
2. Kim, H.K.; Kang, S.T.; Cho, J.H.; Choung, M.G.; Suh, D.Y. Quantitative trait loci associated with oligosaccharide and sucrose contents in soybean (*Glycine max* L.). *J. Plant Biol.* **2005**, *48*, 106–112. [CrossRef]
3. Ollberding, N.J.; Lim, U.; Wilkens, L.R.; Setiawan, V.W.; Shvetsov, Y.B.; Henderson, B.E.; Kolonel, L.N.; Goodman, M.T. Legume, soy, tofu, and isoflavone intake and endometrial cancer risk in postmenopausal women in the multiethnic cohort study. *J. Natl. Cancer Inst.* **2012**, *104*, 67–76. [CrossRef] [PubMed]
4. Jung, Y.S.; Rha, C.S.; Baik, M.Y.; Baek, N.I.; Kim, D.O. A brief history and spectroscopic analysis of soy isoflavones. *Food Sci. Biotechnol.* **2020**, *29*, 1605–1617. [CrossRef] [PubMed]
5. Lim, Y.J.; Lyu, J.I.; Kwon, S.J.; Eom, S.H. Effects of UV-A radiation on organ-specific accumulation and gene expression of isoflavones and flavonols in soybean sprout. *Food Chem.* **2021**, *339*, 128080. [CrossRef]
6. Hoeck, J.A.; Fehr, W.R.; Murphy, P.A.; Welke, J.A. Influence of genotype and environment on isoflavone contents of soybean. *Crop Sci.* **2000**, *40*, 48–51. [CrossRef]
7. Barnes, S.; Peterson, T.G. Biochemical targets of the isoflavone genistein in tumor cell lines. *Proc. Soc. Exp. Biol. Med.* **1995**, *208*, 103–108. [CrossRef] [PubMed]
8. Adlercreutz, H.; Honjo, H.; Higashi, A.; Fotsis, T.; Hämäläinen, E.; Hasegawa, T.; Okada, H. Urinary excretion of lignans and isoflavonoid phytoestrogens in Japanese men and women consuming a traditional Japanese diet. *Am. J. Clin. Nutr.* **1991**, *54*, 1093–1100. [CrossRef]
9. Knight, D.C.; Eden, J.A. A review of the clinical effects of phytoestrogens. *Obstet. Gynecol.* **1996**, *87*, 897–904.
10. Xu, B.; Chang, S.K.C. Total phenolics, phenolic acids, isoflavones, and anthocyanins and antioxidant properties of yellow and black soybeans as affected by thermal processing. *J. Agric. Food Chem.* **2008**, *56*, 7165–7175. [CrossRef]
11. Severson, R.K.; Nomura, A.M.Y.; Grove, J.S.; Stemmermann, G.N. A prospective study of demographics, diet, and prostate cancer among men of Japanese ancestry in Hawaii. *Cancer Res.* **1989**, *49*, 1857–1860. [PubMed]
12. Lee, H.P.; Lee, J.; Gourley, L.; Duffy, S.W.; Day, N.E.; Estève, J. Dietary effects on breast-cancer risk in Singapore. *Lancet* **1991**, *337*, 1197–1200. [CrossRef]
13. Yerramsetty, V.; Gallaher, D.D.; Ismail, B. Malonylglucoside conjugates of isoflavones are much less bioavailable compared with unconjugated β-glucosidic forms in rats. *J. Nutr.* **2014**, *144*, 631–637. [CrossRef] [PubMed]
14. Lee, C.H.; Yang, L.; Xu, J.Z.; Yeung, S.Y.V.; Huang, Y.; Chen, Z.Y. Relative antioxidant activity of soybean isoflavones and their glycosides. *Food Chem.* **2005**, *90*, 735–741. [CrossRef]
15. Izumi, T.; Pikula, M.K.; Osawa, S.; Obata, A.; Tobe, K.; Saito, M.; Kataoka, S.; Kubota, Y.; Kikuchi, M. Soy isoflavone aglycones are absorbed faster and in higher amount than their glucosides in humans. *J. Nutr.* **2000**, *130*, 1695–1699. [CrossRef] [PubMed]
16. Wolf, W.J. Lipoxygenase and flavor of soybean protein products. *J. Agric. Food Chem.* **1975**, *23*, 136–141. [CrossRef]
17. MacLeod, G.; Ames, J.; Betz, N.L. Soy flavor and its improvement. *Crit. Rev. Food Sci. Nutr.* **1989**, *27*, 219–400. [CrossRef]
18. Cai, J.S.; Zh, Y.Y.; Ma, R.H.; Thakur, K.; Zhang, J.G.; Wei, Z.J. Effects of roasting level on physicochemical, sensory, and volatile profiles of soybeans using electronic nose and HS-SPME-GC–MS. *Food Chem.* **2021**, *340*, 127880. [CrossRef] [PubMed]
19. Zhang, Y.; Guo, S.; Liu, Z.; Chang, S.K. Off-flavor related volatiles in soymilk as affected by soybean variety, grinding, and heat-processing methods. *J. Agric. Food Chem.* **2012**, *60*, 7457–7462. [CrossRef]
20. Endo, H.; Ohno, M.; Tanji, K.; Shimada, T.; Kaneko, K. Effect of heat treatment on the lipid peroxide content and aokusami (beany flavor) of soymilk. *Food Sci. Technol. Res.* **2007**, *10*, 328–333. [CrossRef]

21. Villares, A.; Rostagno, M.A.; García-Lafuente, A.; Guillamón, E.; Martínez, J.A. Content and profile of isoflavones in soy-based foods as a function of the production process. *Food Bioprocess Technol.* **2011**, *4*, 27–38. [CrossRef]
22. Muliterno, M.M.; Rodrigues, D.; Lima, F.S.; Ida, E.L.; Kurozawa, L.E. Conversion/degradation of isoflavones and color alterations during the drying of okara. *LWT* **2017**, *75*, 512–519. [CrossRef]
23. Chan, S.G.; Murphy, P.A.; Ho, S.C.; Kreiger, N.; Darlington, G.; So, E.K.F.; Chong, P.Y.Y. Isoflavonoid content of Hong Kong soy foods. *J. Agric. Food Chem.* **2009**, *57*, 5386–5390. [CrossRef] [PubMed]
24. Zhang, Y.; Chang, S.K.; Liu, Z. Isoflavone profile in soymilk as affected by soybean variety, grinding, and heat-processing methods. *J. Food Sci.* **2015**, *80*, C983–C988. [CrossRef] [PubMed]
25. Lee, J.H.; Lee, B.W.; Kim, B.; Kim, H.T.; Ko, J.M.; Baek, I.Y.; Seo, W.T.; Kang, Y.M.; Cho, K.M. Changes in phenolic compounds (Isoflavones and Phenolic acids) and antioxidant properties in high-protein soybean (*Glycine max* L., cv. Saedanbaek) for different roasting conditions. *J. Korean Soc. Appl. Biol. Chem.* **2013**, *56*, 605–612. [CrossRef]
26. Yuan, J.P.; Liu, Y.B.; Peng, J.; Wang, J.H.; Liu, X. Changes of isoflavone profile in the hypocotyls and cotyledons of soybeans during dry heating and germination. *J. Agric. Food Chem.* **2009**, *57*, 9002–9010. [CrossRef]
27. Zhang, Y.C.; Lee, J.H.; Vodovotz, Y.; Schwartz, S.J. Changes in distribution of isoflavones and β-glucosidase activity during soy bread proofing and baking. *Cereal Chem.* **2004**, *81*, 741–745. [CrossRef]
28. Wang, H.J.; Murphy, P.A. Mass balance study of isoflavones during soybean processing. *J. Agric. Food Chem.* **1996**, *44*, 2377–2383. [CrossRef]
29. Jackson, C.J.C.; Dini, J.P.; Lavandier, C.; Rupasinghe, H.P.V.; Faulkner, H.; Poysa, V.; Buzzell, D.; DeGrandis, S. Effects of processing on the content and composition of isoflavones during manufacturing of soy beverage and tofu. *Process Biochem.* **2002**, *37*, 1117–1123. [CrossRef]
30. Yu, X.; Meenu, M.; Xu, B.; Yu, H. Impact of processing technologies on isoflavones, phenolic acids, and antioxidant capacities of soymilk prepared from 15 soybean varieties. *Food Chem.* **2021**, *345*, 128612. [CrossRef] [PubMed]
31. Wang, H.J.; Murphy, P.A. Isoflavone content in commercial soybean foods. *J. Agric. Food Chem.* **1994**, *42*, 1666–1673. [CrossRef]
32. Andrade, J.C.; Mandarino, J.M.G.; Kurozawa, L.E.; Ida, E.I. The effect of thermal treatment of whole soybean flour on the conversion of isoflavones and inactivation of trypsin inhibitor. *Food Chem.* **2016**, *194*, 1095–1101. [CrossRef]
33. Murphy, P.A.; Barua, K.; Hauck, C.C. Solvent extraction selection in the determination of isoflavones in soy foods. *J. Chromatogr. B Biomed. Appl.* **2002**, *777*, 129–138. [CrossRef]
34. Chien, J.T.; Hsieh, H.C.; Kao, T.H.; Chen, B.H. Kinetic model for studying the conversion and degradation of isoflavones during heating. *Food Chem.* **2005**, *91*, 425–434. [CrossRef]
35. Huang, R.Y.; Chou, C.C. Heating affects the content and distribution profile of isoflavones in steamed black soybeans and black soybean koji. *J. Agric. Food Chem.* **2008**, *56*, 8484–8489. [CrossRef] [PubMed]
36. Kumar, V.; Rani, A.; Dixit, A.K.; Bhatnagar, D.; Chauhan, G.S. Relative changes in tocopherols, isoflavones, total phenolic content, and antioxidative activity in soybean seeds at different reproductive stages. *J. Agric. Food Chem.* **2009**, *57*, 2705–2710. [CrossRef] [PubMed]
37. Takahashi, Y.; Sasanuma, T.; Abe, T. Accumulation of gamma-aminobutyrate (GABA) caused by heat-drying and expression of related genes in immature vegetable soybean (edamame). *Breed. Sci.* **2013**, *63*, 205–210. [CrossRef] [PubMed]
38. Simonne, A.; Smith, M.; Weaver, D.B.; Vail, T.; Barnes, S.; Wei, C.I. Retention and changes of soy isoflavones and carotenoids in immature soybean seeds (Edamame) during processing. *J. Agric. Food Chem.* **2000**, *48*, 6061–6069. [CrossRef] [PubMed]
39. Kim, S.L.; Berhow, M.A.; Kim, J.T.; Chi, H.Y.; Lee, S.J.; Chung, I.M. Evaluation of soyasaponin, isoflavone, protein, lipid, and free sugar accumulation in developing soybean seeds. *J. Agric. Food Chem.* **2006**, *54*, 10003–10010. [CrossRef]
40. Simonne, A.H.; Weaver, D.B.; Wei, C.I. Immature soybean seeds as a vegetable or snack food: Acceptability by American consumers. *Innov. Food Sci. Emerg. Technol.* **2000**, *1*, 289–296. [CrossRef]
41. Rubel, A.; Rinne, R.W.; Canvin, D.T. Protein, oil, and fatty acid in developing soybean seeds. *Crop Sci.* **1972**, *12*, 739–741. [CrossRef]
42. Gogoi, N.; Farooq, M.; Barthakur, S.; Baroowa, B.; Paul, S.; Bharadwaj, N.; Ramanjulu, S. Thermal stress impacts on reproductive development and grain yield in grain legumes. *J. Plant Biol.* **2018**, *61*, 265–291. [CrossRef]
43. Sale, P.W.G.; Campbell, L.C. Patterns of mineral nutrient accumulation in soybean seed. *Field Crop Res.* **1980**, *3*, 157–163. [CrossRef]
44. Im, M.H.; Choi, J.D.; Choi, K.S. The oxidation stability and flavor acceptability of oil from roasted soybean. *J. Agric. Food Chem. Biotechnol.* **1995**, *38*, 425–430.
45. Duan, S.; Kwon, S.J.; Eom, S.H. Effect of thermal processing on color, phenolic compounds, and antioxidant activity of Faba bean (*Vicia faba* L.) leaves and seeds. *Antioxidants* **2021**, *10*, 1207. [CrossRef] [PubMed]
46. Lee, S.W.; Lee, J.H. Effects of oven-drying, roasting, and explosive puffing process on isoflavone distributions in soybeans. *Food Chem.* **2009**, *112*, 316–320. [CrossRef]
47. Coward, L.; Smith, M.; Kirk, M.; Barnes, S. Chemical modification of isoflavones in soyfoods during cooking and processing. *Am. J. Clin. Nutr.* **1998**, *68*, 1486S–1491S. [CrossRef] [PubMed]
48. Toda, T.; Sakamoto, A.; Takayagi, T.; Yokotsuka, K. Changes in isoflavone compositions of soybean foods during cooking process. *Food Sci. Technol.* **2000**, *6*, 314–319. [CrossRef]
49. Niamnuy, C.; Nachaisin, M.; Laohavanich, J.; Devahastin, S. Evaluation of bioactive compounds and bioactivities of soybean dried by different methods and conditions. *Food Chem.* **2011**, *129*, 899–906. [CrossRef] [PubMed]

50. Aguiar, C.L.; Haddad, R.; Eberlin, M.N.; Carrão-Panizzi, M.C.; Tsai, S.M.; Park, Y.K. Thermal behavior of malonylglucoside isoflavones in soybean flour analyzed by RPHPLC/DAD and eletrospray ionization mass spectrometry. *LWT* **2012**, *48*, 114–119. [CrossRef]
51. Kao, T.H.; Lu, Y.F.; Hsieh, H.C.; Chen, B.H. Stability of isoflavone glucosides during processing of soymilk and tofu. *Food Res. Int.* **2004**, *37*, 891–900. [CrossRef]
52. Xu, Z.; Wu, Q.; Godber, J.S. Stabilities of daidzin, glycitin, genistin, and generation of derivatives during heating. *J. Agric. Food Chem.* **2002**, *50*, 7402–7406. [CrossRef] [PubMed]
53. Sakthivelu, G.; Akitha Devi, M.K.; Giridhar, P.; Rajasekaran, T.; Ravishankar, G.A.; Nikolova, M.T.; Angelov, G.B.; Todorova, R.M.; Kosturkova, G.P. Isoflavone composition, phenol content, and antioxidant activity of soybean seeds from India and Bulgaria. *J. Agric. Food Chem.* **2008**, *56*, 2090–2095. [CrossRef]
54. Kim, J.J.; Kim, S.H.; Hahn, S.J.; Chung, I.M. Changing soybean isoflavone composition and concentrations under two different storage conditions over three years. *Food Res. Int.* **2005**, *38*, 435–444. [CrossRef]
55. Stintzing, F.C.; Hoffmann, M.; Carle, R. Thermal degradation kinetics of isoflavone aglycones from soy and red clover. *Mol. Nutr. Food Res.* **2006**, *50*, 373–377. [CrossRef]
56. Mathias, K.; Ismail, B.; Corvalan, C.M.; Hayes, K.D. Heat and pH effects on the conjugated forms of genistin and daidzin isoflavones. *J. Agric. Food Chem.* **2006**, *54*, 7495–7502. [CrossRef] [PubMed]
57. Lima, F.S.; Kurozawa, L.E.; Lda, E.L. The effects of soybean soaking on grain properties and isoflavones loss. *LWT* **2014**, *59*, 1274–1282. [CrossRef]
58. Oh, Y.; Kim, K.; Yun, H.; Park, K.; Suh, S.; Moon, J.; Cho, S.; Kim, Y.; Kim, S.; Park, H.; et al. A new soybean cultivar, "Pungwon" for sprout with disease resistance, lodging resistance and high yielding. *Korean J. Breed. Sci.* **2007**, *39*, 502–503.
59. Lim, Y.J.; Lim, B.; Kim, H.Y.; Kwon, S.J.; Eom, S.H. Deglycosylation patterns of isoflavones in soybean extracts inoculated with two enzymatically different strains of lactobacillus species. *Enzym. Microb. Technol.* **2020**, *132*, 109394. [CrossRef] [PubMed]

Influence of Freeze-Dried Phenolic-Rich Plant Powders on the Bioactive Compounds Profile, Antioxidant Activity and Aroma of Different Types of Chocolates

Dorota Żyżelewicz [1,*], Joanna Oracz [1], Martyna Bilicka [1], Kamila Kulbat-Warycha [1] and Elżbieta Klewicka [2]

[1] Institute of Food Technology and Analysis, Faculty of Biotechnology and Food Sciences, Lodz University of Technology, 2/22 Stefanowskiego Street, 90-537 Łódź, Poland; joanna.oracz@p.lodz.pl (J.O.); martyna.bilicka@gmail.com (M.B.); kamila.kulbat-warycha@p.lodz.pl (K.K.-W.)

[2] Institute of Fermentation Technology and Microbiology, Faculty of Biotechnology and Food Sciences, Lodz University of Technology, 171/173 Wólczańska Street, 90-530 Łódź, Poland; elzbieta.klewicka@p.lodz.pl

* Correspondence: dorota.zyzelewicz@p.lodz.pl; Tel.: +48-42-631-34-61

Abstract: In this study, the blueberries (BLUB), raspberries (RASB), blackberries (BLCB), pomegranates pomace (POME) and beetroots (BEET) freeze-dried powders were used as the sources of phenolic compounds to enrich different types of chocolates, substituting a part of the sweetener. It was found that 1% addition of fruit or vegetable powders to chocolates increased the content of total phenolic compounds (flavan-3-ols, phenolic acids and anthocyanins) of enriched dark and milk chocolates compared to the control ones dependent on the powder used. Among the enriched chocolates, the chocolates with the addition of BLUB powder were characterized by the highest total polyphenol content. The highest percentage increase (approximately 80%) in the total polyphenol content was observed in MCH chocolate enriched with BLUB powder. Chocolates incorporated with BLUB, RASB, BLCB and POME powders presented a richer phenolic compound profile than control counterparts. The highest DPPH radical-scavenging capacity was exhibited by the DCH98S chocolate enriched with BEET powder. However, the DCH98ESt chocolates enriched with POME and BEET powders demonstrated the highest FRAP values. An electronic nose analysis confirmed the existence of differences between the profiles of volatile compounds of various types of chocolates enriched with fruit or vegetable powders. Thus, the enrichment of dark and milk chocolates with BLUB, RASB, BLCB, POME and BEET powders seemed to be an interesting approach to enhance bioactivity and to enrich the sensory features of various chocolate types.

Keywords: antioxidants; chocolate; free radical scavenging activity; reducing power; functionalization of food; electronic nose analysis

1. Introduction

In recent years, a rapid development of research on bioactive substances present in plant raw materials and their impact on the human body has been observed. Numerous studies revealed that there was a significant upward trend for the use of the plant-derived natural compounds as antioxidants and functional ingredients. Growing interest in the production and consumption of functional foods with specific pro-health characteristics results from the rationales indicating a close relationship between the consumption of food rich in natural antioxidants and the prevention of degenerative diseases. The main dietary sources of antioxidants are fruits and vegetables, as well as their derived products. The natural antioxidants occurring in plant materials are mainly phenolic compounds, carotenoids, and vitamins [1]. Many of these natural antioxidants, especially phenolic compounds, demonstrate pro-healthy properties. It was confirmed that the presence of these compounds in food plays an important role in the prevention of many civilization diseases, in particular cancer, cardiovascular diseases, as well as diabetes and rheumatoid arthritis [1–3]. However, the biological activity and bioavailability of these compounds highly depend on the molecular weight and chemical structure of these compounds, the matrix of food and their concentration in the consumed products [4].

Generally, cocoa bean and its derived products, such as chocolate and cocoa powder are a good source of natural antioxidants, especially phenolic compounds [5–8]. However, the production of chocolate may result in the loss of up to 80% of phenolic compounds originating from cocoa beans [9]. The largest and the most diverse group of phenolic compounds found in cocoa beans are flavonoids [5,10–12]. The predominant phenolic compounds in raw cocoa beans are proanthocyanidins (58%), monomeric flavan-3-ols (37%) and anthocyanins (4%) [10,11,13]. However, the level of these substances in cocoa beans can vary greatly and depends on a number of factors, mainly the variety, the geographical and environmental conditions during growth, the degree of ripeness, the harvest time, as well as the conditions and duration of storage after harvesting [14–16]. Many studies have shown that the processing of cocoa beans in order to obtain chocolate significantly influences the phenolic compounds content, and thus their activity and bioavailability [10,17–21]. All processing steps, such as fermentation, drying, alkalization and roasting, in addition to beneficial physicochemical, microbiological, and organoleptic changes, cause significant degradation of phenolic compounds [17,18]. During fermentation and drying of the cocoa beans, the phenolic compounds undergo biochemical transformations leading to a reduction in their content. Monomeric flavan-3-ols are enzymatically oxidized to semi-quinones and quinones. Anthocyanins, which are highly unstable and susceptible to various degradation reactions such as enzymatic or non-enzymatic browning, in the presence of the glycosidases are hydrolyzed to anthocyanidins and monosaccharides, mainly arabinose and galactose [13,15,19,22]. Phenolic compound content decreases with thermal processing. Heat exerted during the roasting causes degradation of these substances through non-enzymatic oxidation and polymerization reactions of proteins and protein hydrolysis products, as well as amino acids, polysaccharides and Maillard reaction products leading to the formation of insoluble macromolecular complexes [21,23]. As a result, the concentration of phenolic compounds in raw cocoa beans differs significantly from that in the roasted beans and chocolate [21,24–26].

In recent years, a healthy lifestyle has been promoted. It is mainly manifested by caring for health and taking up physical activity in order to ensure a longer life in a good physical and mental condition. One of the manifestations of caring for health is eating food that is not only of the highest nutritional value, but also has specific health-promoting properties. However, food processing can lead to a reduction in the concentration or even complete loss of many valuable bioactive ingredients positively influencing human health. Hence the efforts of food and nutrition technologists, dieticians and, consequently, many conscious food producers to functionalize (design food products) the aim of which is not only to provide all nutrients, but also to positively influence the body's functions by providing compounds that reduce the risk of developing certain diseases, especially the so-called civilization diseases, or providing compounds that generally improve health and well-being. In the case of chocolate production, the content of bioactive ingredients, such as phenolic compounds, is also reduced. Already at the stage of fermentation of cocoa beans in plantations, their content is reduced by over 50%. Especially anthocyanins and (−)-epicatechin are highly degraded. Drying the beans after fermentation causes a further reduction in the concentration of these compounds. Some authors [5] state that up to 90% of (−)-epicatechin is lost as a result of fermentation and drying of cocoa beans. Further processes leading to obtaining chocolate, especially roasting cocoa beans, only increase the loss of polyphenols. That is why scientists, food technologists and dieticians see the need to enrich food, including chocolate, with an additional portion of bioactive compounds, including antioxidants, and the functional food market is constantly growing and not only small enterprises with niche production but also industrial giants are investing in it [5,16]. The current scientific literature on the subject describes few proposals in this area, starting from the introduction of an additional portion of polyphenols in pure form, in the form of cocoa liquor from raw beans, cocoa liquor or cocoa powder with increased polyphenol content [27–29] to the addition of spices [30], leaves [31,32] or pomaces [33]. These studies have shown that in this way the polyphenol content and antioxidant activity of chocolates can be increased and their sensory profile can be influenced. There are commercially available chocolates with low or unprocessed fruits, e.g., almonds, nuts, raisins, but their shelf life is shorter than chocolate without such additives, due to, among other things, a higher water content in semi-finished fruit products (raisins) or a high content of unsaturated fatty acids (nuts, almonds) [34]. The introduction of freeze-dried fruit or vegetable powder into chocolate recipes eliminates this inconvenience. To the authors' knowledge, no studies have been carried out in terms of the aromatic profile, polyphenol content and antioxidant activity of different kinds of chocolates enriched with freeze-dried fruit or vegetable powders. For this purpose, we used several types of berries (blueberries, raspberries, blackberries), pomegranate pomace and beetroots and we assumed the aim of the presented research to investigate the effect of phenolic-rich plant powders fortification on the bioactive compounds profile, antioxidant activity and aroma (measured by an objective method using an electronic nose) of different types of chocolates. Berries and pomegranates contain significant amounts of flavonoids, mainly anthocyanins, and possess many beneficial properties for human health [35]. Anthocyanins are considered as strong antioxidants and free radical scavengers that have an antioxidant potential twice as high as that of other antioxidants, such as (+)-catechin and α-tocopherol [36]. Therefore, these fruits could be used as a source of phenolic substances with pronounced antioxidant activity. Powdered dried fruits (including berries) and vegetables are new and valuable ingredients for the chocolate industry. European Union regulations allow the introduction of up to 40% of additional foodstuffs to chocolate recipes [37]. In this context, the enrichment of chocolates with freeze-dried fruit (berries, pomegranate) or vegetable (beetroots) powder, which is a rich source of natural antioxidants, including anthocyanins, can greatly improve functional and health-promoting properties of these products. However, the addition of plant powders rich in anthocyanins or other phenolic compounds may have an effect on the organoleptic properties, including aroma, and in consequence consumer acceptance of these novel chocolate products, depending on the source of the bioactive compounds and the type of product in which they are contained.

2. Results and Discussion

2.1. Water Content and Activity and Color of Chocolates

Table 1 shows the water content and activity, as well as the CIE L*a*b* and organoleptic characteristics of the tested chocolates.

Water content is one of the quality parameters of chocolate that affects the properties of this product. The increase in the water content causes the deterioration of the rheological properties of the chocolate. This influences, among other things, an increase in the power consumption of devices during production, problems with pumping of the chocolate mass, coating of cores, forming the product into bars or figures and worse sensory perceptions during its consumption (chocolate sticks to the teeth). The water content of the chocolates should be as low as possible. Bolenz and Glöde (2021) indicate that it should be lower than 0.6% [33]. This is difficult to achieve, especially in the case of white or milk chocolates due to the higher water content in milk powder than in other raw materials used in the production of chocolate. Problems with achieving such a low value of this parameter may also occur in the production of sugar-free chocolates. Sucrose substitutes are often characterized by a higher water content than sugar (sucrose), hence the generally higher moisture content of this type of product. Thus, in practice, it is often aimed at less than 2%. The water content in chocolates also depends on the production technology used, and the type and design of the machines used.

Our results are consistent with the results of other researchers. An example is the study by Godočiková et al. (2019) who studied the antioxidant properties and volatile profile of different kinds and types of chocolates produced in Slovakia with various fruit and nut additions [34]. They found the water content in dark chocolates at 1.1%, in milk chocolates at 1.8% and in white chocolates at 1.6%. Chocolates enriched with plant additives (sea buckthorn, almonds, mulberry, currant, cherry) were characterized by a much higher value of this parameter (8.7–16.6%). In our studies the water content in different types of chocolates varied from 0.93 to 2.19%, with the differences being statistically significant ($p < 0.05$).

Our results indicated that the type of chocolate and functional enrichment affected the water activity of chocolates significantly ($p < 0.05$). The water activity of tested chocolates ranges from 0.378 to 0.490. The present results are within the range reported by other authors [28,34]. Looking at the effect of freeze-dried fruit or vegetable powder on the water activity of chocolates, it was demonstrated that a partial replacement of sweetener in different types of chocolates by 1% freeze-dried phenolic-rich plant powder did not cause an increase of the water activity above the optimal level. Good quality and microbiologically stable chocolates are characterized by low moisture content and water activity of 0.25–0.50 [38]. Interestingly, it can be observed that some chocolate samples enriched with freeze-dried fruit or vegetable powder had lower moisture content and water activity than control ones. The differences in water content and activity could be explained with the changes in the chemical composition of the control and supplemented chocolates.

Table 1. Physicochemical characteristic and organoleptic assessment of different types of chocolates enriched with various freeze-dried phenolic-rich plant powders.

Chocolate Type	Functional Enrichment	Water Content (%)	Water Activity	CIE L*a*b* Color Parameters			Organoleptic Assessment (Point)
				L*	a*	b*	
DCH	CONT	1.15 ± 0.04 [b]	0.408 ± 0.003 [b]	27.79 ± 0.12 [a]	5.30 ± 0.10 [a]	1.15 ± 0.09 [b]	4.8 ± 0.2 [a]
	BLUB	1.63 ± 0.02 [c]	0.426 ± 0.002 [c]	29.88 ± 0.11 [e]	5.33 ± 0.09 [b]	1.63 ± 0.02 [c]	4.9 ± 0.1 [a]
	RASB	2.19 ± 0.09 [f]	0.446 ± 0.005 [d]	29.17 ± 0.11 [b]	5.54 ± 0.05 [d]	2.19 ± 0.06 [f]	4.8 ± 0.2 [a]
	BLCB	1.73 ± 0.08 [d]	0.490 ± 0.002 [f]	29.78 ± 0.12 [d]	5.39 ± 0.09 [c]	1.73 ± 0.02 [d]	4.8 ± 0.2 [a]
	POME	1.83 ± 0.05 [e]	0.400 ± 0.007 [a]	29.58 ± 0.13 [c]	5.50 ± 0.11 [d]	1.83 ± 0.03 [e]	4.7 ± 0.2 [a]
	BEET	0.93 ± 0.04 [a]	0.455 ± 0.003 [e]	31.69 ± 0.10 [f]	5.39 ± 0.08 [c]	0.93 ± 0.04 [a]	4.3 ± 0.3 [b]
DCH98S	CONT	1.63 ± 0.02 [b]	0.409 ± 0.001 [b]	27.70 ± 0.11 [b]	3.75 ± 0.09 [e]	1.63 ± 0.08 [b]	4.5 ± 0.1 [a]
	BLUB	1.97 ± 0.01 [f]	0.378 ± 0.002 [a]	27.74 ± 0.12 [b]	3.51 ± 0.10 [c]	1.97 ± 0.07 [f]	4.6 ± 0.1 [a]
	RASB	1.69 ± 0.04 [c]	0.447 ± 0.003 [d]	28.79 ± 0.14 [e]	3.34 ± 0.12 [a]	1.69 ± 0.02 [c]	4.6 ± 0.2 [a]
	BLCB	1.74 ± 0.07 [d]	0.433 ± 0.006 [c]	27.82 ± 0.11 [c]	3.60 ± 0.03 [d]	1.74 ± 0.06 [d]	4.5 ± 0.2 [a]
	POME	1.26 ± 0.02 [a]	0.408 ± 0.003 [b]	27.98 ± 0.13 [d]	3.53 ± 0.07 [c]	1.26 ± 0.04 [a]	4.5 ± 0.2 [a]
	BEET	1.86 ± 0.08 [e]	0.445 ± 0.005 [d]	27.57 ± 0.12 [a]	3.40 ± 0.09 [b]	1.86 ± 0.02 [e]	4.1 ± 0.3 [b]
DCH98ESt	CONT	1.83 ± 0.05 [c]	0.408 ± 0.002 [b]	27.22 ± 0.10 [a]	3.36 ± 0.07 [e]	1.83 ± 0.03 [c]	4.4 ± 0.2 [a]
	BLUB	1.58 ± 0.04 [a]	0.394 ± 0.003 [a]	27.96 ± 0.10 [c]	3.25 ± 0.10 [d]	1.58 ± 0.02 [a]	4.5 ± 0.1 [a]
	RASB	1.60 ± 0.02 [a]	0.443 ± 0.001 [d]	28.78 ± 0.12 [e]	3.11 ± 0.09 [b]	1.60 ± 0.01 [a]	4.5 ± 0.2 [a]
	BLCB	2.03 ± 0.03 [d]	0.445 ± 0.002 [d]	29.31 ± 0.11 [f]	3.03 ± 0.05 [a]	2.03 ± 0.06 [d]	4.4 ± 0.2 [a,b]
	POME	1.81 ± 0.01 [c]	0.392 ± 0.004 [a]	27.85 ± 0.09 [b]	3.49 ± 0.07 [f]	1.81 ± 0.03 [c]	4.3 ± 0.1 [a,b]
	BEET	1.70 ± 0.04 [b]	0.436 ± 0.003 [c]	28.35 ± 0.13 [d]	3.18 ± 0.09 [c]	1.70 ± 0.02 [b]	3.9 ± 0.3 [c]
MCH	CONT	1.22 ± 0.06 [c]	0.449 ± 0.004 [b]	32.99 ± 0.10 [b]	7.54 ± 0.06 [b]	1.22 ± 0.05 [b]	4.8 ± 0.2 [a]
	BLUB	1.24 ± 0.03 [c]	0.393 ± 0.003 [a]	34.01 ± 0.15 [f]	7.25 ± 0.08 [a]	1.24 ± 0.03 [c]	4.9 ± 0.1 [a]
	RASB	1.17 ± 0.04 [b]	0.441 ± 0.002 [b]	33.16 ± 0.12 [d]	7.60 ± 0.11 [b]	1.17 ± 0.02 [b]	4.8 ± 0.2 [a]
	BLCB	1.19 ± 0.05 [b]	0.475 ± 0.001 [c]	32.29 ± 0.11 [a]	7.55 ± 0.06 [b]	1.19 ± 0.05 [b]	4.8 ± 0.2 [a]
	POME	0.94 ± 0.04 [a]	0.396 ± 0.002 [a]	33.37 ± 0.11 [e]	7.99 ± 0.07 [d]	0.94 ± 0.02 [a]	4.6 ± 0.1 [b]
	BEET	1.24 ± 0.07 [c]	0.446 ± 0.003 [b]	33.08 ± 0.12 [c]	7.70 ± 0.09 [c]	1.24 ± 0.08 [c]	3.8 ± 0.3 [c]

Blueberries (BLUB), raspberries (RASB), blackberries (BLCB), pomegranates pomace (POME), beetroots (BEET), control chocolate, (CONT). Data are presented as mean ± SD of three replications. The values followed by the same lowercase letter (a–f) within each chocolate type in the same column do not differ significantly according to Tukey's HSD test at $p < 0.05$.

The color, next to the characteristic chocolate aroma and taste, is one of the basic attributes influencing the quality of chocolate products. These parameters were dependent on the type of chocolate. In our case, it was influenced by such factors as the content of cocoa liquor and related to this sweetener content, presence of freeze-dried plant powder, as well as the presence of powdered milk in milk chocolates. As can be seen in Table 1, the type of chocolate affected the CIE L*a*b* color parameters of the chocolates significantly

($p < 0.05$). The brightness (L*) of the surface of tested chocolates ranged from 27.22 to 34.01, while the redness (a*) and yellowness (b*) were 3.03–7.99 and 0.93–2.19, respectively. The results suggested that the control chocolates and the supplemented chocolates differed ($p < 0.05$) in terms of values of parameters L*, a* and b*. However, the values of parameter b* remained more similar. Generally, the addition of freeze-dried phenolic-rich plant powder to DCH, DCH98S, DCH98ESt or MCH significantly ($p < 0.05$) brightened the color on the surface of enriched chocolates compared to the control ones, which could be attributed to some changes in the crystal structure of cocoa butter (polymorphism) [32]. On the other hand, there were only slight differences for the a* and b* parameters between the control chocolates and the enriched chocolates of the same type. These results suggested that the addition of 1% freeze-dried phenolic-rich plant powder has no negative effect on the color of the enriched chocolates. Similar results were presented by Muhammad et al. (2018) for milk chocolates supplemented with cinnamon nanoparticles [30].

The organoleptic evaluation of the tested chocolates was in the range of 3.8–4.9 points (Table 1). The DCH chocolates were rated the best, followed by the MCH ones, and the worst were the DCH98Est. The organoleptic quality of the DCH and the MCH chocolates, control and with the addition of BLUB, RASB, BLCB and POME powders was rated as extremely desired. They obtained scores from 4.6 to 4.9 points, while the scores within one group of chocolates, i.e., the DCH or the MCH group, did not differ significantly from each other ($p \geq 0.05$). For example, in the case of the DCH chocolates, their rating was ranging from 4.7 to 4.9 points. Chocolates with BEET powder were rated the worst, though still in the desired organoleptic quality category. This was due to the earthy taste of the chocolates, which was especially noticeable in the case of milk chocolate (3.8 points). Among dark chocolates, chocolates with 98% cocoa were rated worse than the DCH chocolate. Panelists described them as tart and slightly more acidic than the DCH chocolates.

Two-way ANOVA revealed a significant effect of chocolate type ($p < 0.001$), phenolic-rich plant powder ($p < 0.05$) and their interaction ($p < 0.01$) for the water content and activity, the CIE L*a*b* color parameters and organoleptic characteristic of the tested chocolates (Table S1, Supplementary Materials).

2.2. Profile and Concentrations of Bioactive Compounds

The results show that there was considerable diversity between the profile and the levels of bioactive compounds in the control and the enriched chocolates. It is worthwhile noting that raw cocoa beans are known to be a good source of phenolic compounds, mainly flavonoids, but most of them are lost during the production of chocolate and thus even dark chocolate, which contains more cocoa parts than milk chocolate, has a significantly lower level of phenolic compounds. As a result of fermentation and drying, the concentration of phenolic compounds, especially flavonoids, decreases by more than 80% [26]. In the case of unstable anthocyanins, the losses may reach even up to 90% [10]. Heat treatment may also cause the transformation of the remaining anthocyanins into colorless chalcones, which spontaneously degrade to suitable phenolic acids or polymerize and condense with other phenolic compounds to form brown polymeric pigments. Therefore, chocolates obtained in the conventional processing of cocoa beans contain significantly less flavan-3-ols and do not contain anthocyanins. To minimize these losses, various plant extracts (e.g., raspberry leaf and green tea extracts) or dried fruits (e.g., cherry, black mulberry, currant, sea buckthorn) rich in phenolic compounds have been added to the white, milk or dark chocolates for enhancing their functional properties [27,30,31]. The application of freeze-dried fruit (blueberries, raspberries, blackberry, pomegranates pomace) and beetroot powder was exploited to enrich different kinds of chocolates, such as dark (DCH, DCH98S and DCH98ESt) and milk (MCH) chocolates, enhancing their health-promoting properties.

The addition of tested freeze-dried fruit or vegetable powders to different types of chocolates led to a significant ($p < 0.05$) enrichment of these products with phenolic compounds, mainly anthocyanins and phenolic acids (Table 2). It was found that a 1% addition of these powders to chocolates increased the content of total phenolic compounds (flavan-3-ols, phenolic acids and anthocyanins) of enriched dark and milk chocolates compared to the control ones dependent on the powder used. The highest percentage increase (approximately 80%) in the total polyphenol content was observed in the MCH chocolate enriched with BLUB powder (Table 3). The greatest increase in the total content of polyphenols in all obtained chocolates was caused by the addition of BLUB powder followed by the addition of BEET powder. The BLUB powder, in all obtained chocolates, enriched the polyphenol composition by approximately 32.8 mg/100 g DM of anthocyanins, which were absent in the control chocolates. The greatest amount of flavan-3-ols and phenolic acids was introduced into the chocolates also via BLUB powder. Therefore, the profile and concentrations of phenolic compounds in chocolates containing tested freeze-dried plant powders are influenced by the phytochemical composition of cocoa liquor and plant powder used as a functional additive. The contents of individual phenolic compounds detected in the control chocolates and in the chocolates made with 1% addition of the fruit or vegetable powder in the product recipe are presented in Table 3 (powders were added instead of part of sweetener).

Table 2. Phenolic compounds content and antioxidant properties of studied freeze-dried phenolic-rich plant powders.

Compounds and Antioxidant Activity	BLUB	RASB	BLCB	POME	BEET
Phenolic Content					
Flavan-3-ols (mg/100 g DM)					
Cat	35.41 ± 0.12 [e]	30.70 ± 0.14 [d]	10.09 ± 0.09 [a]	11.56 ± 0.11 [b]	21.87 ± 0.15 [c]
Ecat	57.45 ± 0.24 [d]	52.23 ± 0.19 [b]	48.34 ± 0.18 [a]	55.34 ± 0.26 [c]	58.50 ± 0.31 [e]
PC B2	39.34 ± 0.17 [d]	20.46 ± 0.19 [c]	43.24 ± 0.21 [e]	16.78 ± 0.13 [b]	13.65 ± 0.10 [a]
PC C1	11.98 ± 0.08 [e]	0.06 ± 0.02 [a]	0.12 ± 0.03 [c]	0.09 ± 0.02 [b]	0.05 ± 0.02 [a]
Total	144.18 ± 0.56 [e]	103.45 ± 0.25 [d]	101.79 ± 0.21 [c]	83.77 ± 0.14 [a]	94.07 ± 0.18 [b]
Anthocyanins (mg/100 g DM)					
Cy-3-Glu	nd	3730.65 ± 10.87 [a]	4370.09 ± 12.44 [b]	nd	nd
Cy-3-Rut	nd	nd	59.76 ± 0.21	nd	nd
Cy-3,5-diGlu	10,280.60 ± 32.51 [b]	nd	nd	98.69 ± 0.36 [a]	nd
Cy-3-Xyl	4195.67 ± 14.41 [b]	nd	164.86 ± 0.41 [a]	nd	nd
Cy-3-(6″-Mal-Glu)	nd	nd	315.46 ± 0.65 [b]	nd	nd
Del-3,5-diGlu	7697.48 ± 26.54 [b]	nd	nd	31.56 ± 0.21 [a]	nd
Del-3-Glu	nd	nd	nd	8.49 ± 0.07	nd
Pel-3,5-diGlu	10,759.88 ± 36.38	nd	nd	nd	nd
Total	32,933.63 ± 61.89 [d]	3730.65 ± 10.87 [b]	4910.17 ± 13.70 [c]	138.74 ± 0.39 [a]	nd
Phenolic Acids (mg/100 g DM)					
GA	9.36 ± 0.09 [b]	nd	2.57 ± 0.05 [a]	nd	nd
PA	6.14 ± 0.05 [c]	3.19 ± 0.05 [b]	2.24 ± 0.04 [a]	nd	26.48 ± 0.11 [d]
p-HBA	1.83 ± 0.03 [a]	10.29 ± 0.08 [b]	18.48 ± 0.12 [d]	11.80 ± 0.06 [c]	70.40 ± 0.19 [e]
Total	17.33 ± 0.25 [c]	13.48 ± 0.08 [b]	23.29 ± 0.22 [d]	11.80 ± 0.05 [a]	96.88 ± 0.36 [e]
Total phenolics (mg/100 g DM)	33,095.14 ± 62.70 [e]	3847.58 ± 11.20 [c]	5035.25 ± 14.13 [d]	234.31 ± 0.58 [b]	190.95 ± 0.54 [a]
Antioxidant Activity					
DPPH EC$_{50}$ (mg/mg DPPH)	0.15 ± 0.02 [a]	0.62 ± 0.03 [b]	1.17 ± 0.05 [c]	1.49 ± 0.04 [d]	0.15 ± 0.02 [a]
FRAP (µmol TE/g DM)	761.27 ± 0.13 [e]	646.86 ± 0.16 [c]	629.61 ± 0.09 [b]	671.25 ± 0.12 [d]	498.34 ± 0.18 [a]

Blueberries (BLUB), raspberries (RASB), blackberries (BLCB), pomegranates pomace (POME), beetroots (BEET), control chocolate, (CONT). Data are presented as mean ± SD of three replications. The values followed by the same lowercase letter (a–e) in the same row do not differ significantly according to Tukey's HSD test at $p < 0.05$. nd—not detected.

Table 3. The content of individual phenolic compounds in different types of chocolates enriched with various freeze-dried phenolic-rich plant powders (mg/100 g DM).

Phenolic Compounds	Functional Enrichment					
	CONT	BLUB	RASB	BLCB	POME	BEET
DCH						
Flavan-3-ols						
Cat	14.15 ± 0.09 [a]	18.66 ± 0.08 [e]	16.60 ± 0.07 [d]	14.18 ± 0.11 [b]	15.16 ± 0.12 [c]	17.89 ± 0.09 [e]
Ecat	77.23 ± 0.48 [a]	97.32 ± 0.43 [f]	85.24 ± 0.47 [c]	80.68 ± 0.38 [b]	88.67 ± 0.34 [d]	96.54 ± 0.51 [e]
PC B2	23.30 ± 0.11 [a]	43.19 ± 0.15 [d]	43.35 ± 0.16 [d]	45.49 ± 0.12 [e]	40.41 ± 0.18 [c]	34.89 ± 0.15 [b]
PC C1	10.47 ± 0.06 [a]	17.79 ± 0.07 [e]	11.80 ± 0.08 [b]	14.71 ± 0.09 [d]	11.86 ± 0.07 [b]	14.40 ± 0.06 [c]
Total flavan-3-ols	125.15 ± 0.54 [a]	176.96 ± 0.59 [d]	156.99 ± 0.66 [b]	156.06 ± 0.65 [b]	156.10 ± 0.58 [b]	163.72 ± 0.63 [c]
Anthocyanins						
Cy-3-Glu	nd	nd	3.73 ± 0.05 [a]	4.37 ± 0.04 [b]	nd	nd
Cy-3-Rut	nd	nd	nd	0.06 ± 0.01 [a]	nd	nd
Cy-3,5-diGlu	nd	10.28 ± 0.15 [b]	nd	nd	0.10 ± 0.04 [a]	nd
Cy-3-Xyl	nd	4.20 ± 0.07 [b]	nd	0.16 ± 0.07 [a]	nd	nd
Cy-3-(6″-Mal-Glu)	nd	nd	nd	0.32 ± 0.03	nd	nd
Del-3,5-diGlu	nd	7.70 ± 0.10 [b]	nd	nd	0.03 ± 0.05 [a]	nd
Del-3-Glu	nd	nd	nd	nd	0.01 ± 0.01	nd
Pel-3,5-diGlu	nd	10.76 ± 0.09	nd	nd	nd	nd
Total anthocyanins	nd	32.93 ± 0.31 [d]	3.73 ± 0.05 [b]	4.91 ± 0.15 [c]	0.14 ± 0.09 [a]	nd
Phenolic acids						
GA	7.23 ± 0.09 [b]	8.77 ± 0.11 [c]	7.42 ± 0.10 [b]	7.12 ± 0.12 [a]	9.25 ± 0.10 [d]	8.88 ± 0.11 [c]
PA	1.34 ± 0.04 [a]	4.24 ± 0.10 [e]	2.86 ± 0.07 [c]	2.41 ± 0.06 [b]	2.91 ± 0.08 [c]	3.07 ± 0.05 [d]
p-HBA	7.69 ± 0.09 [a]	8.25 ± 0.11 [c]	8.60 ± 0.05 [d]	7.90 ± 0.09 [b]	7.96 ± 0.10 [b]	8.90 ± 0.03 [e]
Total phenolic acids	16.26 ± 0.21 [a]	21.26 ± 0.24 [f]	18.88 ± 0.21 [c]	17.43 ± 0.18 [b]	20.12 ± 0.26 [d]	20.85 ± 0.19 [e]
Total phenolics	**141.41 ± 0.74 [a]**	**231.16 ± 0.63 [d]**	**179.60 ± 0.64 [b]**	**177.40 ± 0.70 [b]**	**176.36 ± 0.71 [b]**	**184.57 ± 0.84 [e]**
DCH98S						
Flavan-3-ols						
Cat	28.48 ± 0.10 [c]	31.73 ± 0.08 [d]	28.21 ± 0.14 [c]	23.14 ± 0.12 [a]	25.77 ± 0.09 [b]	33.00 ± 0.14 [e]
Ecat	152.29 ± 0.51 [a]	165.44 ± 0.45 [e]	164.91 ± 0.31 [d]	154.30 ± 0.39 [b]	155.17 ± 0.43 [c]	173.70 ± 0.23 [f]
PC B2	39.61 ± 0.12 [a]	63.42 ± 0.11 [e]	53.69 ± 0.14 [c]	48.43 ± 0.09 [b]	70.96 ± 0.10 [f]	59.39 ± 0.19 [d]
PC C1	21.20 ± 0.08 [b]	29.25 ± 0.10 [e]	20.05 ± 0.06 [a]	27.95 ± 0.07 [c]	21.23 ± 0.09 [b]	28.73 ± 0.11 [d]
Total flavan-3-ols	241.58 ± 0.78 [a]	289.84 ± 0.69 [e]	266.86 ± 0.58 [c]	253.82 ± 0.72 [b]	273.13 ± 0.73 [d]	294.82 ± 0.63 [f]
Anthocyanins						
Cy-3-Glu	nd	nd	3.73 ± 0.06 [a]	4.37 ± 0.05 [b]	nd	nd
Cy-3-Rut	nd	nd	nd	0.06 ± 0.02	nd	nd
Cy-3,5-diGlu	nd	10.28 ± 0.11 [b]	nd	nd	0.10 ± 0.02 [a]	nd
Cy-3-Xyl	nd	4.20 ± 0.08 [b]	nd	0.16 ± 0.04 [a]	nd	nd
Cy-3-(6″-Mal-Glu)	nd	nd	nd	0.32 ± 0.03	nd	nd
Del-3,5-diGlu	nd	7.70 ± 0.12 [b]	nd	nd	0.03 ± 0.01 [a]	nd
Del-3-Glu	nd	nd	nd	nd	0.01 ± 0.01	nd
Pel-3,5-diGlu	nd	10.76 ± 0.17	nd	nd	nd	nd
Total anthocyanins	nd	32.94 ± 0.34 [d]	3.73 ± 0.06 [b]	4.91 ± 0.14 [c]	0.14 ± 0.04 [a]	nd
Phenolic acids						
GA	11.29 ± 0.11 [a]	14.91 ± 0.09 [e]	12.61 ± 0.10 [b]	13.53 ± 0.12 [d]	16.28 ± 0.11 [f]	12.95 ± 0.08 [c]
PA	2.58 ± 0.04 [a]	7.21 ± 0.06 [f]	4.86 ± 0.05 [d]	4.59 ± 0.06 [c]	5.20 ± 0.07 [e]	3.72 ± 0.05 [b]
p-HBA	9.78 ± 0.10 [b]	14.02 ± 0.12 [f]	10.41 ± 0.08 [c]	11.21 ± 0.11 [d]	13.53 ± 0.10 [e]	8.59 ± 0.07 [a]
Total phenolic acids	23.65 ± 0.24 [a]	36.14 ± 0.27 [f]	27.88 ± 0.23 [c]	29.33 ± 0.28 [d]	35.01 ± 0.28 [e]	25.26 ± 0.20 [b]
Total phenolics	**265.23 ± 1.02 [a]**	**358.92 ± 1.32 [f]**	**298.47 ± 0.87 [c]**	**288.06 ± 0.94 [b]**	**308.28 ± 0.95 [d]**	**320.08 ± 0.82 [e]**
DCH98Est						
Flavan-3-ols						
Cat	27.73 ± 0.13 [d]	26.90 ± 0.12 [c]	25.92 ± 0.14 [b]	25.62 ± 0.11 [a]	25.62 ± 0.13 [a]	27.97 ± 0.11 [e]
Ecat	149.37 ± 0.49 [d]	140.24 ± 0.40 [b]	139.79 ± 0.35 [a]	139.84 ± 0.47 [a]	141.54 ± 0.21 [b]	147.25 ± 0.31 [c]
PC B2	33.18 ± 0.17 [a]	53.76 ± 0.16 [e]	45.52 ± 0.15 [c]	41.05 ± 0.14 [b]	60.15 ± 0.21 [f]	50.35 ± 0.16 [d]
PC C1	17.76 ± 0.15 [b]	24.80 ± 0.11 [e]	17.00 ± 0.10 [a]	23.70 ± 0.12 [d]	18.00 ± 0.13 [c]	24.35 ± 0.10 [d]
Total flavan-3-ols	228.04 ± 0.66 [a]	245.70 ± 0.55 [c]	228.23 ± 0.61 [a]	230.21 ± 0.59 [b]	245.31 ± 0.69 [c]	249.92 ± 0.53 [d]
Anthocyanins						
Cy-3-Glu	nd	nd	3.74 ± 0.05 [a]	4.38 ± 0.04 [b]	nd	nd
Cy-3-Rut	nd	nd	nd	0.06 ± 0.02	nd	nd
Cy-3,5-diGlu	nd	10.30 ± 0.12 [b]	nd	nd	0.10 ± 0.01 [a]	nd
Cy-3-Xyl	nd	4.20 ± 0.09 [b]	nd	0.17 ± 0.03 [a]	nd	nd
Cy-3-(6″-Mal-Glu)	nd	nd	nd	0.32 ± 0.04	nd	nd
Del-3,5-diGlu	nd	7.71 ± 0.11 [b]	nd	nd	0.03 ± 0.01 [a]	nd
Del-3-Glu	nd	nd	nd	nd	0.01 ± 0.01	nd

81

Table 3. Cont.

Phenolic Compounds	Functional Enrichment					
	CONT	BLUB	RASB	BLCB	POME	BEET
Pel-3,5-diGlu	nd	10.78 ± 0.09	nd	nd	nd	nd
Total anthocyanins	nd	32.99 ± 0.35 [d]	3.74 ± 0.05 [b]	4.93 ± 0.13 [c]	0.14 ± 0.03 [a]	nd
Phenolic acids						
GA	11.14 ± 0.08 [c]	12.64 ± 0.10 [e]	10.69 ± 0.09 [a]	11.47 ± 0.11 [d]	13.80 ± 0.09 [f]	10.98 ± 0.09 [b]
PA	2.16 ± 0.04 [a]	6.11 ± 0.03 [f]	4.12 ± 0.05 [d]	3.89 ± 0.06 [c]	4.41 ± 0.07 [e]	3.15 ± 0.05 [b]
p-HBA	10.70 ± 0.09 [c]	11.89 ± 0.10 [f]	11.74 ± 0.06 [e]	9.50 ± 0.08 [b]	11.47 ± 0.11 [d]	7.29 ± 0.06 [a]
Total phenolic acids	24.00 ± 0.21 [b]	30.64 ± 0.23 [f]	26.55 ± 0.22 [d]	24.86 ± 0.24 [c]	29.68 ± 0.19 [e]	21.42 ± 0.20 [a]
Total phenolics	**252.04 ± 0.86 [a]**	**309.33 ± 0.83 [e]**	**258.52 ± 0.72 [b]**	**260.00 ± 0.81 [b]**	**275.13 ± 0.90 [d]**	**271.34 ± 0.73 [c]**
	MCH					
Flavan-3-ols						
Cat	4.44 ± 0.03 [a]	5.54 ± 0.04 [b]	11.83 ± 0.03 [d]	11.35 ± 0.04 [c]	12.01 ± 0.05 [e]	14.65 ± 0.11 [f]
Ecat	45.58 ± 0.16 [a]	60.00 ± 0.17 [e]	58.72 ± 0.18 [d]	56.92 ± 0.18 [b]	58.21 ± 0.21 [c]	64.64 ± 0.16 [f]
PC B2	23.41 ± 0.12 [a]	31.59 ± 0.11 [e]	31.03 ± 0.10 [d]	27.55 ± 0.13 [b]	28.40 ± 0.11 [c]	34.05 ± 0.14 [f]
PC C1	6.23 ± 0.05 [c]	18.90 ± 0.04 [f]	5.90 ± 0.07 [b]	7.36 ± 0.06 [d]	15.93 ± 0.07 [e]	2.20 ± 0.05 [a]
Total flavan-3-ols	79.66 ± 0.36 [a]	116.03 ± 0.36 [f]	107.48 ± 0.38 [c]	103.18 ± 0.41 [b]	114.55 ± 0.44 [d]	115.54 ± 0.46 [e]
Anthocyanins						
Cy-3-Glu	nd	nd	3.77 ± 0.03 [a]	4.40 ± 0.04 [b]	nd	nd
Cy-3-Rut	nd	nd	nd	0.60 ± 0.02	nd	nd
Cy-3,5-diGlu	nd	10.38 ± 0.15 [b]	nd	nd	0.10 ± 0.02 [a]	nd
Cy-3-Xyl	nd	4.24 ± 0.04 [b]	nd	0.17 ± 0.03 [a]	nd	nd
Cy-3-(6″-Mal-Glu)	nd	nd	nd	0.32 ± 0.02	nd	nd
Del-3,5-diGlu	nd	7.77 ± 0.12 [b]	nd	nd	0.03 ± 0.01 [a]	nd
Del-3-Glu	nd	nd	nd	nd	0.01 ± 0.01	nd
Pel-3,5-diGlu	nd	10.08 ± 0.13	nd	nd	nd	nd
Total anthocyanins	nd	32.47 ± 0.24 [d]	3.77 ± 0.03 [b]	5.49 ± 0.11 [c]	0.14 ± 0.04 [a]	nd
Phenolic acids						
GA	6.08 ± 0.10 [a]	7.18 ± 0.11 [b]	7.56 ± 0.12 [c]	7.99 ± 0.09 [d]	7.34 ± 0.13 [b]	8.09 ± 0.05 [d]
PA	1.52 ± 0.04 [a]	2.04 ± 0.05 [c]	1.87 ± 0.03 [b]	2.00 ± 0.03 [c]	1.81 ± 0.05 [b]	2.53 ± 0.10 [d]
p-HBA	1.98 ± 0.06 [a]	2.96 ± 0.07 [c]	3.05 ± 0.02 [d]	3.01 ± 0.05 [d]	2.81 ± 0.04 [b]	3.92 ± 0.04 [e]
Total phenolic acids	9.58 ± 0.20 [a]	12.18 ± 0.23 [b]	12.48 ± 0.17 [b,c]	13.00 ± 0.17 [c]	11.96 ± 0.22 [b]	14.54 ± 0.19 [d]
Total phenolics	**89.24 ± 0.56 [a]**	**160.68 ± 0.83 [f]**	**123.73 ± 0.58 [c]**	**121.67 ± 0.69 [b]**	**126.65 ± 0.70 [d]**	**130.08 ± 0.65 [e]**

nd—not detected. Blueberries (BLUB), raspberries (RASB), blackberries (BLCB), pomegranates pomace (POME), beetroots (BEET), control chocolate, (CONT). Data are presented as mean ± SD of three replications. The values followed by the same lowercase letter (a–f) within each chocolate type in the same row do not differ significantly according to Tukey's HSD test at $p < 0.05$.

The addition of plant powders made the chocolates differ in the total phenolics content and the qualitative and quantitative composition of polyphenols (Table 3). The feature that distinguished them is primarily the content and concentration of anthocyanins. The control and chocolates with BEET powder did not contain anthocyanins. Chocolates with the addition of BLUB powder included in their composition four anthocyanins: cyanidin-3,5-O-diglucoside (Cy-3,5-diGlu), cyanidin-3-O-xyloside (Cy-3-Xyl), delphinidin-3,5-O-diglucoside (Del-3,5-diGlu) and pelargonidin-3,5-O-diglucoside (Pel-3,5-diGlu), whose total concentration was approximately 33 mg/100 g DM. Cy-3,5-di Glu and Pel-3,5-diGlu were present in the highest amounts, each at concentrations of above 10 mg/100 g DM. Chocolates with the addition of RASB powder included only one anthocyanin—cyanidin-3-O-glucoside (Cy-3-Glu) in a concentration of approximately 3.7 mg/100 g DM. There were four anthocyanins in the chocolates with BLCB powder, i.e., Cy-3-Glu, cyanidin-3-O-rutinoside (Cy-3-Rut), Cy-3-Xyl and cyanidin-3-(6″-malonyl)-glucoside (Cy-3-(6″-Mal-Glu)), the total concentration of which was approximately 5 mg/100 g DM, with Cy-3-Glu being the highest amount of 4.4 mg/100 g DM. On the other hand, in chocolates with POME powder there were three anthocyanins, i.e., Cy-3,5-diGlu, Del-3,5-diGlu and delphinidin-3-O-glucoside (Del-3-Glu), with a total concentration of 0.14 mg/100 g DM, with Cy-3,5-diGlu being the highest amount of 0.1 mg/100 g DM.

Seven phenolic compounds were identified in all types of control chocolates and chocolates enriched with BEET powder, including four flavan-3-ols (catechin—Cat, epicatechin—Ecat, procyanidin B2—PC B2 and procyanidin C1—PC C1) and three phenolic acids (gallic acid—GA, protocatechuic acid—PA and p-hydroxybenzoic acid—p-HBA). The presence of these compounds in chocolates has already been described by other authors [29,39,40]. Chocolates enriched with RASB powder showed eight phenolic compounds, seven of which were present in the control chocolates and in chocolates made with vegetable powder in addition to Cy-3-Glu. The dark and milk chocolates containing BLCB powder showed the presence of eleven phenolic compounds and eight of these phenolics were identified in raspberry-enriched chocolates in addition to Cy-3-Rut, Cy-3-Xyl and Cy-3-(6''-Mal-Glu). The samples of DCH, DCH98S, DCH98Est and MCH made with BLUB powder also showed eleven phenolic compounds, eight of which were present in chocolates with BLCB powder in addition to Cy-3,5-diGlu, Del-3,5-diGlu and Pel-3,5-diGlu. The different types of chocolates containing POME powder showed the presence of ten phenolic compounds and nine of these phenolics were identified in BLUB-enriched chocolates in addition to Del-3-Glu. The predominant phenolic compound in all tested chocolates was Ecat. The second most abundant compound was PC B2, followed by Cat, PC C1, GA and p-HBA. Moreover, Cy-3,5-diGlu, Pel-3,5-diGlu, Cy-3-Glu and Cy-3-Xyl were found in significant quantities but only in chocolates made with berry powders. Depending on the evaluated chocolate types and functional enrichment, the concentrations of individual phenolic compounds varied significantly ($p < 0.05$) within tested chocolates.

As can be seen in Table 3, the sum of phenolic compounds differed significantly ($p < 0.05$) between control and enriched chocolates of different types, with the highest total phenolics found for DCH98S chocolate enriched with BLUB powder and the lowest for control MCH (the results ranged from 89.24 to 358.92 mg/100 g DM).

The major phenolic compounds in both control and chocolates enriched with fruit or vegetable powders were flavan-3-ols, which represented approximately 72–92% of total phenolics levels. The total amount of the investigated flavan-3-ols within the different chocolate types ranged from 79.66 mg/100 g DM in control milk chocolate to 294.82 mg/100 g DM in DCH98S chocolate enriched with BEET powder. The content of these compounds was similar to the amount reported by other authors [29,39,40] in different kinds of chocolates. Considerable amounts of phenolic acids were also found in tested chocolates. The concentrations of these phenolics represented approximately 8–11% of the average amounts of total phenolics. Among investigated samples, the highest phenolic acids levels were found in DCH98S chocolate enriched with either BLUB or POME powders. In turn, significant quantities of anthocyanins were found in chocolates enriched with fruit powders but mainly in those made with berry powders. Depending on the evaluated chocolate types and functional enrichment, the concentrations of anthocyanins varied significantly ($p < 0.05$) within chocolates enriched with fruit powders and ranged from 0.14 to 32.99 mg/100 g DM. In this study, no anthocyanins were found in the control chocolates. Moreover, chocolates with the addition of POME powder were characterized by very small amounts of these compounds.

The results indicated that the addition of all fruit and vegetable powders to different types of chocolates led to substantial changes in the levels of phenolic compounds of enriched chocolates (Table 3). A two-way ANOVA revealed that the content of all phenolic compounds, apart from anthocyanins, varied significantly with the type of chocolate ($p < 0.001$), phenolic-rich plant powder ($p < 0.001$) and their interaction ($p < 0.001$) (Table S2, Supplementary Materials). In addition, the total anthocyanins, Cy-3-Glu, Cy-3-Rut, Cy-3,5-diGlu, Cy-3-Xyl, Cy-3-(6''-Mal-Glu), Del-3,5-diGlu and Del-3-Glu concentrations were significantly affected by phenolic-rich plant powder, but there was not a statistically significant interaction between the effects of the type of chocolate and the phenolic-rich plant powder. The addition of all tested fruit and vegetable powders increased considerably the total content of phenolic compounds of all chocolate types compared to the control ones. Irrespective of the chocolate type, there was a significant increase in the level of flavan-3-ols and phenolic acids of the enriched chocolates. It was also observed that the addition of berry powders also caused a significant ($p < 0.05$) increase in the total anthocyanins content in both dark and milk chocolates with respect to control chocolates, while the amount of these pigments in chocolates made with POME powder only slightly increased compared to control ones. Overall, the greatest increment in the total contents of three classes of phenolic compounds of all types of chocolates was caused by the supplementation of BLUB powder. The increase in phenolic contents in fruit- or vegetable-supplemented chocolates reflects the addition of specific functional enrichment. Godočiková et al. (2017) reported also that specific types of dried fruits, for example black mulberry, rich in anthocyanins, was also suitable to enhance the concentration of bioactive substances of chocolate even with a lower cocoa solids content [41]. Recently, Martini, Conte and Tagliazucchi (2018) demonstrated that the enrichment of dark chocolates with Sakura green tea leaves or turmeric powder is an effective technique to improve the health-enhancement of the final product [42].

Our data supported the possible application of berries and POME powders to the formulation of both dark and milk chocolates with increased phenolic compounds, mainly anthocyanins, which are never found in a given type of cocoa bean or are lost during their processing.

2.3. Antioxidant Activity

In order to evaluate the freeze-dried phenolic-rich plant powders' contribution to the antioxidant properties of the different types of chocolates, the DPPH radical scavenging activity and the ferric-reducing ability in control and enriched chocolates were determined and the results have been presented in Figure 1I and II, respectively.

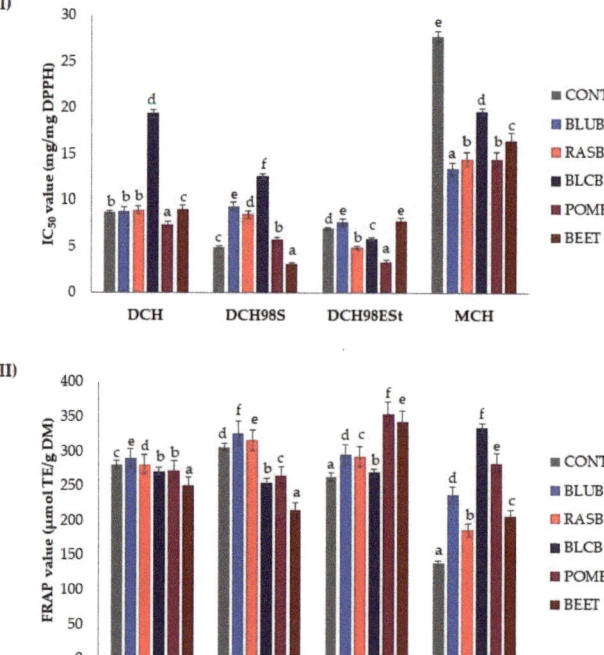

Figure 1. (**I**) DPPH radical scavenging activity of different types of chocolates enriched with various freeze-dried phenolic-rich plant powders, expressed as IC50 values. (**II**) Ferric reducing antioxidant power (FRAP value) of different types of chocolates enriched with various freeze-dried phenolic-rich plant powders. Data are expressed as the mean of triplicate ± SD. Bars with the same lowercase letter (a–f) within each type of chocolate do not differ significantly according to Tukey's HSD test at $p < 0.05$. Blueberries (BLUB), raspberries (RASB), blackberries (BLCB), pomegranates pomace (POME), beetroots (BEET), control (CONT).

The DPPH• scavenging capacity was expressed as IC_{50} values, the concentration at which 50% inhibition of free radical scavenging activity is observed. The range of IC_{50} values of the analyzed chocolates was 3.05–28.12 mg/mg DPPH (Figure 1I). Two-way ANOVA revealed the significant effect of chocolate type ($p < 0.001$), freeze-dried phenolic-rich plant powders ($p < 0.001$) and their interaction for the DPPH radical scavenging activity (Table S2).

Overall, dark chocolates revealed better antioxidant properties than milk chocolates, which agrees with the higher content of phenolic compounds found in the dark chocolates. The antioxidant activity of chocolates is usually attributed to the presence of monomeric flavan-3-ols, polymeric procyanidins and Maillard reaction products (e.g., melanoidins) that are well known to possess effective scavenging activity of free radicals [43].

The results indicated that the enrichment of chocolates with various fruit or vegetable powders can improve the antioxidant activity of chocolates, depending on the chocolate type and plant powder used as a functional additive. As compared to control chocolates, the supplementation with almost all freeze-dried fruit and vegetable powders caused significant ($p < 0.05$) decreases in the DPPH free radical scavenging activity in many types of obtained chocolates. Interestingly, among all studied chocolates, the highest DPPH radical scavenging capacity was exhibited by the DCH98S chocolate enriched with BEET powder. Nevertheless, the results indicated that the addition of BEET powder to DCH and DCH98ESt chocolates reduced DPPH radical scavenging activity significantly ($p < 0.05$) compared to the control. The observed differences in the free radical scavenging capacity of chocolates of different types with the same additive and different sweeteners may be due to different reaction mechanisms occurring during the preparation of the chocolates, including the Maillard reaction, the degradation of phenolic compounds of higher molecular weight to smaller phenolics and/or various transformations of flavan-3-ols and phenolic acids. In addition, other authors reported that supplementation of a sour cherry puree with sucrose or erythritol significantly declines its free radical scavenging activity [44]. They showed that the addition of natural sweeteners to a sour cherry puree resulted in a significant reduction in phenolic compounds, mainly flavan-3-ols. These phenomena may be due to the intermolecular interactions between the hydroxyl group from phenolic compounds in chocolate and phenolic-rich plant powders and a hydroxyl group in sucrose or sugar alcohol molecules [44,45].

It was observed that dark chocolates (98%) sweetened with erythritol and stevia instead of sucrose supplemented with RASB, BLCB and POME powders exhibited a higher DPPH radical-scavenging activity as compared to control DCH98ESt samples. Regarding the DCH chocolates, the enrichment with POME powder significantly increased ($p < 0.05$) the DPPH antioxidant capacity compared to the control sample. The obtained data highlighted, moreover, that the addition of freeze-dried berries, POME and BEET powders to MCH samples caused a significant ($p < 0.05$) increase in DPPH radical scavenging activity. As expected, the lowest free radical scavenging abilities was exhibited by the control milk chocolate. Our results also show that the partial sweetener substitution by BLCB powder caused the most pronounced reduction of the DPPH radical-scavenging potential of all dark chocolates. This result may be attributed to the synergistic and antagonistic interaction that results from the coexistence of many antioxidant compounds in enriched chocolates [41]. Some reports revealed that interactions between flavan-3-ols and anthocyanins might accelerate the degradation of anthocyanin pigments that further react giving rise to polymeric brown pigments [44]. It should be understood that the antioxidant activity of a mix is not the sum of the antioxidant activities of each of the components, due to interactions between the components. Therefore, it is difficult to predict in advance the result of food functionalization into components with antioxidant properties, e.g., the antioxidant potential of the product, inhibition of the growth of cancer cells or other biological properties. The effects can be surprising. Godočikova et al. (2017) observed that dark chocolates enriched with mulberry and sea buckthorn exhibited higher DPPH scavenging activity than control ones.

Antioxidant capacities significantly increased with the addition of capsules of bioactive compounds [41].

The addition of freeze-dried phenolic-rich plant powders led to significant ($p < 0.001$) differences in the reducing capacity of all types of chocolates (Table S2). The ferric-reducing antioxidant power of the tested chocolate samples varied from 140.15 to 354.38 μmol TE/g DM (Figure 1II).

Among investigated samples, the DCH98ESt chocolates enriched with POME and BEET powders demonstrated the highest FRAP values. The obtained results indicated that the reducing capacity of dark chocolates made with sucrose noticeably decreases after supplementation of BLCB, POME and BEET powders. While in the case of dark chocolate sweetened with erythritol and stevia instead of sucrose, the addition of all functional powders led to a considerable increase in the reducing power compared to the control ones. This phenomenon may be ascribed to the interaction of phenolic compounds with sucrose. For example, Shalaby et al. (2016) showed that the introduction of sucrose to green tea significantly decreased its antioxidant potential [45]. In the present study, irrespective of the functional enrichment type, there was a significant increase in the ferric-reducing ability of all supplemented milk chocolates. Other authors have also observed that the addition of different sweeteners to fruit puree and green or black tea affects their antioxidant properties in different ways [44,45]. Therefore, we can conclude that the observed differences in DPPH and FRAP values of dark chocolates (98%) with the same powders and different sweeteners may be due to different reaction mechanisms occurring between phenolic compounds and sucrose and erythritol with stevia glycosides. Interestingly, unlike dark chocolates, the addition of BLCB powder caused the greatest increase in the reducing capacity of milk chocolate. Our results also showed that the addition of anthocyanin-rich BLUB powder caused an increase in reducing power regardless of the type of chocolate. This increase may be attributed to the fact that anthocyanins can act as reducing agents mainly through the electron-transfer mechanism [36].

Other studies have also reported that the addition of fruit or other phenolic-rich plants to chocolates either increase or decrease antioxidant activity evaluated by FRAP and DPPH assays [32,33,41,46]. These distinct differences may be attributed to the increased interaction between phenolics and other compounds, including carbohydrates, sweeteners, and proteins, present in chocolate and in fruits or vegetables. It is well known that both non-oxidized and oxidized phenolic compounds have a strong affinity to proteins, polysaccharides, alkaloids and Maillard reaction products, and may form insoluble complexes [46]. The results provide strong evidence that the interactions of mixtures of antioxidant compounds might generate synergic or inhibitor effects and can enhance or inhibit the antioxidant activity or even modify their reaction mechanisms [41].

2.4. Electronic Nose Analysis of Chocolates

Chocolate aroma depends on the combination of many volatile compounds (VCs) derived from cocoa beans and other ingredients, such as sucrose (sweetener), milk, and flavors, formed or modified during the roasting, alkalization and conching stages. It is well known that the typical chocolate flavor is mainly formed due to the Maillard reactions and the Strecker degradation of flavor precursors, such as free amino acids, short-chain peptides, and reducing sugars (e.g., glucose) during roasting [47,48]. However, it has to be noticed that functional additives rich in phenolic compounds having a positive effect on biological activity of enriched chocolates, can also affect the sensory properties of the final product. For example, phenolic compounds are responsible for the specific astringent and bitter taste of the raw beans and influence the stability and digestibility of the products obtained from them as a result of the formation of complexes mainly with polysaccharides, proteins, methylxanthines and Maillard reaction products. Therefore, these compounds are playing an important role in shaping the sensory characteristics of chocolates, fruits, and vegetables, as well as products obtained from them [48].

In our study, volatile compounds in chocolates were determined by using an electronic nose. A total of twenty-six VCs were identified, including alcohols, phenols, aldehydes, ketones, esters, acids, pyrazines, furfural, lactone, and sulfide compound in the all-enriched chocolates (Table 4). The results revealed that the addition of berries, POME and BEET powders significantly ($p < 0.05$) influenced the sensory attributes of the resultant chocolates. A two-way ANOVA revealed that the content of all VCs, apart from vanillin, varied significantly with chocolate type ($p < 0.001$), freeze-dried phenolic-rich plant powders ($p < 0.001$) and their interaction ($p < 0.001$) (Table S3, Supplementary Materials). The most important compounds of control and supplemented chocolates were acetic acid, benzaldehyde, 2-methylpropanal, 3-methylbutanal, 2-furfural, 2,5-dimethylpyrazine, pentanal and phenylethylacetate. The compound found in the highest concentration in all samples was acetic acid, which is associated with sour, pungent, and unpleasant notes. This compound is the highest odor-active compound in unroasted cocoa beans. Despite the fact that during further processing of cocoa beans acetic acid concentration decreases by over 70%, it is still the highest odor-active compound in roasted cocoa beans, cocoa mass and chocolates obtained from them [47–50]. The second compound found in the highest concentration in all tested chocolates is benzaldehyde. This compound has a pleasant fruity-type odor and a fruity-type flavor.

Table 4. The content of volatile compounds in different types of chocolates.

Volatile Compounds	Functional Enrichment					
	CONT	BLUB	RASB	BLCB	POME	BEET
	DCH					
Alcohols and Phenols						
2,3-Butanediol	0.25 ± 0.04 [a]	0.69 ± 0.05 [e]	0.43 ± 0.03 [c]	0.58 ± 0.06 [d]	0.37 ± 0.08 [b]	0.40 ± 0.02 [c]
2-Phenylethanol	0.03 ± 0.01 [a]	0.11 ± 0.03 [b]	0.04 ± 0.02 [a]	0.04 ± 0.01 [a]	0.03 ± 0.02 [a]	0.03 ± 0.02 [a]
Aldehydes and Ketones						
2-Methylpropanal	3.49 ± 0.03 [c]	2.84 ± 0.06 [a]	4.09 ± 0.04 [e]	3.68 ± 0.02 [d]	2.99 ± 0.02 [b]	4.66 ± 0.04 [f]
Benzaldehyde	18.91 ± 0.13 [d]	12.74 ± 0.14 [a]	19.93 ± 0.10 [e]	17.55 ± 0.15 [c]	15.50 ± 0.13 [b]	22.39 ± 0.19 [f]
Butan-2-one	0.47 ± 0.06 [b]	0.54 ± 0.02 [c]	0.45 ± 0.03 [b]	0.56 ± 0.04 [c]	0.46 ± 0.06 [b]	0.40 ± 0.02 [a]
3-Methylbutanal	1.01 ± 0.07 [e]	0.88 ± 0.09 [d]	0.70 ± 0.06 [b]	0.90 ± 0.04 [d]	0.81 ± 0.03 [c]	0.52 ± 0.04 [a]
2,3-Pentanedione	0.63 ± 0.04 [a]	1.18 ± 0.10 [e]	0.87 ± 0.04 [c]	1.03 ± 0.04 [d]	0.76 ± 0.04 [b]	0.84 ± 0.05 [c]
Pentanal	0.08 ± 0.02 [a]	0.67 ± 0.06 [c]	0.29 ± 0.04 [b]	1.13 ± 0.04 [d]	0.11 ± 0.04 [a]	0.09 ± 0.04 [a]
(Z)-4-Heptenal	0.08 ± 0.01 [a]	0.10 ± 0.05 [a]	0.08 ± 0.02 [a]	0.06 ± 0.01 [a]	0.08 ± 0.02 [a]	0.07 ± 0.03 [a]
Octanal	0.02 ± 0.01 [a]	0.10 ± 0.06 [b]	0.02 ± 0.01 [a]	0.02 ± 0.01 [a]	0.01 ± 0.01 [a]	0.01 ± 0.01 [a]
Butanal	0.04 ± 0.01 [b]	0.08 ± 0.03 [c]	0.03 ± 0.01 [a]	0.03 ± 0.01 [a]	0.03 ± 0.01 [a]	0.01 ± 0.01 [a]
Nonan-2-one	0.06 ± 0.03	0.06 ± 0.01	0.07 ± 0.01	0.05 ± 0.04	0.07 ± 0.01	0.07 ± 0.02
(Z)-2-Nonenal	0.10 ± 0.04 [b]	0.08 ± 0.02 [a]	0.07 ± 0.02 [a]	0.07 ± 0.02 [a]	0.11 ± 0.04 [b]	0.06 ± 0.02 [a]
(E,E)-2,4-Nonadienal	0.02 ± 0.01 [a]	0.09 ± 0.02 [c]	0.06 ± 0.04 [b]	0.05 ± 0.04 [b]	0.03 ± 0.01 [a]	0.07 ± 0.01 [b]
(Z)-2-Decenal	0.04 ± 0.01 [a]	0.57 ± 0.10 [c]	0.10 ± 0.02 [b]	0.02 ± 0.01 [a]	0.04 ± 0.01 [a]	0.04 ± 0.01 [a]
Vanillin	0.06 ± 0.02	0.06 ± 0.01	0.07 ± 0.02	0.06 ± 0.01	0.06 ± 0.02	0.07 ± 0.02
Acids						
Pentanoic acid	0.02 ± 0.01	0.01 ± 0.01	0.02 ± 0.01	0.02 ± 0.01	0.04 ± 0.02	0.02 ± 0.01
Acetic acid	60.86 ± 0.13 [b]	69.34 ± 0.14 [e]	60.13 ± 0.11 [b]	62.73 ± 0.16 [c]	66.99 ± 0.09 [d]	57.29 ± 0.12 [a]
Phenylacetic acid	0.49 ± 0.02 [d]	0.40 ± 0.03 [b]	0.46 ± 0.01 [c]	0.30 ± 0.02 [a]	0.51 ± 0.03 [d]	0.50 ± 0.04 [d]
Furfurals						
2-Furfural	2.17 ± 0.04 [d]	1.11 ± 0.05 [a]	1.77 ± 0.07 [b]	1.14 ± 0.03 [a]	1.92 ± 0.05 [c]	1.92 ± 0.04 [c]
Pyrazines						
2,5-Dimethylpyrazine	10.85 ± 0.12	7.54 ± 0.11	9.80 ± 0.10	9.47 ± 0.13	8.60 ± 0.11	10.01 ± 0.12
Trimethylpyrazine	0.08 ± 0.03 [b]	0.07 ± 0.02 [b]	0.05 ± 0.01 [a]	0.06 ± 0.02 [a,b]	0.05 ± 0.02 [a]	0.04 ± 0.01 [a]
Tetramethylpyrazine	0.06 ± 0.01 [a]	0.15 ± 0.05 [c]	0.07 ± 0.02 [a,b]	0.09 ± 0.03 [b]	0.06 ± 0.02 [a]	0.05 ± 0.01 [a]
Esters						
Ethyl octanoate	0.03 ± 0.01 [a]	0.05 ± 0.01 [a]	0.07 ± 0.02 [a,b]	0.07 ± 0.03 [a,b]	0.07 ± 0.02 [a,b]	0.08 ± 0.01 [b]
Phenylethylacetate	0.13 ± 0.03 [b]	0.31 ± 0.06 [c]	0.16 ± 0.04 [b]	0.07 ± 0.02 [a]	0.13 ± 0.03 [b]	0.16 ± 0.04 [b]
Lactones						
γ-Nonalactone	nd	0.08 ± 0.02	0.08 ± 0.02	0.11 ± 0.04	0.08 ± 0.03	0.10 ± 0.05
Sulfur Compounds						
Dimethyl trisulfide	0.02 ± 0.01 [a]	0.13 ± 0.03 [c]	0.08 ± 0.01 [b]	0.09 ± 0.02 [b]	0.08 ± 0.03 [b]	0.10 ± 0.04 [b]
	DCH98S					
Alcohols and Phenols						
2,3-Butanediol	0.28 ± 0.05 [a]	1.13 ± 0.03 [e]	0.61 ± 0.04 [c]	0.92 ± 0.07 [d]	0.50 ± 0.05 [b,c]	0.47 ± 0.03 [b]

Table 4. Cont.

Volatile Compounds	Functional Enrichment					
	CONT	BLUB	RASB	BLCB	POME	BEET
2-Phenylethanol	0.06 ± 0.02 [b]	0.19 ± 0.05 [c]	0.05 ± 0.02 [a,b]	0.06 ± 0.02 [b]	0.03 ± 0.01 [a]	0.03 ± 0.01 [a]
Aldehydes and Ketones						
2-Methylpropanal	3.57 ± 0.07 [c]	2.19 ± 0.06 [a]	4.69 ± 0.08 [e]	3.87 ± 0.03 [d]	2.48 ± 0.07 [b]	5.24 ± 0.08 [f]
Benzaldehyde	17.34 ± 0.15 [d]	6.58 ± 0.09 [a]	20.95 ± 0.17 [e]	16.18 ± 0.09 [c]	12.09 ± 0.11 [b]	24.13 ± 0.18 [f]
Butan-2-one	0.35 ± 0.04 [a]	0.60 ± 0.07 [c]	0.43 ± 0.05 [b]	0.65 ± 0.06 [c]	0.46 ± 0.03 [b]	0.36 ± 0.05 [a]
3-Methylbutanal	0.51 ± 0.03 [c]	0.75 ± 0.05 [e]	0.40 ± 0.06 [b]	0.80 ± 0.05 [e]	0.61 ± 0.04 [d]	0.28 ± 0.03 [a]
2,3-Pentanedione	0.93 ± 0.07 [b]	1.72 ± 0.08 [e]	1.10 ± 0.05 [c]	1.42 ± 0.09 [d]	0.88 ± 0.08 [a]	0.93 ± 0.07 [b]
Pentanal	0.13 ± 0.06 [b]	1.26 ± 0.07 [d]	0.50 ± 0.03 [c]	2.18 ± 0.04 [e]	0.13 ± 0.03 [b]	0.09 ± 0.03 [a]
(Z)-4-Heptenal	0.06 ± 0.02 [b]	0.11 ± 0.05 [c]	0.07 ± 0.02 [b]	0.04 ± 0.01 [a]	0.07 ± 0.02 [b]	0.07 ± 0.02 [b]
Octanal	0.02 ± 0.01 [a]	0.18 ± 0.03 [b]	0.03 ± 0.01 [a]	0.03 ± 0.01 [a]	0.01 ± 0.01 [a]	0.01 ± 0.01 [a]
Butanal	0.02 ± 0.01 [a]	0.13 ± 0.04 [b]	0.02 ± 0.01 [a]	0.03 ± 0.01 [a]	0.03 ± 0.01 [a]	0.01 ± 0.01 [a]
Nonan-2-one	0.02 ± 0.01 [a]	0.07 ± 0.02 [b]	0.07 ± 0.01 [b]	0.04 ± 0.02 [a]	0.08 ± 0.02 [b]	0.08 ± 0.03 [b]
(Z)-2-Nonenal	0.02 ± 0.01 [a]	0.06 ± 0.02 [b]	0.04 ± 0.02 [a,b]	0.02 ± 0.01 [a]	0.12 ± 0.04 [c]	0.03 ± 0.01 [a]
(E,E)-2,4-Nonadienal	0.12 ± 0.05 [c]	0.16 ± 0.06 [d]	0.11 ± 0.03 [b,c]	0.08 ± 0.02 [b]	0.03 ± 0.01 [a]	0.10 ± 0.03 [b,c]
(Z)-2-Decenal	0.03 ± 0.01 [a]	1.10 ± 0.04 [d]	0.17 ± 0.05 [c]	0.02 ± 0.01 [a]	0.04 ± 0.01 [a,b]	0.05 ± 0.02 [b]
Vanillin	0.06 ± 0.02	0.06 ± 0.02	0.07 ± 0.02	0.06 ± 0.02	0.06 ± 0.01	0.07 ± 0.03
Acids						
Pentanoic acid	0.02 ± 0.01 [a]	0.01 ± 0.01 [a]	0.02 ± 0.01 [a]	0.02 ± 0.01 [a]	0.06 ± 0.02 [b]	0.03 ± 0.01 [a]
Acetic acid	67.02 ± 0.12 [d]	77.90 ± 0.15 [f]	59.48 ± 0.11 [b]	64.68 ± 0.10 [c]	73.20 ± 0.13 [e]	55.54 ± 0.16 [a]
Phenylacetic acid	0.02 ± 0.01 [a]	0.32 ± 0.05 [c]	0.43 ± 0.04 [d]	0.10 ± 0.03 [b]	0.53 ± 0.07 [e]	0.50 ± 0.06 [e]
Furfurals						
2-Furfural	1.63 ± 0.04 [d]	0.05 ± 0.01 [a]	1.36 ± 0.09 [c]	0.11 ± 0.03 [b]	1.68 ± 0.07 [d]	1.79 ± 0.05 [e]
Pyrazines						
2,5-Dimethylpyrazine	7.60 ± 0.10 [c]	4.14 ± 0.09 [a]	8.67 ± 0.07 [e]	8.01 ± 0.08 [d]	6.28 ± 0.11 [b]	9.54 ± 0.14 [f]
Trimethylpyrazine	0.02 ± 0.01 [a]	0.06 ± 0.02 [b]	0.03 ± 0.01 [a]	0.04 ± 0.02 [a]	0.03 ± 0.01 [a]	0.03 ± 0.01 [a]
Tetramethylpyrazine	0.06 ± 0.02 [a]	0.25 + 0.06 [d]	0.09 ± 0.03 [b]	0.13 ± 0.04 [c]	0.06 ± 0.02 [a]	0.05 ± 0.02 [d]
Esters						
Ethyl octanoate	0.03 ± 0.01 [a]	0.08 ± 0.02 [b]	0.10 ± 0.03 [c]	0.12 ± 0.04 [c]	0.11 ± 0.03 [c]	0.11 ± 0.02 [c]
Phenylethylacetate	0.02 ± 0.01 [a]	0.49 ± 0.07 [d]	0.19 ± 0.05 [c]	0.02 ± 0.01 [a]	0.13 ± 0.03 [b]	0.17 ± 0.05 [c]
Lactones						
γ-Nonalactone	nd	0.16 ± 0.03 [a]	0.16 ± 0.05 [a]	0.21 ± 0.07 [b]	0.16 ± 0.05 [a]	0.15 ± 0.03 [a]
Sulfur Compounds						
Dimethyl trisulfide	0.08 ± 0.03 [a]	0.25 ± 0.06 [c]	0.15 ± 0.02 [b]	0.16 ± 0.03 [b]	0.15 ± 0.04 [b]	0.13 ± 0.02 [b]
	DCH98ESt					
Alcohols and Phenols						
2,3-Butanediol	0.29 ± 0.05 [a]	0.71 ± 0.06 [d]	0.53 ± 0.04 [b]	0.60 ± 0.03 [c]	0.51 ± 0.03 [b]	0.50 ± 0.04 [b]
2-Phenylethanol	0.06 ± 0.02 [b]	0.12 ± 0.03 [c]	0.04 ± 0.02 [a]	0.06 ± 0.02 [b]	0.04 ± 0.01 [a]	0.03 ± 0.01 [a]
Aldehydes And Ketones						
2-Methylpropanal	2.78 ± 0.04 [b]	2.48 ± 0.04 [a]	4.14 ± 0.06 [d]	3.32 ± 0.04 [c]	3.31 ± 0.05 [c]	4.69 ± 0.05 [e]
Benzaldehyde	17.67 ± 0.11 [d]	12.12 ± 0.10 [a]	19.05 ± 0.09 [e]	16.93 ± 0.11 [c]	15.57 ± 0.12 [b]	21.59 ± 0.12 [f]
Butan-2-one	0.31 ± 0.02 [a]	0.46 ± 0.03 [c]	0.42 ± 0.04 [b]	0.48 ± 0.04 [c]	0.44 ± 0.05 [b,c]	0.39 ± 0.04 [b]
3-Methylbutanal	0.43 ± 0.03 [b]	0.59 ± 0.03 [d]	0.43 ± 0.03 [b]	0.61 ± 0.04 [d]	0.52 ± 0.05 [c]	0.35 ± 0.03 [a]
2,3-Pentanedione	1.48 ± 0.03 [c]	1.60 ± 0.04 [d]	0.98 ± 0.03 [b]	1.45 ± 0.04 [c]	0.93 ± 0.04 [a]	0.95 ± 0.04 [a,b]
Pentanal	1.59 ± 0.05 [d]	1.42 ± 0.04 [c]	0.24 ± 0.03 [b]	1.89 ± 0.05 [e]	0.18 ± 0.04 [a]	0.17 ± 0.03 [a]
(Z)-4-Heptenal	0.04 ± 0.01 [a]	0.08 ± 0.04 [b]	0.07 ± 0.04 [b]	0.04 ± 0.01 [a]	0.07 ± 0.04 [b]	0.07 ± 0.02 [b]
Octanal	0.02 ± 0.01 [a]	0.10 ± 0.02 [b]	0.01 ± 0.01 [a]	0.02 ± 0.01 [a]	0.01 ± 0.01 [a]	0.01 ± 0.01 [a]
Butanal	0.02 ± 0.01 [a]	0.08 ± 0.02 [b]	0.02 ± 0.01 [a]	0.03 ± 0.01 [a]	0.02 ± 0.01 [a]	0.01 ± 0.01 [a]
Nonan-2-one	0.02 ± 0.01 [a]	0.04 ± 0.01 [a]	0.08 ± 0.01 [b]	0.03 ± 0.01 [a]	0.08 ± 0.01 [b]	0.08 ± 0.02 [b]
(Z)-2-Nonenal	0.02 ± 0.01 [a]	0.04 ± 0.01 [a,b]	0.06 ± 0.01 [a]	0.03 ± 0.01 [a]	0.09 ± 0.02 [c]	0.05 ± 0.01 [a]
(E,E)-2,4-Nonadienal	0.03 ± 0.01 [a]	0.10 ± 0.03 [b]	0.08 ± 0.02 [b]	0.05 ± 0.02 [a]	0.05 ± 0.01 [a]	0.09 ± 0.01 [b]
(Z)-2-Decenal	0.04 ± 0.01 [a]	0.57 ± 0.05 [c]	0.09 ± 0.02 [b]	0.02 ± 0.01 [a]	0.07 ± 0.02 [b]	0.07 ± 0.02 [b]
Vanillin	0.06 ± 0.01	0.06 ± 0.01	0.07 ± 0.02	0.06 ± 0.02	0.06 ± 0.01	0.07 ± 0.01
Acids						
Pentanoic acid	0.02 ± 0.01 [a]	0.01 ± 0.01 [a]	0.04 ± 0.01 [a,b]	0.01 ± 0.01 [a]	0.05 ± 0.01 [b]	0.03 ± 0.01 [a]
Acetic acid	67.46 ± 0.14 [d]	72.69 ± 0.15 [e]	62.74 ± 0.17 [b]	66.08 ± 0.15 [c]	67.97 ± 0.17 [d]	59.14 ± 0.16 [a]
Phenylacetic acid	0.03 ± 0.01 [a]	0.17 ± 0.03 [b]	0.49 ± 0.04 [c]	0.07 ± 0.01 [b]	0.51 ± 0.06 [c]	0.49 ± 0.05 [c]
Furfurals						
2-Furfural	0.06 ± 0.01 [a]	0.05 ± 0.01 [a]	1.61 ± 0.06 [b]	0.08 ± 0.02 [a]	1.64 ± 0.05 [b]	1.70 ± 0.08 [c]
Pyrazines						
2,5-Dimethylpyrazine	7.38 ± 0.13 [b]	5.69 ± 0.12 [a]	8.16 ± 0.14 [d]	7.62 ± 0.12 [c]	7.22 ± 0.12 [b]	8.85 ± 0.13 [e]
Trimethylpyrazine	0.02 ± 0.01	0.04 ± 0.01	0.03 ± 0.01	0.03 ± 0.01	0.03 ± 0.01	0.03 ± 0.01
Tetramethylpyrazine	0.06 ± 0.01 [a]	0.15 ± 0.03 [c]	0.07 ± 0.02 [a]	0.09 ± 0.01 [a,b]	0.06 ± 0.01 [a]	0.06 ± 0.01 [a]

Table 4. Cont.

Volatile Compounds	Functional Enrichment					
	CONT	BLUB	RASB	BLCB	POME	BEET
Esters						
Ethyl octanoate	0.02 ± 0.01 [a]	0.05 ± 0.01 [b]	0.11 ± 0.03 [c]	0.07 ± 0.01 [b]	0.11 ± 0.02 [c]	0.11 ± 0.01 [c]
Phenylethylacetate	0.03 ± 0.01 [a]	0.26 ± 0.07 [c]	0.16 ± 0.03 [b]	0.02 ± 0.01 [a]	0.15 ± 0.03 [b]	0.17 ± 0.04 [b]
Lactones						
γ-Nonalactone	nd	0.15 ± 0.02	0.16 ± 0.03	0.18 ± 0.04	0.16 ± 0.03	0.15 ± 0.03
Sulfur Compounds						
Dimethyl trisulfide	0.07 ± 0.02 [a]	0.16 ± 0.03 [b]	0.14 ± 0.03 [b]	0.12 ± 0.02 [b]	0.15 ± 0.03 [b]	0.14 ± 0.02 [b]
MCH						
Alcohols and Phenols						
2,3-Butanediol	0.29 ± 0.03 [a]	0.79 ± 0.06 [e]	0.53 ± 0.06 [d]	0.58 ± 0.08 [d]	0.36 ± 0.04 [b]	0.41 ± 0.03 [c]
2-Phenylethanol	0.03 ± 0.01 [a]	0.10 ± 0.02 [b]	0.05 ± 0.01 [a]	0.04 ± 0.01 [a]	0.03 ± 0.01 [a]	0.03 ± 0.01 [a]
Aldehydes and Ketones						
2-Methylpropanal	3.42 ± 0.07 [b]	2.83 ± 0.05 [a]	4.37 ± 0.07 [c]	3.41 ± 0.06 [b]	3.10 ± 0.04 [b]	4.63 ± 0.07 [d]
Benzaldehyde	17.96 ± 0.10 [c]	11.88 ± 0.08 [a]	20.20 ± 0.12 [d]	16.08 ± 0.11 [b]	16.00 ± 0.09 [b]	22.07 ± 0.10 [e]
Butan-2-one	0.45 ± 0.04 [b]	0.55 ± 0.05 [c]	0.43 ± 0.05 [b]	0.53 ± 0.06 [c]	0.45 ± 0.04 [b]	0.39 ± 0.03 [a]
3-Methylbutanal	0.69 ± 0.05 [c,d]	0.72 ± 0.06 [d]	0.47 ± 0.05 [b]	0.71 ± 0.07 [d]	0.66 ± 0.07 [c]	0.41 ± 0.05 [a]
2,3-Pentanedione	1.22 ± 0.06 [c]	1.40 ± 0.07 [d]	1.13 ± 0.06 [b]	1.24 ± 0.07 [c]	1.11 ± 0.06 [b]	1.04 ± 0.05 [a]
Pentanal	0.30 ± 0.02 [c]	1.03 ± 0.05 [e]	0.45 ± 0.03 [d]	1.02 ± 0.06 [e]	0.24 ± 0.03 [b]	0.16 ± 0.03 [a]
(Z)-4-Heptenal	0.11 ± 0.03 [b]	0.09 ± 0.03 [a]	0.08 ± 0.02 [a]	0.07 ± 0.04 [a]	0.09 ± 0.03 [a]	0.08 ± 0.02 [a]
Octanal	0.02 ± 0.01 [a]	0.08 ± 0.04 [b]	0.02 ± 0.01 [a]	0.02 ± 0.01 [a]	0.01 ± 0.01 [a]	0.01 ± 0.01 [a]
Butanal	0.03 ± 0.01 [a]	0.07 ± 0.04 [b]	0.02 ± 0.01 [a]	0.03 ± 0.01 [a]	0.03 ± 0.01 [a]	0.01 ± 0.01 [a]
Nonan-2-one	0.06 ± 0.03	0.06 ± 0.03	0.07 ± 0.03	0.06 ± 0.04	0.07 ± 0.04	0.07 ± 0.03
(Z)-2-Nonenal	0.11 ± 0.04 [c]	0.08 ± 0.03 [a,b]	0.06 ± 0.03 [a]	0.08 ± 0.04 [a,b]	0.11 ± 0.04 [c]	0.06 ± 0.03 [a]
(E,E)-2,4-Nonadienal	0.02 ± 0.01 [a]	0.09 ± 0.04 [b]	0.08 ± 0.03 [b]	0.04 ± 0.01 [a]	0.02 ± 0.01 [a]	0.07 ± 0.03 [b]
(Z)-2-Decenal	0.15 ± 0.05 [b]	0.48 ± 0.07 [c]	0.17 ± 0.04 [b]	0.07 ± 0.02 [a]	0.11 ± 0.06 [a]	0.08 ± 0.03 [a]
Vanillin	0.06 ± 0.02	0.06 ± 0.02	0.07 ± 0.04	0.06 ± 0.04	0.06 ± 0.03	0.07 ± 0.04
Acids						
Pentanoic acid	0.05 ± 0.01	0.03 ± 0.01	0.03 ± 0.01	0.04 ± 0.02	0.05 ± 0.03	0.04 ± 0.02
Acetic acid	64.84 ± 0.17 [b]	71.71 ± 0.19 [e]	60.82 ± 0.15 [a]	66.45 ± 0.16 [c]	67.64 ± 0.15 [d]	58.64 ± 0.12 [a]
Phenylacetic acid	0.15 ± 0.04 [a]	0.29 ± 0.04 [c]	0.36 ± 0.05 [b]	0.21 ± 0.04 [b]	0.28 ± 0.04 [c]	0.38 ± 0.05 [b]
Furfurals						
2-Furfural	1.93 ± 0.08 [e]	0.76 ± 0.07 [a]	1.51 ± 0.08 [c]	1.15 ± 0.07 [b]	1.85 ± 0.09 [d]	1.84 ± 0.04 [d]
Pyrazines						
2,5-Dimethylpyrazine	7.44 ± 0.12 [c]	6.00 ± 0.11 [a]	8.37 ± 0.11 [d]	7.44 ± 0.10 [c]	7.06 ± 0.09 [b]	8.83 ± 0.12 [e]
Trimethylpyrazine	0.02 ± 0.01	0.03 ± 0.01	0.03 ± 0.01	0.03 ± 0.01	0.02 ± 0.01	0.02 ± 0.01
Tetramethylpyrazine	0.06 ± 0.01 [a]	0.16 ± 0.03 [b]	0.08 ± 0.01 [a]	0.08 ± 0.02 [a]	0.06 ± 0.02 [a]	0.05 ± 0.01 [a]
Esters						
Ethyl octanoate	0.03 ± 0.01	0.08 ± 0.01 [b]	0.08 ± 0.02 [b]	0.08 ± 0.02 [b]	0.05 ± 0.01 [a]	0.08 ± 0.01 [b]
Phenylethylacetate	0.49 ± 0.05 [d]	0.32 ± 0.04 [b,c]	0.26 ± 0.04 [b]	0.22 ± 0.04 [a]	0.37 ± 0.05 [c]	0.28 ± 0.04 [b]
Lactones						
γ-Nonalactone	nd	0.14 ± 0.03 [b]	0.12 ± 0.02 [b]	0.12 ± 0.01 [b]	0.05 ± 0.01 [a]	0.11 ± 0.02 [b]
Sulfur Compounds						
Dimethyl trisulfide	0.08 ± 0.01 [a]	0.18 ± 0.02 [c]	0.13 ± 0.03 [b]	0.13 ± 0.02 [b]	0.10 ± 0.01 [a,b]	0.12 ± 0.02 [b]

nd—not detected. Blueberries (BLUB), raspberries (RASB), blackberries (BLCB), pomegranates pomace (POME), beetroots (BEET), control (CONT). Data are expressed as the relative peak area (in percentage) of each compound and presented as mean ± SD of three replications. The values followed by the same lowercase letter (a–f) within each chocolate type in the same row do not differ significantly according to Tukey's HSD test at $p < 0.05$.

The presence of pyrazines, aldehydes and furfural was attributed to Maillard reactions. Among the aldehydes characteristic of the Strecker degradation, which is one of the main stages of the Maillard reaction, 3-methylbutanal, 2-methylpropanal and dimethyl disulfide derived from the decomposition of leucine, valine, and methionine, respectively, were determined. 3-Methylbutanal and 2-methylpropanal are very important compounds that have a positive effect on the development of the characteristic chocolate aroma of cocoa products [47–50].

The principal component analysis (PCA) showed that dark and milk chocolates made with the addition of different functional additives are markedly different in terms of their VCs and thus clustered separately (Figure 2).

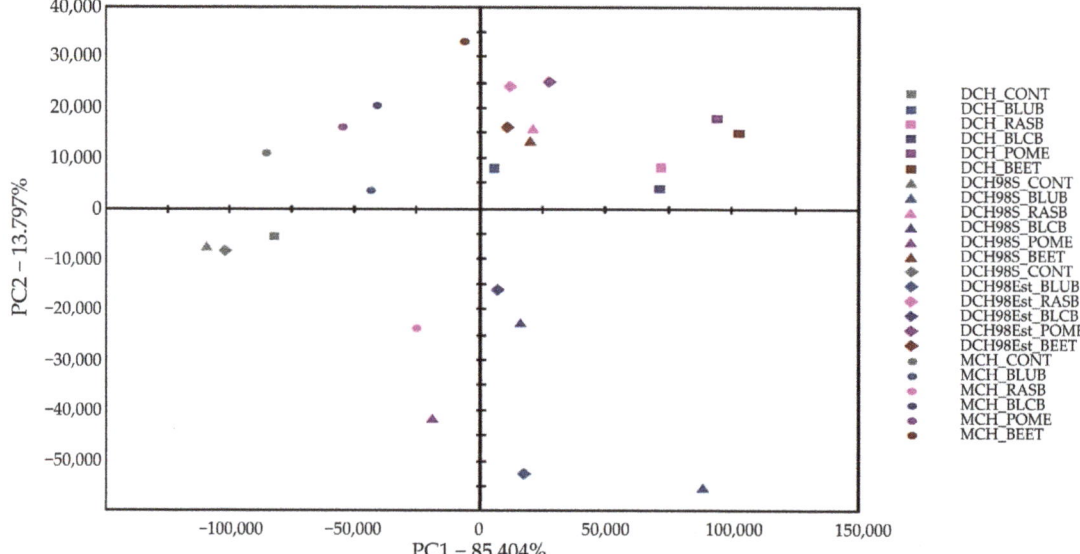

Figure 2. Principal component analysis (PCA) scores plot of aroma signals of different types of chocolate enriched with different freeze-dried phenolic-rich plant powders: DCH (**square**), DCH98S (**triangle**), DCH98ESt (**diamond**) and MCH (**dot**). Blueberries (BLUB—blue), raspberries (RASB—pink), blackberries (BLCB—dark blue), pomegranates pomace (POME—violet), beetroots (BEET—dark red), control (CONT—gray).

It is clear that each type of chocolate enriched with various functional additives was clearly distinguished by PC1 into two clusters, which suggested that the substitution of sweetener by 1% of fruit or vegetable powder resulted in the majority of the variance in the VCs composition compared to the corresponding control chocolate. It was demonstrated that almost all enriched chocolates could be distinguished from the control chocolates due to the abundance of some aldehydes, ketones, alcohols and acetic acid contents and the emergence of γ-nonalactone, which was not present in the control chocolates. In all chocolates enriched with berries, pomegranates pomace and beetroot powders the same classes of VCs were observed which were identified in control chocolates, in addition to γ-nonalactone. From the detected VCs, mainly 3-methylbutanal, phenylethylacetate, 2-phenylethanol, 2,5-dimethylpyrazine, 2,3-butanediol were positively correlated with chocolate aroma. However, the presence of benzaldehyde and pentanal with bitter and pungent notes origin from lipid oxidation was negatively correlated with chocolate flavor quality [47–49].

3-Methylbutanal produce key cocoa aromas such as malty and chocolate notes. Phenylethylacetate and 2-phenylethanol confer pleasant flowery and honey flavor notes enhancing flavor impression. 2,3-Butanediol, with the natural odor of cocoa butter, has been considered an important compound that could alter the overall aroma of chocolate [47–49].

Generally, the concentration of 2,3-pentanedione, γ-nonalactone and dimethyl trisulfide benzaldehyde, pentanal was significantly increased by the addition of fruit or vegetable powder. As demonstrated in Table 4, significant differences ($p < 0.05$) in the content of acetic acid were found between chocolates with different functional additives. The results showed that, depending on the functional ingredient type, a substantial change in the content of acetic acid was observed in all samples. Interestingly, all chocolates supplemented with RASB and BEET powder contained significantly lower amounts of acetic acid while those enriched with BLUB and POME powder had higher amounts of acetic acid than control chocolates. Independent of chocolate type, chocolates supplemented with BLUB and POME powders showed the highest content of acetic acid, while those enriched with

RASB and BEET powders exhibited the highest content of benzaldehyde. On the other hand, the concentrations of 3-methylbutanal were higher in the control than in almost all enriched chocolates, mainly those made with BLUB or POME powder. Nevertheless, almost all of the enriched chocolates showed higher levels of alcohols, such as 2-phenylethanol and 2,3-butanediol, which are desirable to obtain cocoa products with flowery and honey aromas [49]. Thus, chocolates made with the addition of berries, pomegranates pomace and beetroot powders may have a good consumer acceptability when compared to control dark and milk chocolates.

3. Materials and Methods

3.1. Materials

The research materials were chocolates supplemented with lyophilized fruits and vegetables rich in flavonoids, including anthocyanins and phenolic acids. Chocolates were obtained from the following raw materials: Cocoa liquor (with 55% w/w of fat) and butter were purchased from Barry Callebaut (Łódź, Poland). Sugar, alkalized cocoa powder (with 10% w/w of fat), skimmed milk powder (with 1.5% w/w of fat), soy lecithin, polyglycerol polyricinoleate—PGPR emulsifier and ethyl vanillin were obtained from WIEPOL Zakład Pracy Chronionej Ireneusz Wielimborek (Sierpc, Poland). Erythritol with the addition of stevia (99% erythritol and 1% stevia) was purchased from Domos Polska Sp. z o.o. (Czosnów, Polska). Plants, such as blueberries (BLUB), raspberries (RASB), blackberries (BLCB), pomegranates (POME), and beetroots (BEET) were bought on the local market.

3.2. Chemicals and Reagents

Standards of catechin (Cat), epicatechin (ECat), procyanidin B2 (PC B2), procyanidin C1 (PC C1), gallic acid (GA), protocatechuic acid (PA), p-hydroxybenzoic acid (p-HBA), cyanidin-3-O-glucoside (Cy-3-Glu), 6-hydroxy-2,5,7,8-tetramethylchroman-2-carboxylic acid (Trolox), 2,2′-azino-bis (3-ethylbenzothiazoline-6-sulfonic acid) diammonium salt (ABTS), 2,2-diphenyl-1-(2,4,6-trinitrophenyl) hydrazyl (DPPH), 2,4,6-tri(2-pyridyl)-s-triazine (TPTZ), sodium acetate, ferric chloride hexahydrate, ferrozine, and ammonium acetate were purchased from Sigma-Aldrich (St. Louis, MO, USA). HPLC grade methyl tert-butyl ether (MTBE) and methanol were purchased from J.T. Baker (Deventer, The Netherlands). All other reagents were of analytical grade and were purchased from Chempur (Piekary Śląskie, Poland). Chromacol PTFE syringe filters (0.2 μm pore size) were purchased from Shim-Pol (Izabelin, Poland). Ultrapure water (resistivity 18.2 MΩ cm), obtained from a Milli-Q purification system (Millipore, Bedford, MA, USA), was used for all analyses.

3.3. Lyophilization of Fruits and Vegetables

Plant materials, i.e., pomegranates pomace, whole berries and beetroots cut into cubes, were frozen at −80 °C for 48 h. Then they were freeze-dried in a BETTA2-8LSC plus Christ freeze drier (Osterode am Harz, Germany) for 24 h. The initial parameters of the process were—pressure: 1 millibar, shelf temperature: 5 °C, while final parameters—pressure: 0.1 millibar, shelf temperature: 5 °C. The obtained freeze-dried products were then ground to a fine powder in an XB-9103 MPM PRODUCT knife mill (Milanówek, Poland) and stored in glass containers.

3.4. Preparation of Chocolates

Four types of chocolate with 1% addition of fruit or vegetable powders were prepared during the study: dark chocolate 53% (~53% cocoa) with the total fat content of 35% (w/w) and sweetened with sucrose (DCH), dark chocolate 98% (~98% cocoa) with the total fat content of 51% (w/w) sweetened with sucrose (DCH98S), dark chocolate 98% (~98% cocoa) with the total fat content of 51% (w/w) sweetened with erythritol with stevia (DCH98ESt), milk chocolate (~40% cocoa, 20% skimmed milk powder) with the total fat content of 36% (w/w) and sweetened with sucrose (MCH). Recipes of chocolates are given in Table 5.

Table 5. Recipes of examined chocolates.

Raw Material	Content (%)							
	Control DCH	DCH	Control DCH98S	DCH98S	Control DCH98ESt	DCH98ESt	Control MCH	MCH
Cocoa liquor	40.00	40.00	92.00	92.00	92.00	92.00	20.00	20.00
Milk powder	-	-	-	-	-	-	20.00	20.00
Cocoa butter	13.40	13.40	0.80	0.80	0.80	0.80	19.80	19.80
Alkalized cocoa powder	-	-	5.00	5.00	5.00	5.00	-	-
Lecithin	0.50	0.50	0.50	0.50	0.50	0.50	0.50	0.50
PGPR	0.50	0.50	0.50	0.50	0.50	0.50	0.50	0.50
Ethyl vanillin	0.01	0.01	0.01	0.01	0.01	0.01	0.01	0.01
Sugar (sucrose)	45.59	44.59	1.19	0.19	-	-	39.19	38.19
Erythritol+stevia	-	-	-	-	1.19	0.19	-	-
Lyophilizate of fruits or vegetables	-	1.00	-	1.00	-	1.00	-	1.00

DCH—dark chocolate with 53% cocoa content sweetened with sucrose, DCH98S—dark chocolate with 98% cocoa content sweetened with sucrose, DCH98ESt—dark chocolate with 98% cocoa content sweetened with erythritol with stevia, MCH—milk chocolate with 40% cocoa content sweetened with sucrose.

Furthermore, control chocolates were obtained in which an additional portion of the sweetener was added to the chocolates instead of the freeze-dried fruits or vegetables. For example, in the DCH, the sucrose percentage was then 45.59% instead of 44.59%.

The preparation process of chocolates consisted of the following basic stages: grinding in the ball mill type M-5 (Promet, Łódź, Poland; loading up to 6 kg), conching in the K-5 type conch (Promet, Łódź, Poland; loading up to 6 kg), tempering in the temperer model T8 type Temperatrice containing a closed cooling system with an additional AC current heat exchanger (Pomati Group Srl, Zona Ind. Mirandolina, Italy; loading up to 8 kg), moulding, cooling and wrapping.

The cocoa butter, liquor and eventually cocoa powder were liquefied in the preheated to 70 °C ball mill. Next, sugar, milk powder (in the case of MCH) and 50% of the amount of lecithin were dosed into the ball mill. The grinding was carried out at 70 °C for 50 min (DCH), at 85 °C for 90 min (DCH98S and DCH98ESt) or at 55 °C for 60 min (MCH) with a rotational velocity of 75 rpm to obtain a particle size in the range of 20–25 μm, which was measured using the micrometric screw NSK Digitrix-MARK II ELECTRONIC MICROMETER with the electronic readout of the results (Japan Micrometer MFG. Co., Ltd., Tokyo, Japan). After this time, the obtained cocoa mass was transferred to preheated to 50 °C conch for further homogenization and emulsification. Then, freeze-dried phenolic-rich plant powders were introduced into the conch. After 45 min of conching, ethyl vanillin, PGPR emulsifier and the remaining part of the lecithin were added to the mass, and then conching was continued for 15 min. Next, the mass was subjected to tempering. For this purpose, the temperature of the mass was lowered in the temperer from 50 to 32 °C in the case of dark chocolates and to 28 °C in the case of milk chocolate. These temperatures were maintained for 15 min. Finally, chocolate masses were poured to preheated to 30 °C (dark chocolates) or 27 °C (milk chocolate) forms, cooled to 18 °C in a cooling tunnel (Promet, Łódź, Poland), and removed from the forms. Chocolate bars were wrapped in aluminum foil and subjected to analysis. All chocolates were obtained in triplicate.

3.5. Water Content and Water Activity Determination

Water content was determined by drying the ground chocolate samples mixed with sand at 102–105 °C to constant weight [28].

The water activity of the chocolates was determined by using HYGROPALM AW1 meter (Rotronic, Helvetia, Switzerland) equipped with a digital probe AW-DIO [28].

3.6. Color Determination

The color was determined using a trichromatic reflection colorimeter Konica Minolta CR-400 with Spectra Magic NX 1.3 software (Konica Minolta Sensing INC., Osaka, Japan). The results were expressed in accordance with CIE L*a*b* system (D65 illuminant and 10° viewing angle) [51].

3.7. UHPLC-DAD-ESI–MS/MS Analysis of Phenolic Compounds

The phenolic compounds were extracted according to the method described by Żyżelewicz et al. (2018), with some modifications [28]. Briefly, the accurately weighed defatted chocolate samples were extracted 3 times in an orbital shaker at room temperature for 30 min at 150× g with a mixture of acetone/water/acetic acid (70/29.5/0.5, $v/v/v$). The mixture was centrifuged at 4000× g for 10 min and the supernatant from each extraction were combined and evaporated under a stream of nitrogen. The residues were dissolved in methanol and filtered through a 0.20 µm pore size PTFE syringe filters. Finally, the samples were analyzed for the content of phenolic compounds using a UHPLC+ Dionex UltiMate 3000 system equipped with a UV–Vis diode array detector (Thermo Fisher Scientific Inc., Waltham, MA, USA), and a Transcend™ TLX-2 multiplexed LC system equipped with Q-Exactive Orbitrap mass spectrometer (Thermo Scientific, Hudson, NH, USA) using a heated electrospray ionization (ESI) interface (HESI–II). Samples (10 µL) were injected on an Accucore™ C18 column (150 mm × 2.1 mm i.d., 2.6 µm; Thermo Fisher Scientific Inc., Waltham, MA, USA). The column temperature was set at 30 °C. The mobile phase and gradient program were used as previously described by Oracz, Nebesny and Żyżelewicz (2019), with some modifications [52]. The 2-phase solvent system used for phenolic compounds separation was composed of 0.1% formic acid in water as solvent A and 0.1% formic acid in acetonitrile as solvent B. The flow rate was 0.35 mL/min and the gradient was as follows: 0–8 min, 1–5% B; 8–15 min, 5–8% B; 15–20 min, 8–10% B; 20–25 min, 10–15% B; 25–35 min, 15–20% B; 35–40 min, 20–25% B; 40–50 min, 25–90% B; 50–53 min, 90% B; 53–58 min, 90–1% B. Finally, the initial conditions were held for 7 min for column re-equilibration and for 5 min as a re-equilibration step. UV–Vis detection was performed at 280 nm for flavan-3-ols and phenolic acids and at 520 nm for anthocyanins. Instrument control, data acquisition, and evaluation were conducted with Chromeleon 6.8 Chromatography Data System, Qexactive Tune 2.1, Aria 1.3.6, and Thermo Xcalibur 2.2 software, respectively. Phenolic compounds were identified by comparing their retention times, UV–Vis absorbance spectra, full scan mass spectra, and MS/MS fragmentation patterns with their corresponding standards analyzed under identical conditions and previous literature reports [53,54]. Quantification was carried out using an external standard method. The concentration of individual flavan-3-ols and phenolic acids was determined based on peak area and calibration curves derived from corresponding reference compounds. For the quantification of anthocyanins, the calibration curves of Cy-3-Glu were used. All measurements were conducted in triplicate and results were expressed as mg phenolic compound per 100 g chocolate dry mass (mg/100 g DM).

3.8. Free Radical Scavenging Assay

The free radical scavenging activity was determined using the DPPH assay [28]. The analytical samples were prepared using serial dilutions of chocolate extracts in methanol. For each sample, experiments were conducted in triplicate. Finally, the mean concentration of the test chocolate extracts at which the concentration of the DPPH free radicals was reduced by 50% (IC_{50}) was calculated.

3.9. Ferric Reducing Antioxidant Power Assay

The ferric reducing ability (FRAP) was evaluated using the method of Oracz and Żyżelewicz (2019) [55]. For each sample, experiments were conducted in triplicate. The results were expressed as μmol Trolox equivalents per gram of chocolate DM (μmol TE/g DM).

3.10. Electronic Nose Analysis of Tested Chocolates

Electronic nose (E-nose) analysis of volatile flavor compounds was carried out according to the method of Rottiers et al. (2019), with some modifications [50]. The E-nose analyses were performed using a commercial Heracles II electronic nose (Alpha MOS, Toulouse, France), equipped with an HS-100 autosampler, a sensor array unit, and 2 columns working in parallel mode: a non-polar column (MXT5: 5% diphenyl, 95% methylpolysiloxane, 10 m length and 180 lm diameter) and a slightly polar column (MXT1701: 14% cyanopropylphenyl, 86% methylpolysiloxane, 10 m length and 180 lm diameter). An accurately weighed 1.0 g chocolate sample was put into 20-mL screw vials sealed with a magnetic cap with polytetrafluorethylene-silicone septa and placed in the auto-sampler. The vials were incubated in a shaker oven for 20 min at 50 °C and shaken at 500 rpm. Next, a syringe sampled 1000 μL of the headspace and then injected it into the gas chromatograph with 2 flame ionization detectors. The thermal program started at 50 °C (held for 2 s) and increased up to 250 °C at 3 °C/s and held for 21 s. The total separation time was 100 s. The calibration of the apparatus was carried out using a solution of alkanes (from *n*-hexane to *n*-hexadecane). The retention times of *n*-alkanes were used to determine the Kovats indices and identify the volatile compounds using AromaChemBase software (Alpha MOS, Toulouse, France). Each sample was measured in triplicate. Instrument control, data acquisition, and evaluation were conducted with Alphasoft 14.2 and AroChembase (Alpha MOS, Toulouse, France) softwares. The principal component analysis (PCA) was performed using AlphaSoft software (Alpha MOS, Toulouse, France) to determine the dissimilarities among the same types of chocolates in terms of volatile components.

3.11. Organoleptic Evaluation of Chocolates

The organoleptic evaluation of chocolates was carried out according to Żyżelewicz et al. (2018) [28] in our specialist sensory analysis laboratory. The evaluation was made by ten panelists using a 5-point scale with the relevant significance coefficients, in which 5 points corresponded to the best quality and 1 point to the worst. The sensory attributes of the chocolates, i.e., appearance in the packet, shape, color, consistency (hardness, smoothness), conchoidal fracture, aroma, taste, and upper and lower surface glossiness were evaluated. Final assessments were presented on a 5-point scale, according to which 5 meant extremely desirable quality, 4 was desirable quality, 3 was tolerable quality, 2 represented dislike, and 1 was for a defective product.

3.12. Statistical Analysis

The results are presented as mean ± standard deviations of 3 replicates. The one-way analysis of variance (ANOVA) was used to determine if there were significant differences between the physicochemical properties, phenolic compounds and antioxidant activity observed in the control and enriched chocolate samples. Where effects of supplementation of anthocyanin-rich were significant, the means were compared with Tukey's HSD (Honestly Significant Difference) at $p < 0.05$, using the Statistica 13.0 software (StatSoft, Inc., Tulsa, OK, USA). The effects of the types of chocolates and different freeze-dried phenolic-rich plant powders and their interaction on phenolic content, antioxidant activity and volatile compounds content in chocolates were tested by means of two-way ANOVA.

4. Conclusions

The results of the present study revealed that the enrichment of dark and milk chocolates with berries, pomegranates pomace and beetroot powders caused an increase in the amount of phenolic compounds, including flavan-3-ols, anthocyanins and phenolic acids.

Chocolates enriched with BLUB powder were characterized by the highest total polyphenol content. Our findings were further supported by the enhanced free radical scavenging activity and reducing capacity of different types of chocolates supplemented with fruit or vegetable powders. All chocolates with the addition of BLUB and RASB powders obtained an extremely desirable assessment in the organoleptic evaluation. The analysis of aroma compounds (volatile compounds) with the use of an electronic nose showed that berries, pomegranates pomace and beetroot powders have been successfully added to produce both dark and milk chocolates with acceptable sensory quality.

The physicochemical and sensory analysis results indicated that up to 1% of tested freeze-dried phenolic-rich plant powders can be successfully added to produce milk and dark chocolates with increased contents of polyphenols and good sensory properties.

Supplementary Materials: The following are available online, Table S1: Two-way ANOVA analysis of physicochemical characteristic and organoleptic assessment of different types of chocolates enriched with various freeze-dried phenolic-rich plant powders; Table S2: Two-way ANOVA analysis of the content of individual phenolic compounds and antioxidant properties of different types of chocolates enriched with various freeze-dried phenolic-rich plant powders; Table S3: Two-way ANOVA analysis of the content of volatile compounds in different types of chocolates enriched with various freeze-dried phenolic-rich plant powders.

Author Contributions: Conceptualization, D.Ż. and J.O.; methodology, D.Ż. and J.O.; validation, D.Ż. and J.O.; formal analysis, D.Ż., J.O. and M.B.; investigation, D.Ż., J.O. and M.B.; resources, D.Ż., J.O. and E.K.; data curation, D.Ż. and J.O.; writing—original draft preparation, D.Ż., J.O. and K.K.-W.; writing—review and editing, D.Ż.; supervision, D.Ż.; project administration, D.Ż.; funding acquisition, D.Ż. All authors have read and agreed to the published version of the manuscript.

Funding: This research was funded by Lodz University of Technology, Institute of Food Technology and Analysis, grant number 501/5-54-1-2.

Institutional Review Board Statement: Not applicable.

Informed Consent Statement: Not applicable.

Data Availability Statement: All the data are included in the present study.

Conflicts of Interest: The authors declare no conflict of interest.

Abbreviations

BEET	beetroots
BLCB	blackberries
BLUB	blueberries
Cat	catechin
CONT	control chocolates without the addition of freeze-dried phenolic-rich plant powders
Cy-3-(6″-Mal-Glu)	cyanidin-3-(6″-malonyl)-glucoside
Cy-3,5-diGlu	cyanidin-3,5-O-diglucoside
Cy-3-Glu	cyanidin-3-O-glucoside
Cy-3-Rut	cyanidin-3-O-rutinoside
Cy-3-Xyl	cyanidin-3-O-xyloside
DCH	dark chocolate with 53% cocoa and the total fat content of 35% (w/w) sweetened with sucrose
DCH98Est	dark chocolate with 98% cocoa and the total fat content of 51% (w/w) sweetened with erythritol with stevia
DCH98S	dark chocolate with 98% cocoa and the total fat content of 51% (w/w) sweetened with sucrose
Del-3,5-diGlu	delphinidin-3,5-O-diglucoside
Del-3-Glu	delphinidin-3-O-glucoside
Ecat	epicatechin
GA	gallic acid

MCH	milk chocolate with the total fat content of 36% (w/w) sweetened with sucrose
PA	protocatechuic acid
PC B2	procyanidin B2
PC C1	procyanidin C1
PCA	principal component analysis
Pel-3,5-diGlu	pelargonidin-3,5-O-diglucoside
p-HBA	p-hydroxybenzoic acid
POME	pomegranates pomace
RASP	raspberries
VCs	volatile compounds

References

1. Xu, D.P.; Li, Y.; Meng, X.; Zhou, T.; Zhou, Y.; Zheng, J.; Zhang, J.J.; Li, H.B. Natural antioxidants in foods and medicinal plants: Extraction, assessment and resources. *Int. J. Mol. Sci.* **2017**, *18*, 96. [CrossRef]
2. Valls, J.; Millán, S.; Marti, M.P.; Borràs, E.; Arola, L. Advanced separation methods of food anthocyanins, isoflavones, and flavanols. *J. Chromatogr. A* **2009**, *1216*, 7143–7172. [CrossRef]
3. Li, Y.; Zhang, J.J.; Xu, D.P.; Zhou, T.; Zhou, Y.; Li, S.; Li, H. Bioactivities and health benefits of wild fruits. *Int. J. Mol. Sci.* **2016**, *17*, 1258. [CrossRef]
4. Minatel, I.O.; Borges, C.V.; Ferreira, M.I.; Gomez, H.A.G.; Chen, C.Y.O.; Lima, G.P.P. Phenolic Compounds: Functional properties, impact of processing and bioavailability. In *Phenolic Compounds—Biological Activity*; Soto-Hernandez, M., Palma-Tenango, M., del Rosario Garcia-Mateos, M., Eds.; IntechOpen: London, UK, 2017. [CrossRef]
5. Cienfuegos-Jovellanos, E.; Quiñones, M.M.; Muguerza, B.; Moulay, L.; Miguel, M.; Aleixandre, A. Antihypertensive effect of a polyphenol-rich cocoa powder industrially processed to preserve the original flavonoids of the cocoa beans. *J. Agric. Food Chem.* **2009**, *57*, 6156–6162. [CrossRef] [PubMed]
6. Arranz, S.; Valderas-Martinez, P.; Chiva-Blanch, G.; Casas, R.; Urpi-Sarda, M.; Lamuela-Raventos, R.M.; Estruch, R. Cardioprotective effects of cocoa: Clinical evidence from randomized clinical intervention trials in humans. *Mol. Nutr. Food Res.* **2013**, *57*, 936–947. [CrossRef] [PubMed]
7. Ioannone, F.; Di Mattia, C.D.; De Gregorio, M.; Sergi, M.; Serafini, M.; Sacchetti, G. Flavanols, proanthocyanidins and antioxidant activity changes during cocoa (*Theobroma cacao* L.) roasting as affected by temperature and time of processing. *Food Chem.* **2015**, *174*, 256–262. [CrossRef]
8. Fernández-Romero, E.; Chavez-Quintana, S.G.; Siche, R.; Castro-Alayo, E.M.; Cardenas-Toro, F.P. The kinetics of total phenolic content and monomeric flavan-3-ols during the roasting process of Criollo cocoa. *Antioxidants* **2020**, *9*, 146. [CrossRef] [PubMed]
9. Medeiros, N.D.; Marder, R.K.; Wohlenberg, M.F.; Funchal, C.; Dani, C. Total phenolic content and antioxidant activity of different types of chocolate, milk, semisweet, dark, and soy, in cerebral cortex, hippocampus, and cerebellum of wistar rats. *Biochem. Res. Int.* **2015**, *2015*, 294659. [CrossRef]
10. Wollgast, J.; Anklam, E. Review on polyphenols in *Theobroma cacao*: Changes in composition during the manufacture of chocolate and methodology for identification and quantification. *Food Res. Int.* **2000**, *33*, 423–447. [CrossRef]
11. Tomas-Barberan, F.A.; Cienfuegos-Jovellanos, E.; Marín, A.; Muguerza, B.; Gil-Izquierdo, A.; Cerda, B.; Zafrilla, P.; Morillas, J.; Mulero, J.; Ibarra, A.; et al. A new process to develop a cocoa powder with higher flavonoid monomer content and enhanced bioavailability in healthy humans. *J. Agric. Food Chem.* **2007**, *55*, 3926–3935. [CrossRef]
12. Aprotosoaie, A.C.; Miron, A.; Trifan, A.; Luca, V.S.; Costache, I.I. The cardiovascular effects of cocoa polyphenols—An overview. *Diseases* **2016**, *4*, 39. [CrossRef]
13. Andres-Lacueva, C.; Monagas, M.; Khan, N.; Izquierdo-Pulido, M.; Urpi-Sarda, M.; Permanyer, J.; Lamuela-Raventtos, R.M. Flavanol and flavonol contents of cocoa powder products: Influence of manufacturing process. *J. Agric. Food Chem.* **2008**, *56*, 3111–3117. [CrossRef] [PubMed]
14. Suazo, Y.; Davidov-Pardo, G.; Arozarena, I. Effect of fermentation and roasting on the phenolic concentration and antioxidant activity of cocoa from Nicaragua. *J. Food Qual.* **2014**, *37*, 50–56. [CrossRef]
15. Voigt, J.; Lieberei, R. Biochemistry of cocoa fermentation. In *Cocoa and Coffee Fermentation*; CRC Press: Boca Raton, FL, USA, 2014; pp. 193–227.
16. Oracz, J.; Żyżelewicz, D.; Nebesny, E. The content of polyphenolic compounds in cocoa beans (*Theobroma cacao* L.), depending on variety, growing region and processing operations: A review. *Crit. Rev. Food Sci. Nutr.* **2015**, *55*, 1176–1192. [CrossRef] [PubMed]
17. Counet, C.; Ouwerx, C.; Rosoux, D.; Collin, S. Relationship between procyanidin and flavor contents of cocoa liquors from different origins. *J. Agric. Food Chem.* **2004**, *52*, 6243–6249. [CrossRef]
18. Schinella, G.; Mosca, S.; Cienfuegos-Jovellanos, E.; Pasamar, M.A.; Muguerza, B.; Ramon, D.; Rios, J.L. Antioxidant properties of polyphenol-rich cocoa products industrially processed. *Food Res. Int.* **2010**, *43*, 1614–1623. [CrossRef]
19. Afoakwa, E. Roasting effects on phenolic content and free radical scavenging activities of pulp preconditioned and fermented (*Theobroma cacao*) beans. *Afr. J. Food Agric. Nutr. Dev.* **2015**, *15*, 9635–9650.

20. Teh, Q.T.M.; Tan, G.L.Y.; Loo, S.M.; Azhar, F.Z.; Menon, A.S.; Hii, C.L. The drying kinetics and polyphenol degradation of cocoa beans: Cocoa drying and polyphenol degradation. *J. Food Proc. Eng.* **2016**, *39*, 484–491. [CrossRef]
21. Sacchetti, G.; Ioannone, F.; De Gregorio, M.; Di Mattia, C.; Serafini, M.; Mastrocola, D. Non enzymatic browning during cocoa roasting as affected by processing time and temperature. *J. Food Eng.* **2016**, *169*, 44–52. [CrossRef]
22. Niemenak, N.; Rohsius, C.; Elwers, S.; Omokolo Ndoumou, D.; Lieberei, R. Comparative study of different cocoa (*Theobroma cacao* L.) clones in terms of their phenolics and anthocyanins contents. *J. Food Compost. Anal.* **2006**, *19*, 612–619. [CrossRef]
23. Jumnongpon, R.; Chaiseri, S.; Hongsprabhas, P.; Healy, J.P.; Meade, S.J.; Gerrard, J.A. Cocoa protein crosslinking using Maillard chemistry. *Food Chem.* **2012**, *134*, 375–380. [CrossRef]
24. Belščak, A.; Komes, D.; Horzic, D.; Kovacević Ganić, K.; Karlović, D. Comparative study of commercially available cocoa products in terms of their bioactive composition. *Food Res. Int.* **2009**, *42*, 707–716. [CrossRef]
25. Żyżelewicz, D.; Krysiak, W.; Oracz, J.; Sosnowska, D.; Budryn, G.; Nebesny, E. The influence of the roasting process conditions on the polyphenol content in cocoa beans, nibs and chocolates. *Food Res. Int.* **2016**, *89*, 918–929. [CrossRef]
26. Di Mattia, C.D.; Sacchetti, G.; Mastrocola, D.; Serafini, M. From cocoa to chocolate: The impact of processing on in vitro antioxidant activity and the effects of chocolate on antioxidant markers in vivo. *Front. Immunol.* **2017**, *8*, 1207. [CrossRef]
27. Mursu, J.; Voutilainen, S.; Nurmi, T.; Rissanen, T.H.; Virtanen, J.K.; Kaikkonen, J.; Nyyssönen, K.; Salonen, J.T. Dark chocolate consumption increases HDL cholesterol concentration and chocolate fatty acids may inhibit lipid peroxidation in healthy humans. *Free Radic. Biol. Med.* **2004**, *37*, 1351–1359. [CrossRef] [PubMed]
28. Żyżelewicz, D.; Budryn, G.; Oracz, J.; Antolak, H.; Kręgiel, D.; Kaczmarska, M. The effect on bioactive components and characteristics of chocolate by functionalization with raw cocoa beans. *Food Res. Int.* **2018**, *113*, 234–244. [CrossRef]
29. González-Barrio, R.; Nuñez-Gomez, V.; Cienfuegos-Jovellanos, E.; García-Alonso, F.J.; Periago-Castón, M.J. Improvement of the flavanol profile and the antioxidant capacity of chocolate using a phenolic rich cocoa powder. *Foods* **2020**, *9*, 189. [CrossRef] [PubMed]
30. Muhammad, D.M.; Saputro, A.D.; Rottiers, H.; Van de Walle, D.; Dewettinck, K. Physicochemical properties and antioxidant activities of chocolates enriched with engineered cinnamon nanoparticles. *Eur. Food Res. Tech.* **2018**, *244*, 1185–1202. [CrossRef]
31. Belščak-Cvitanović, A.; Komes, D.; Benković, M.; Karlović, S.; Hečimović, D.J.; Bauman, I. Innovative formulations of chocolates enriched with plant polyphenols from *Rubus idaeus* L. leaves and characterization of their physical, bioactive and sensory properties. *Food Res. Int.* **2012**, *48*, 820–830. [CrossRef]
32. Lončarević, I.; Pajin, B.; Tumbas Šaponjac, V.; Petrović, J.; Vulić, J.; Fišteš, A.; Jovanović, P. Physical, sensorial and bioactive characteristics of white chocolate with encapsulated green tea extract. *J. Sci. Food Agric.* **2019**, *99*, 5834–5841. [CrossRef]
33. Bolenz, S.; Glöde, L. Technological and nutritional aspects of milk chocolate enriched with grape pomace products. *Eur. Food Res. Tech.* **2021**, *247*, 623–636. [CrossRef]
34. Godočiková, L.; Ivanišová, E.; Noguera-Artiaga, L.; Carbonell-Barrachina, Á.A.; Kačániová, M. Biological activity, antioxidant capacity and volatile profile of enriched Slovak chocolates. *J. Sci. Food Agric.* **2019**, *58*, 283–293.
35. Khoo, H.E.; Azlan, A.; Tang, S.T.; Lim, S.M. Anthocyanidins and anthocyanins: Colored pigments as food, pharmaceutical ingredients, and the potential health benefits. *Food Nutr. Res.* **2017**, *61*, 1361779. [CrossRef] [PubMed]
36. Martín, J.; Kuskoski, E.M.; Navas, J.M.; Asuero, A.G. Antioxidant capacity of anthocyanin pigments. In *Flavonoids—From Biosynthesis to Human Health*; Justino, G.C., Ed.; IntechOpen: London, UK, 2017. [CrossRef]
37. European Council Directive 2000/36/EG Relating to Cocoa and Chocolate Products Intended for Human Consumption. *Off. J. Eur. Communities* **2000**, *L 197/19*. Available online: https://eur-lex.europa.eu/eli/dir/2000/36/oj (accessed on 3 October 2021).
38. Toker, O.S.; Zorlucan, F.T.; Konar, N.; Dağlıoglu, O.; Sagdic, O.; Sener, S. Investigating the effect of production process of ball mill refiner on some physical quality parameters of compound chocolate: Response surface methodology approach. *Int. J. Food Sci. Tech.* **2017**, *52*, 788–799. [CrossRef]
39. Miller, K.B.; Stuart, D.A.; Smith, N.L.; Lee, C.Y.; Mc Hale, N.L.; Flanagan, J.A.; Ou, B.; Hurst, W.J. Antioxidant activity and polyphenol and procyanidin contents of selected commercially available cocoa-containing and chocolate products in the United States. *J. Agric. Food Chem.* **2006**, *54*, 4062–4068. [CrossRef]
40. Todorovic, V.; Radojcic, I.; Todorovic, Z.; Jankovic, G.; Dodevska, M.; Sobajic, S. Polyphenols, methylxanthines, and antioxidant capacity of chocolates produced in Serbia. *J. Food Compost. Anal.* **2015**, *41*, 137–143. [CrossRef]
41. Godočiková, L.; Ivanišová, E.; Kačániová, M. The influence of fortification of dark chocolate with sea buckthorn and mulberry on the content of biologically active substances. *Adv. Res. Life Sci.* **2017**, *1*, 26–31. [CrossRef]
42. Martini, S.; Conte, A.; Tagliazucchi, D. Comprehensive evaluation of phenolic profile in dark chocolate and dark chocolate enriched with Sakura green tea leaves or turmeric powder. *Food Res. Int.* **2018**, *112*, 1–16. [CrossRef]
43. Batista, N.N.; de Andrade, D.P.; Ramos, C.L.; Dias, D.R.; Schwan, R.F. Antioxidant capacity of cocoa beans and chocolate assessed by FTIR. *Food Res. Int.* **2016**, *90*, 313–319. [CrossRef]
44. Nowicka, P.; Wojdyło, A. Bioactive compounds and sensory attributes of sour cherry puree sweetened with natural sweeteners. *Int. J. Food Sci. Technol.* **2015**, *50*, 585–591. [CrossRef]
45. Shalaby, E.A.; Mahmoud, G.I.; Shanab, S.M.M. Suggested mechanism for the effect of sweeteners on radical scavenging activity of phenolic compounds in black and green tea. *Front. Life Sci.* **2016**, *9*, 241–251. [CrossRef]

46. Belščak-Cvitanović, A.; Komes, D.; Dujmović, M.; Karlović, S.; Biškić, M.; Brnčić, M.; Ježek, D. Physical, bioactive and sensory quality parameters of reduced sugar chocolates formulated with natural sweeteners as sucrose alternatives. *Food Chem.* **2015**, *167*, 61–70. [CrossRef] [PubMed]
47. Bertazzo, A.; Comai, S.; Brunato, I.; Zancato, M.; Costa, C.V.L. The content of protein and non-protein (free and protein-bound) tryptophan in *Theobroma cacao* beans. *Food Chem.* **2011**, *124*, 93–96. [CrossRef]
48. Aprotosoaie, A.C.; Luca, S.V.; Miron, A. Flavor chemistry of cocoa and cocoa products—An overview. *Compr. Rev. Food Sci. Food Saf.* **2016**, *15*, 73–91. [CrossRef] [PubMed]
49. Rodriguez-Campos, J.; Escalona-Buendía, H.B.; Orozco-Avila, I.; Lugo-Cervantes, E.; Jaramillo-Flores, M.E. Dynamics of volatile and non-volatile compounds in cocoa (*Theobroma cacao* L.) during fermentation and drying processes using principal components analysis. *Food Res. Int.* **2011**, *44*, 250–258. [CrossRef]
50. Rottiers, H.; Sosa, D.A.T.; Van de Vyver, L.; Hinneh, M.; Everaert, H.; De Wever, J.; Messens, K.; Dewettinck, K. Discrimination of cocoa liquors based on their odor fingerprint: A fast GC electronic nose suitability study. *Food Anal. Methods* **2019**, *12*, 475–488. [CrossRef]
51. Żyżelewicz, D.; Krysiak, W.; Nebesny, E.; Budryn, G. Application of various methods for determination of the color of cocoa beans roasted under variable process parameters. *Eur. Food Res. Tech.* **2014**, *238*, 549–563. [CrossRef]
52. Oracz, J.; Nebesny, E.; Żyżelewicz, D. Identification and quantification of free and bound phenolic compounds contained in the high-molecular weight melanoidin fractions derived from two different types of cocoa beans by UHPLC-DAD-ESI-HR-MS^n. *Food Res. Int.* **2019**, *115*, 135–149. [CrossRef]
53. Fischer, U.A.; Carle, R.; Kammerer, D.R. Identification and quantification of phenolic compounds from pomegranate (*Punica granatum* L.) peel, mesocarp, aril and differently produced juices by HPLC-DAD-ESI/MS. *Food Chem.* **2011**, *127*, 807–821. [CrossRef]
54. Yang, H.; Kim, H.W.; Kwon, Y.S.; Kim, H.K.; Sung, S.H. Fast and simple discriminative analysis of anthocyanins-containing berries using LC/MS spectral data. *Phytochem. Anal.* **2017**, *28*, 416–423. [CrossRef]
55. Oracz, J.; Żyżelewicz, D. In vitro antioxidant activity and FTIR characterization of high-molecular weight melanoidin fractions from different types of cocoa beans. *Antioxidants* **2019**, *8*, 560. [CrossRef] [PubMed]

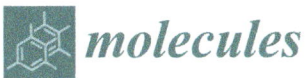

Article

Effect of Inoculated Lactic Acid Fermentation on the Fermentable Saccharides and Polyols, Polyphenols and Antioxidant Activity Changes in Wheat Sourdough

Ewa Pejcz [1,*], Sabina Lachowicz-Wiśniewska [1], Paulina Nowicka [2], Agata Wojciechowicz-Budzisz [1], Radosław Spychaj [1] and Zygmunt Gil [1]

[1] Department of Fermentation and Cereals Technology, Wrocław University of Environmental and Life Sciences, 51-630 Wrocław, Poland; sabina.lachowicz@upwr.edu.pl (S.L.-W.); agata.wojciechowicz-budzisz@upwr.edu.pl (A.W.-B.); radoslaw.spychaj@upwr.edu.pl (R.S.); zygmunt.gil@upwr.edu.pl (Z.G.)
[2] Department of Fruit, Vegetable and Nutraceutical Technology, Wrocław University of Environmental and Life Sciences, 51-630 Wrocław, Poland; paulina.nowicka@upwr.edu.pl
* Correspondence: ewa.pejcz@upwr.edu.pl

Abstract: Inoculation of sourdough allows the fermentation medium to be dominated by desired microorganisms, which enables determining the kinetics of the conversion of chemical compounds by individual microorganisms. This knowledge may allow the design of functional food products with health features dedicated to consumers with special needs. The aim of the study was to assess the dynamics of transformations of fermentable oligosaccharide, disaccharide, monosaccharide and polyol (FODMAP) compounds from wheat flour as well as their antioxidant activity during inoculated and spontaneous sourdough fermentation. The FODMAP content in grain products was determined by the fructan content with negligible amounts of sugars and polyols. To produce a low-FODMAP cereal product, the fermentation time is essential. The 72 h fermentation time of *L. plantarum*-inoculated sourdough reduced the FODMAP content by 91%. The sourdough fermentation time of at least 72 h also positively influenced the content of polyphenols and antioxidant activity, regardless of the type of fermentation. The inoculation of both *L. plantarum* and *L. casei* contributed to a similar degree to the reduction in FODMAP in sourdough compared to spontaneous fermentation.

Keywords: sourdough fermentation; inoculation; lactic acid bacteria; FODMAP; fructans; antioxidant activity

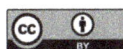

1. Introduction

Sourdough is traditionally prepared by mixing flour with water, and subjecting this mixture to a multi-stage spontaneous fermentation, which is carried out by exogenous flour microflora, including mainly 10^4–10^7 CFU/g of bacteria and yeast [1]. In order to shorten the technological process and increase its repeatability, it is an increasingly common practice to add starter cultures to sourdough. A group of lactic acid bacteria (LAB) plays a key role in these processes and has a long and safe history of use and consumption in fermented foods and beverages [2]. Another solution is to inoculate fermented products, including bakery sourdoughs, with pure cultures of bacteria or yeast proliferated to a desired number of colony-forming units [3,4]. Sourdough fermentation allows the fermentation medium to be dominated by desired microorganisms, which enables determining the kinetics of the conversion of chemical compounds of flour by individual microorganisms, and their targeted selection [5].

Cereal products make up a significant proportion of food consumed by the worldwide population. Wheat bread is considered a rich source of fermentable oligosaccharides, disaccharides, monosaccharides and polyols (FODMAPs) due to a high content of fructans, formed by the aggregation of fructose molecules. FODMAPs are easily fermentable, highly osmotic carbohydrates, including fructooligosaccharides (FOSs), galactooligosaccharides (GOSs), lactose, fructose and polyols (notably sorbitol and mannitol) [6–8].

The effect of FODMAPs on human health is determined by the amount of sugar delivered to the body within food. The appropriate intake of FODMAPs has a positive impact on human health because certain FODMAP sugars exhibit prebiotic effects [9,10]. The excess intake of FODMAP-rich products (above 20 g/day) can lead to sugar accumulation in the intestines, which in turn may induce various gastric ailments, which are acute in people suffering from irritable bowel syndrome [6,8].

Irritable bowel syndrome (IBS) is a gastrointestinal disorder that can appear in persons of various ages, genders and ethnical origins. It affects 4–20% of the population. Its typical symptoms usually appear after the intake of FODMAP-containing food products and include abdominal discomfort and stomachache, accompanied by flatulence, constipation or diarrhea [11,12]. Simple sugars and polyols exhibit a stronger osmotic effect, whereas saccharides such as fructans, FOSs and GOSs are more susceptible to fermentation by the intestinal microbiome [8,13].

Research has shown that FODMAP components trigger clinical symptoms in IBS patients [14–16]. One of the diets most often recommended by dietitians to help combat IBS symptoms is the low-FODMAP diet. Its principle is to reduce the intake of food products containing short-chain carbohydrates, which are rapidly absorbable in the human gastrointestinal tract [17]. In addtion, dietitians advise paying attention to the fructose:glucose ratio in consumed food products and recommend that their levels are similar or a higher glucose content. This can help improve the intestine's capability to absorb fructose [6]. Food products rich in these compounds include cereal products rich in fructans [11].

Fructans are not digested nor absorbed in the human digestive tract [6]. When ingested in small amounts, fructans have some health benefits but their excess can cause various ailments of the digestive tract [9]. The low-FODMAP dietary guidelines recommend substituting traditional bread with gluten-free products [11,14,18]. Wheat bakery products have significantly higher contents of protein, dietary fiber, minerals and vitamins than the gluten-free ones. Therefore, the exclusive consumption of gluten-free products can lead to deficiencies of these compounds in the body [19].

The FODMAP content in bread depends on both flour type and bread-making method [20]. The content in bread can be reduced in many ways, one of which is to use sourdough in the bread-making process. Another means is to appropriately select microorganisms responsible for the fermentation and degradation of sugars that trigger the gastrointestinal disorders [8]. In wheat bread, the above goal can also be achieved by extending fermentation time, which not only improves the flavor values of bread but also effectively decreases FODMAP content [20]. Fructans present in high quantities in cereal kernels can be degraded during sourdough fermentation. The consumption of sourdough bread has been proved to have a beneficial effect on mitigating irritable bowel syndrome symptoms [8]. In order to produce a low-FODMAP bread, LAB should also be added to the sourdough as they enhance the metabolic activity of fermenting flora. Apart from their capability to metabolize fructans, LAB can also convert free fructose to mannitol. In addition, they produce α-galactosidase, i.e., an enzyme responsible for breaking the bonds between the molecules of sugars constituting GOSs [8]. In turn, the enzymes capable of mannitol conversion are secreted by, e.g., *Lactobacillus delbrueckii*, *Lactobacillus casei*, *Lactobacillus plantarum* and *Lactobacillus salivarius* [7,21]. Bread produced with sourdough requires longer fermentation, which entails multiple changes in the carbohydrate composition. Microbial invertase rapidly degrades flour saccharose into glucose and fructose. Afterward, glucose is consumed as a source of energy, whereas fructose can be reduced by heterofermentative LAB to mannitol. All fermentable carbohydrates are rapidly depleted in the first hours of fermentation, whereas the carbohydrates featuring a high degree of polymerization (like fructans) are consumed later [8,22].

Sourdough fermentation used in bread making improves the nutritional value and antioxidative properties of bread, as well as its taste, aroma, texture and stability, and finally the bioaccessibility of its elements [23]. The antioxidant activity of the components of sourdough depends on the type of inoculum used for fermentation [24] and sourdough fermentation time [25]. The aim of the study was to assess the dynamics of transformations of FODMAP compounds from wheat flour as well as the antioxidant activity of nutrients of flour during inoculated and spontaneous sourdough fermentation.

2. Results and Discussion

2.1. Dynamics of pH Changes during Fermentation

Table 1 shows the results of the pH measurement of spontaneously fermented and lactobacilli-inoculated wheat sourdoughs. In each type of sourdough, the greatest decrease in pH was observed after the first 24 h of fermentation. During fermentation, LAB produce lactic acid, which results in a lower pH level [26]. In spontaneously fermenting and *L. casei*-inoculated sourdough after the first day of fermentation, pH remained at a similar level. A further slight decrease in pH was observed in *L. plantarum*-inoculated sourdough when the fermentation time was extended to 72 h. The study by Menezes et al. [8] also showed the greatest decrease in the pH level in the first hours of wheat dough fermentation, until relatively stable values were achieved after several stages. Fluctuations in the pH level affect the action of amylases. A study by Struyf et al. [27], showed that lowering the pH level has an effect on maltose release but has no effect on other saccharides.

Table 1. pH of wheat sourdough during fermentation.

Fermentation Time [h]/Sourdough Type	Spontaneous Fermentation	*Lactobacillus casei*	*Lactobacillus plantarum*
0	6.159 a	6.159 a	6.159 a
24	3.410 c	3.592 b	3.566 b
48	3.441 b	3.506 c	3.437 c
72	3.410 c	3.593 b	3.416 d

Values represent the means of four replicates. Mean values in columns with different letters are significantly different according to Duncan test at $p \leq 0.05$.

2.2. Dynamics of FODMAP Content Change during Fermentation

Changes in the FODMAP content in the sourdoughs during their fermentation are presented in Table 2. Fructans constituted the majority of these compounds in the tested samples. The content of fructans in the sourdough was influenced by the fermentation time and the type of LAB used. Each extension of the fermentation time resulted in a significant decrease in the content of fructans in the sourdough compared to the control, which was non-fermented sourdough. For each of the sourdough types, the content of fructans decreased with the fermentation time and reached the lowest values after 72 h of fermentation. A similar relationship between the extension of the fermentation time and the decrease in the content of fructans was observed by Struyf et al. [28], where after 1 h of fermentation, more than half of the fructans were degraded in the dough compared to the content of fructans present in the flour. In the study by Gélinas et al. [29], it was found that 20% of fructans were degraded after the dough-mixing process. Then, by fermenting the dough with yeast for 180 min, the fructan content was reduced by 82% compared to the amount of fructans present after mixing the dough. For fermentation lasting 24 h, the sourdough fermented with *L. plantarum* achieved the lowest content of fructans among the analyzed sourdoughs. However, in the case of 48 h and 72 h fermentation, the lowest fructan content was observed in sourdoughs inoculated with *L. casei*. Fraberger et al. [30] tested 13 strains of microorganisms for their ability to reduce fructans and found that the metabolism of microflora contributed to a significant reduction in the content of fructans in the dough compared to the control sample. Sourdough fermented with *L. casei* bacteria reached a lower content of fructans faster compared to sourdough fermented with *L. plantarum* and this could be due to the higher activity of *L. casei* enzymes than *L. plantarum* [7].

Table 2. The content of FODMAP components (g/100 g d.m.) in wheat sourdough.

Sourdough Type	Fermentation Time [h]	Fructan	Glucose	Fructose	Mannitol	Sum of FODMAPs
unfermented sourdough	0	1.15 a	0.00 e	nd	0.000 d	1.15 a
spontanous fermentation	24	0.42 b	0.06 c	nd	0.000 d	0.48 b
	48	0.28 d	0.08 b	nd	0.000 d	0.35 c
	72	0.18 e	0.00 e	nd	0.007 a	0.19 d
Lactobacillus casei	24	0.39 bc	0.20 a	nd	0.000 d	0.45 b
	48	0.11 ef	0.00 e	nd	0.006 b	0.12 de
	72	0.07 f	0.00 e	nd	0.002 c	0.08 e
Lactobacillus plantarum	24	0.31 cd	0.05 d	nd	0.000 d	0.36 c
	48	0.31 cd	0.05 d	nd	0.000 d	0.36 c
	72	0.10 ef	0.00 e	nd	0.000 d	0.10 de

Nd: not detected. Values represent the means of two replicates. Mean values in columns with different letters are significantly different according to Duncan test at $p \leq 0.05$.

The non-fermented sourdough control sample did not contain free glucose (Table 2). After 24 h of spontaneous fermentation, the glucose content was 0.06 g/100 g d.m., then after 48 h its value increased to 0.08 g/100 g d.m., and after 72 h it dropped back to 0. In the case of sourdough inoculated with *L. plantarum*, after 24 h and after 48 h of fermentation, the glucose content was 0.05 g/100 g, and after 72 h, its content in the sourdough decreased to 0. In the case of sourdough fermented with *L. casei*, the content of glucose increased to 0.2 g/100 g d.m. after 24 h of fermentation, and after both 48 and 72, its value dropped to 0. The glucose level in sourdough is determined by the content of damaged starch and the activity of β-amylase and amyloglucosidase [22]. It was also found that it is a factor blocking the transformations of, among others, sucrose, raffinose and mannitol. A fermentation time of 72 h led to a complete reduction of glucose in the sourdough. Further changes in glucose may result in the formation of CO_2, lactate, acetate and ethanol [7,21,27]. No fructose content was observed in any of the analyzed sourdough. It is consumed quickly and can also be converted into mannitol by lactobacilli [7].

The presence of mannitol was not found in any of the analyzed sourdough during the first 24 h of fermentation, because mannitol is formed from the degradation of fructose, which is transformed in the later stages of fermentation [31]. No mannitol was detected in the spontaneously fermented sourdough for 24 as well as 48 h, and after 72 h its value increased to 0.007 g/100 g d.m. In the sourdough with the addition of *L. casei* bacteria, after 48 h, the mannitol content was found at the level of 0.006 g/100 g of dry matter, and after 72 h, the content decreased to 0.002 g/100 g d.m. In sourdough fermented with *L. plantarum*, the level of mannitol remained at 0 during 72 h of fermentation. Gänzle [21] claims that the degradation of mannitol requires the enzymes of lactobacilli found, among others, in *L. casei* bacteria. In the spontaneously fermented sourdough, mannitol was present only after 72 h of fermentation, which results from the metabolism of fructose. It is converted into mannitol by lactobacilli, therefore in pure bacterial cultures fructose was degraded to mannitol faster than in the case of spontaneously fermenting sourdough. Mannitol metabolism, however, may be inhibited by the presence of glucose [7,21].

The total FODMAP content before fermentation was 1.153% d.m. and was determined by the fructan content of the flour. The FODMAP content of wheat is influenced by its variety. Ziegler et al. [20] studied the content of compounds from the FODMAP group in two wheat flour varieties and showed that it is from 1.24 ± 0.38 to 2.01 ± 0.42 g/100 g d.m. The fermentation of the flour always resulted in a significant decrease in the FODMAP content, but with a different effect depending on the type of sourdough used and its duration. In the spontaneously fermenting sourdough, the FODMAP content decreased with the extension of the fermentation time, and it reached the lowest value after 72 h. The FODMAP content in the spontaneously fermenting sourdough in the study by Menezes et al. [8] was

0.553 g/100 g d.m. and 0.603 g/100 g d.m. depending on various parameters of sourdough fermentation. A similar effect was observed in *L. casei*-inoculated sourdough, but with slight difference in FODMAP content after 48 and 72 h of fermentation. Sourdough fermentation with the addition of *L. plantarum* resulted in the lowest FODMAP content after 72 h and was constant after 24 and 48 h. In the study of Menezes et al. [8], it is claimed that the sourdough biotechnology requires a longer fermentation time than is usually used in bread making (0.5–3 h). Carbohydrates such as sucrose, maltose, glucose and fructose are depleted quickly during the first hours of fermentation, while higher-polymerized carbohydrates such as fructans are used later, so longer fermentation of sourdough will degrade all FODMAP components more efficiently. Comparing sourdoughs after 24 h of fermentation, the one with the addition of *L. plantarum* had the lowest content of FODMAP, while after 48 and 72 h of fermentation, the lowest FODMAP concentration was in sourdough with *L. casei*. Finally, after 72 h of fermentation with the addition of *L. casei*, the lowest FODMAP level of 0.076 g/100 g d.m. was achieved, which is a reduction of their content by 93%. It is important to select the microorganisms responsible for the fermentation of the sourdough. Appropriate LAB have enzymes that degrade FODMAP components, and they also have the ability to lower the pH of the environment, thanks to which the activity of the enzymes increases, which leads to a reduction in the FODMAP content. By lowering the FODMAP content in wheat bread, it is possible to reduce the symptoms of irritable bowel syndrome [7,8,30].

2.3. Dynamics of Polyphenolic Compounds and Antioxidant Activity Changes during Fermentation

The total content of polyphenols and the antioxidant activity of sourdoughs are presented in Table 3. The content of polyphenols in the sourdough was higher after each type of fermentation than before. However, the content of polyphenols in the analyzed material did not totally change. The matrix of the components of flour and sourdough was loosened during fermentation and water-extractable polyphenols were released. The fermentation process may increase the antioxidant activity by increasing the amount of easily extractable phenolic compounds [24]. Spontaneously fermenting sourdough reached the highest content of polyphenols after 24 h of fermentation, after which their amount remained on a similar level. *L. casei*-inoculated sourdough contained the highest amounts of polyphenols after 48 and 72 h of fermentation. The content of polyphenols in *L. plantarum*-inoculated sourdough increased significantly after 24 h of fermentation and then again after 72 h. Chiș et al. [32] observed an increase in the content of polyphenols with the fermentation time with the addition of *L. plantarum*, which is explained by their proteolytic activity's influence on the polyphenol profile. LAB can affect polyphenols, improving their solubility [33].

The antioxidant activity measured by both ABTS and FRAP methods of the spontaneously fermenting sourdough increased significantly after 24 h of fermentation and then after 72 h. In the study of Banu et al., 2010 [24], the addition of starter cultures containing *Lactobacillus rhamnosus* to the dough increased the antioxidant activity compared to spontaneous fermentation. In this study, the sourdough inoculated with *L. casei* showed a higher antioxidant activity against the ABTS radical after 24 h fermentation than before, and the highest value was achieved after 72 h of fermentation. A significant increase in the ability to reduce iron ions of this sourdough took place only after 72 h of fermentation. The antioxidant activity of *L. plantarum*-inoculated sourdough increased significantly after 72 h of fermentation. In the study of Banu et al. [24], antioxidant activity (measured with ABTS and DPPH methods) of 20 h spontaneously fermented dough was almost two times higher than before fermentation. Colosimo et al. [25] observed a significant increase in polyphenols and antioxidant activity with the fermentation time of the sourdough, which should last 72 h and preferably 96 h. In a study by Rodríguez et al. [34], *L. plantarum* was able to increase the antioxidant activity and improve the aroma profile of the product by degrading certain phenolic components through the metabolic activity of the LAB. The metabolic activity of LAB influences the levels of bioactive ingredients, which allows for an increase in antioxidant activity. During fermentation with their participation, antioxidant peptides are released, which increases the amount of phenols and antioxidant activity by acidification and hydrolysis of more complex and glycosylated forms [24,35]. Extending fermentation to 72 h resulted in an increase in the antioxidant activity of sourdoughs by 83 to 98% compared to the samples before fermentation, regardless of the type of sourdough fermentation. Sourdough fermentation can remove peptides associated with human intolerance to grain products. It can also lead to the production of bioactive peptides with antioxidant potential, which may affect the bioavailability of nutrients [25].

Table 3. The content of polyphenolic compounds and antioxidant activity of wheat sourdough.

Sourdough Type	Fermentation Time [h]	Polyphenolic Compounds [mg/100 g d.m.]	ABTS [mmol Trolox/100 g d.m.]	FRAP [mmol Trolox/100 g d.m.]
unfermented sourdough	0	208.30 c	1.95 c	0.96 c
spontaneous fermentation	24	273.74 ab	2.16 bc	1.36 b
	48	270.54 ab	2.18 bc	1.27 b
	72	262.35 b	3.88 a	1.80 a
Lactobacillus casei	24	263.13 b	2.48 bc	1.06 c
	48	270.65 ab	2.01 c	1.03 c
	72	295.96 ab	3.60 a	1.85 a
Lactobacillus plantarum	24	251.38 b	1.96 c	1.09 c
	48	260.07 b	1.91 c	1.11 c
	72	309.59 a	3.58 a	1.89 a

Values represent the means of three replicates. Mean values in columns with different letters are significantly different according to Duncan test at $p \leq 0.05$.

3. Materials and Methods

3.1. Material

Wheat flour type 650 was supplied from GoodMills (Stradunia, Poland). The flour particle size was 93 ± 0.3 μm, it had falling number of 390.5 ± 1.0 and contained $14.72 \pm 0.02\%$ protein (data not shown). Lyophilizates of two safe and well-described species of lactic acid bacteria: *Lactobacillus casei*, catalogue number 20,011 and *Lactobacillus plantarum*, catalogue number 20,174, were purchased from DSMZ—German Collection of Microorganisms and Cell Cultures (Leibniz, Germany).

Lactobacilli were grown in Man, Rogosa and Sharp medium (MRS) (Sigma-Aldrich, Hamburg, Germany) and incubated under aerobic conditions at 37 °C until the late exponential growth phase was reached (about 24 h). Cells were harvested by centrifugation at 10,000 rpm for 10 min at 4 °C. Dilutions were made in saline solution plated on MRS 273 agar, resulting in a concentration of about 10^9 CFU/mL.

The next multiplication of microorganisms took place by preparing a mixture of 100 g of flour, 300 mL of water and 20 mL of liquid microorganism culture (*L. casei* and *L. plantarum*). A mixture without the addition of bacteria was prepared based on the spontaneous fermentation of microorganisms found naturally in the flour. The fermentation lasted three days at 28 °C.

Sourdoughs were made from a combination of flour (500 g), water (500 mL) and the appropriate liquid sourdough prepared in the previous step (50 mL). The fermentation of sourdoughs was carried out for 24, 48 and 72 h at a temperature of 28 °C.

3.2. Methods

3.2.1. Dynamic of Fermentation

The pH of the sourdoughs was determined in four replicates after 24, 48 and 72 h of fermentation using the potentiometric method. The pH of the non-fermented sourdough was used as a control. The samples were frozen, freeze dried, ground and vacuum packed for further determinations.

3.2.2. Determination of Fructans

The content of fructans in the freeze-dried sourdough samples was determined using the fructan determination kit based on AOAC Method 999.03 [36], which is based on the determination of the fructose content in the samples resulting from the enzymatic breakdown of fructans. Using a spectrophotometer, the fructose content was measured at a wavelength of $\lambda = 410$ nm. The determination was performed in duplicate.

3.2.3. Determination of Sugar and Polyol Content by HPLC-ELSD

Preparation of samples for the determination of sugar and polyol content consisted of adding 10 g of the analyzed sample into a volumetric flask, filling the volumetric flask to 50 mL and boiling and shaking the samples in a boiling water bath for 20 min. Then, 100 mL of cooled samples was made up with distilled water, 10 mL of the extract was centrifuged (10,000 rpm, 10 min) and the samples were filtered on a Sep-Pak C-18.

The content of sugars and polyols was determined by the HPLC method coupled with a light scattering detector. A 40 µL sample was injected by an autosampler (L-7200) onto a Unison UK-Amino 3 µL (3 mm × 250 mm) column (Imtakt, Kyoto, Japan). Detection was performed using an evaporative light scattering detector (PL-ELS 1000) with the following input parameters: evaporator temperature $-80\ °C$; nebulizer temperature $-80\ °C$; nitrogen flow -1.2 SLM. The elution was performed at 30 $°C$ in an isocratic flow using 85% acetonitrile solution at a flow rate of 0.7 mL/min. FODMAP content was identified by comparing with standard HPLC area measurements. The measurements were performed in duplicate and the results were expressed in grams/100 g dry weight of the product. The sum of the FODMAPs was calculated from the fructan content and those identified in the samples: fructose, mannitol and glucose.

3.2.4. Determination of Polyphenolic Compounds and Antioxidant Activity

The extraction for the antioxidant capacity was conducted following a protocol described by Lachowicz et al. [37]. The total polyphenolic content of the sourdough samples was determined using the Folin–Ciocalteu spectrophotometric method [38]. The absorbance at 765 nm was measured after 1 h, using the UV-2401 PC spectrophotometer (Shimadzu, Kyoto, Japan). The results were expressed as mg of gallic acid equivalents (GAE) per 100 g of dry sourdough. Data were expressed as the mean value for three measurements. The ABTS and FRAP methods were carried out with the methods described by Re et al. [39] and Benzie and Strain [40]. The absorbance was measured at 734 nm and 593 nm using the UV-2401 PC spectrophotometer (Shimadzu, Kyoto, Japan). The results of antiradical capacity were expressed as Trolox equivalents in mmol per 100 g of dry sample. Data were expressed as the mean value for three measurements.

3.3. Statistic Analysis

The results were statistically analyzed with the Statistica 13.3 software package (StatSoft, Tulsa, OK, USA). One-way ANOVA at $p \leq 0.05$ was calculated and homogeneous groups according to the Duncan test were estimated.

4. Conclusions

The FODMAP content in grain products turned out to be determined by the fructan content with negligible amounts of sugars and polyols. To produce a low-FODMAP cereal product, the fermentation time is essential, and its extension to 72 h or more allows for a strong reduction in the content of these compounds. A sourdough fermentation time of at least 72 h also positively influences the content of polyphenols and antioxidant activity, regardless of the type of fermentation. The inoculation of both *L. plantarum* and *L. casei* contributed to a similar degree to the reduction of FODMAPs in sourdough compared to spontaneous fermentation. Knowledge of the processes that take place during the fermentation of inoculated sourdoughs may allow the production of food products designed according to the needs of consumers.

Author Contributions: Conceptualization, E.P. and Z.G.; methodology, E.P., S.L.-W. and P.N.; investigation, E.P., S.L.-W., P.N.; writing—original draft preparation, E.P.; writing—review and editing, R.S. and A.W.-B. All authors have read and agreed to the published version of the manuscript.

Funding: This research was funded by Wrocław University of Environmental and Life Sciences; grant name "Innovative scientist", grant number N060/0033/20.

Institutional Review Board Statement: Not applicable.

Informed Consent Statement: Not applicable.

Data Availability Statement: Results will be available from the corresponding author.

Acknowledgments: The authors thank Patrycja Jurczyk for contributing to the research.

Conflicts of Interest: The authors declare no conflict of interest.

Sample Availability: Sourdough lyophilisates are available from the authors upon reasonable request.

References

1. De Vuyst, L.; Neysens, P. The sourdough microflora: Biodiversity and metabolic interactions. *Trends Food Sci. Technol.* **2005**, *16*, 43–56. [CrossRef]
2. Marco, M.L.; Heeney, D.; Binda, S.; Cifelli, C.J.; Cotter, P.D.; Foligné, B.; Gänzle, M.; Kort, R.; Pasin, G.; Pihlanto, A.; et al. Health benefits of fermented foods: Microbiota and beyond. *Curr. Opin. Biotechnol.* **2017**, *44*, 94–102. [CrossRef] [PubMed]
3. Bertsch, A.; Roy, D.; LaPointe, G. Fermentation of Wheat Bran and Whey Permeate by Mono-Cultures of Lacticaseibacillus rhamnosus Strains and Co-culture with Yeast Enhances Bioactive Properties. *Front. Bioeng. Biotechnol.* **2020**, *8*, 956. [CrossRef]
4. Ferraz, R.; Hickmann Flores, S.; Frazzon, J.; CruzSilveira Thys, R. The Effect of co-Fermentation on Sourdough Breadmaking using Different Viable Cell Concentrations of Lactobacillus plantarum and Saccharomyces cerevisiae as Starter Cultures. *J. Culin. Sci. Technol.* **2019**, *19*, 1–17. [CrossRef]
5. Acín Albiac, M.; Di Cagno, R.; Filannino, P. How fructophilic lactic acid bacteria may reduce the FODMAPs content in wheat-derived baked goods: A proof of concept. *Microb. Cell* **2020**, *19*, 182. [CrossRef]
6. Gibson, P.R.; Shepherd, S.J. Evidence-based dietary management of functional gastrointestinal symptoms: The FODMAP approach. *J. Gastroenterol. Hepatol.* **2010**, *25*, 252–258. [CrossRef] [PubMed]
7. Loponen, J.; Gänzle, M.G. Use of Sourdough in Low FODMAP Baking. *Foods* **2018**, *7*, 96. [CrossRef]
8. Menezes, L.A.A.; Minervini, F.; Filannin, P.; Sardaro, M.L.S.; Gatti, M.; De Dea Lindner, J. Effects of Sourdough on FODMAPs in Bread and Potential Outcomes on Irritable Bowel Syndrome Patients and Healthy Subjects. *Front. Microbiol.* **2018**, *9*, 1–7. [CrossRef] [PubMed]
9. Whelan, K.; Abrahmsohn, O.; David, G.J.P.; Staudacher, H.; Irving, P.; Lomer, M.C.E.; Ellis, P.R. Fructan content of commonly consumed wheat, rye and gluten-free breads. *Int. J. Food Sci. Nutr.* **2011**, *62*, 498–503. [CrossRef]
10. Yan, Y.L.; Hu, Y.; Gänzle, M.G. Prebiotics, FODMAPs and dietary fibre-conflicting concepts in development of functional food products? *Curr. Opin. Food Sci.* **2018**, *20*, 30–37. [CrossRef]
11. El-Salhy, M.; Gundersen, D.; Hatlebakk, J.G.; Hausken, T. Diet and Irritable Bowel Syndrome, with a Focus on Appetite-Regulating Gut Hormones. In *Nutrition in the Prevention and Treatment of Abdominal Obesity*; Watson, R.R., Ed.; Academic Press: Amsterdam, The Netherlands, 2014; pp. 5–16.
12. Shah, S.L.; Lacy, B.E. Dietary Interventions and Irritable Bowel Syndrome: A Review of the Evidence. *Curr. Gastroenterol. Rep.* **2016**, *18*, 1–6. [CrossRef]
13. Biesiekierski, J.R.; Rosella, O.; Rose, R.; Liels, K.; Barrett, J.S.; Shepherd, S.J.; Gibson, P.R.; Muir, J.G. Quantification of fructans, galacto-oligosaccharides and other short-chain carbohydrates in processed grains and cereals. *J. Hum. Nutr. Diet.* **2011**, *24*, 154–176. [CrossRef]
14. Halmos, E.P.; Power, V.A.; Shepherd, S.J.; Gibson, P.R.; Muir, J.G. A Diet Low in FODMAPs Reduces Symptoms of Irritable Bowel Syndrome. *Gastroenterology* **2014**, *146*, 67–75. [CrossRef]
15. Shepherd, S.J.; Gibson, P.R. Fructose Malabsorption and Symptoms of Irritable Bowel Syndrome: Guidelines for Effective Dietary Management. *J. Am. Diet. Assoc.* **2006**, *106*, 1631–1639. [CrossRef]
16. Shepherd, S.J.; Lomer, M.C.E.; Gibson, P.R. Short-Chain Carbohydrates and Functional Gastrointestinal Disorders. *Am. J. Gastroenterol.* **2013**, *108*, 707–717. [CrossRef] [PubMed]
17. Mansueto, P.; Seidita, A.; D'Alcamo, A.; Carroccio, A. Role of FODMAPs in Patients with Irritable Bowel Syndrome: A Review. *Nutr. Clin. Pract.* **2015**, *30*, 665–682. [CrossRef]

18. El-Salhy, M.; Gundersen, D. Diet in irritable bowel syndrome. *Nutr. J.* **2015**, *14*, 1–11. [CrossRef] [PubMed]
19. Calderon de la Barca, A.M.; Mejia-Leon, M.E. Are Gluten-Free Foods Just for Patients with a Gluten-Related Disease? In *Celiac Disease and Non-Celiac*; Rodrigo, L., Ed.; IntechOpen: London, UK, 2017; pp. 59–72.
20. Ziegler, J.U.; Steiner, D.; Longin, C.F.H.; Würschum, T.; Schweiggert, R.M.; Carle, R. Wheat and the irritable bowel syndrome-FODMAP levels of modern and ancient species and their retention during bread making. *J. Funct. Foods* **2016**, *25*, 257–266. [CrossRef]
21. Gänzle, M.G. Lactic metabolism revisited: Metabolism of lactic acid bacteria in food fermentations and food biotechnology. *Curr. Opin. Food Sci.* **2015**, *2*, 106–117. [CrossRef]
22. Gänzle, M.G. Enzymatic and bacterial conversions during sourdough fermentation. *Food Microbiol.* **2014**, *37*, 2–10. [CrossRef]
23. Gänzle, M.G.; Vermeulen, N.; Vogel, R.F. Carbohydrate, peptide and lipid metabolism of lactic acid bacteria in sourdough. *Food Microbiol.* **2007**, *24*, 128–138. [CrossRef] [PubMed]
24. Banu, I.; Vasilean, I.; Aprodu, I. Effect of Lactic Fermentation on Antioxidant Capacity of Rye Sourdough and Bread. *Food Sci. Technol. Res.* **2010**, *16*, 571–576. [CrossRef]
25. Colosimo, R.; Gabriele, M.; Cifelli, M.; Longo, V.; Domenici, V.; Pucci, L. The effect of sourdough fermentation on Triticum dicoccum from Garfagnana: ^{1}H NMR characterization and analysis of the antioxidant activity. *Food Chem.* **2020**, *305*, 125510. [CrossRef]
26. Galle, S.; Arendt, E.K. Exopolysaccharides from sourdough lactic acid bacteria. *Food Sci. Nutr.* **2014**, *54*, 891–901. [CrossRef]
27. Struyf, N.; Laurent, J.; Lefevere, B.; Verspreet, J.; Verstrepen, K.J.; Courtin, C.M. Establishing the relative importance of damaged starch and fructan as sources of fermentable sugars in wheat flour and whole meal bread dough fermentations. *Food Chem.* **2017**, *218*, 89–98. [CrossRef]
28. Struyf, N.; Laurent, J.; Verspreet, J.; Verstrepen, K.J.; Courtin, C.M. *Saccharomyces cerevisiae* and *Kluyveromyces marxianus* co-cultures allow to reduce FODMAP levels in whole wheat bread. *J. Agric. Food Chem.* **2017**, *65*, 8704–8713. [CrossRef]
29. Gélinas, P.; McKinnon, C.; Gagnon, F. Fructans, water-soluble fibre and fermentable sugars in bread and pasta made with ancien and modern wheat. *Int. J. Food Sci. Technol.* **2016**, *51*, 555–564. [CrossRef]
30. Fraberger, V.; Call, L.M.; Domin, K.J.; D'Amico, S. Applicability of Yeast Fermentation to Reduce Fructans and Other FODMAPs. *Nutrients* **2018**, *10*, 1247. [CrossRef] [PubMed]
31. Wisselink, H.W.; Moers, A.P.; Mars, A.E.; Hoefnagel, M.H.; de Vos, W.M.; Hugenholtz, J. Overproduction of heterologous mannitol 1-phosphatase: A key factor for engineering mannitol production by Lactococcus lactis. *Appl. Environ. Microbiol.* **2005**, *71*, 1507–1514. [CrossRef]
32. Chiș, M.S.; Păucean, A.; Stan, L.; Mureșan, V.; Vlaic, R.A.; Man, S.; Biriș-Dorhoi, E.S.; Muste, S. *Lactobacillus plantarum* ATCC 8014 in quinoa sourdough adaptability and antioxidant potential. *Rom. Biotechnol. Lett.* **2018**, *23*, 13581–13591.
33. Curiel, A.; Curri, N.; Curiel, J.A.; Di Cagno, R.; Pontonio, E.; Cavoski, I.; Gobbetti, M.; Rizzello, C.G. Exploitation of Albanian wheat cultivars: Characterization of the flours and lactic acid bacteria microbiota and selection of starters for sourdough fermentation. *Food Microbiol.* **2014**, *44*, 96–107.
34. Rodríguez, H.; Curiel, J.A.; Landete, J.M.; De Las Rivas, B.; Felipe, F.L.; Gómezcordovés, C. Food phenolics and lactic acid bacteria. *Int. J. Food Microbiol.* **2009**, *132*, 79–90. [CrossRef] [PubMed]
35. Rizzello, C.G.; Lorusso, A.; Russo, V.; Pinto, D.; Marzani, B.; Gobbetti, M. Improving the antioxidant properties of quinoa flour through fermentation with selected autochthonous lactic acid bacteria. *Int. J. Food Microbiol.* **2017**, *241*, 252. [CrossRef] [PubMed]
36. McCleary, B.V.; Murphy, A.; Mugford, D.C. Measurement of total fructan in foods by enzymatic/spectrophotometric method: Collaborative study. *J AOAC Int.* **2000**, *83*, 356–364. [CrossRef] [PubMed]
37. Lachowicz, S.; Świeca, M.; Pejcz, E. Biological activity, phytochemical parameters, and potential bioaccessibility of wheat bread enriched with powder and microcapsules made from Saskatoon berry. *Food Chem.* **2021**, *338*. [CrossRef]
38. Prior, R.L.; Wu, X.; Schaich, K. Standardized methods for the determination of antioxidant capacity and phenolics in foods and dietary supplements. *J. Agric. Food Chem.* **2005**, *53*, 4290–4302. [CrossRef]
39. Re, R.; Pellegrini, N.; Proteggente, A.; Pannala, A.; Yang, M. Antioxidant activity applying an improved abts radical cation decolorization assay. *Free Radic. Biol. Med.* **1999**, *26*, 1231–1237. [CrossRef]
40. Benzie, I.F.F.; Strain, J.J. The ferric reducing Ability of plasma (FRAP) as a measure of "Antioxidant Power": The FRAP assay. *Anal. Biochem.* **1996**, *239*, 70–76. [CrossRef]

Article

The Effect of Brewing Process Parameters on Antioxidant Activity and Caffeine Content in Infusions of Roasted and Unroasted Arabica Coffee Beans Originated from Different Countries

Anna Muzykiewicz-Szymańska *, Anna Nowak, Daria Wira and Adam Klimowicz

Chair and Department of Cosmetic and Pharmaceutical Chemistry, Pomeranian Medical University in Szczecin, Powstańców Wielkopolskich Ave. 72, 70-111 Szczecin, Poland; anna.nowak@pum.edu.pl (A.N.); daria.wira@pum.edu.pl (D.W.); adam.klimowicz@pum.edu.pl (A.K.)
* Correspondence: anna.muzykiewicz@pum.edu.pl

Abstract: Coffee is one of the most often consumed beverages almost all over the world. The multiplicity of beans, as well as the methods and parameters used to brew, encourages the optimization of the brewing process. The study aimed to analyze the effect of roasting beans, the brewing technique, and its parameters (time and water temperature) on antioxidant activity (determined using several in vitro methods), total polyphenols, flavonoids, and caffeine content. The infusions of unroasted and roasted Arabica beans from Brazil, Colombia, India, Peru, and Rwanda were analyzed. In general, infusions prepared from roasted beans had higher antioxidant activity and the content of above-mentioned compounds. The hot brew method was used to obtain infusions with a higher antioxidant activity, while the cold brew with higher caffeine content. The phenolic compound content in infusions prepared using both techniques depended on the roasting process. Moreover, the bean's origin, roasting process, and brewing technique had a significant effect on the tested properties, in contrary to brewing time and water temperature (below and above 90 °C), which had less impact. The results confirm the importance of coffee brewing optimization.

Keywords: coffee Arabica; roasting process; brewing methods; antioxidant activity; polyphenols; flavonoids; caffeine; pH of infusions; tannins

1. Introduction

Coffee trees belong to the constantly green trees and shrubs of the Rubiaceae family [1]. The optimal conditions for the growth of different coffee varieties occur in so-called the Coffee Belt located in the intertropical areas [2]. Ninety-five percent of global production of Coffea Arabica and Coffea Robusta are used for consumption, especially Coffea Arabica due to its delicate and less bitter taste [3]. An annual production of green coffee beans is about nine million tons. Even though Ethiopia is the cradle of Coffea Arabica [4], Brazil is the greatest world coffee exporter [1]. Other major suppliers of coffee beans are South American countries (Colombia and Peru) as well as African and Asian, such as Rwanda, above-mentioned Ethiopia, and Vietnam, Indonesia, and India [4].

After harvesting, the coffee beans are selected, shelled, and roasted at 200–250 °C [5]. The desired aroma and flavor of coffee are related to the volatile and non-volatile compounds. Their content is affected by the selection of appropriate roasting parameters and the subsequent Maillard reaction, which additionally leads to a change of beans color as a result of the production of melanoidins [6]. There are many techniques of coffee brewing. Generally, they can be divided into high- and low-temperature processes. The most popular methods of hot coffee brewing are the Turkish technique, French press, Aeropress, espresso, and simple infusion method [7,8]. Turkish coffee preparation involves boiling a mixture of coffee with water. The brew cannot be filtered [8]. A simple infusion based on pouring the ground grains with hot water (~85–95 °C) and macerated for about 5 min [7,9]. During the preparation of espresso, the roast ground coffee is briefly pressurizing with hot water using a percolator to obtain a small concentrated cup of coffee. The pressure is one of the most important parameters of the coffee brewing process [10]. Aeropress created in 2005 by Adler is a device that uses pressure, overflow, and French press techniques. Hot water and the short brewing time (~2 min) are used to prepare infusions [7,9]. Methods of cold coffee extraction include direct and indirect immersion methods, dripping, and the French press [10]. To prepare cold brew coffee using the direct method, water at room temperature is applied, as in the cold drip case. Then, the ground coffee beans are immersed in a proper amount of water for at least 6–8 up to 24 h followed by filtration [11,12]. In the cold drip method, water at a temperature of 20–25 °C is slowly dripped onto coffee powder placed in the filter to obtain a relatively intensive coffee extract in the beaker. For this purpose, one drop of water is added usually every 5 or 10 s. Recently, a French press method, the so-called plunger pot, has gained interest. This technique uses the pot with the plunger, to which hot or cold water is poured inside [7,10]. It allows to get fresh unfiltered infusion immediately. French press coffee maker enables to depress the plunger to separate coarsely ground coffee beans from the liquid [13].

Many researchers confirmed the health-promoting properties of consuming coffee brew. The most important benefits are summarized in Table 1. In addition to the taste, coffee beans are a valuable source of bioactive compounds, whose profile depends on coffee species, thermal processing, cultivating conditions, and harvesting time [11,14]. Due to the content of antioxidants, as well as caffeine, the brews of coffee belong to the functional food sector [14]. The caffeine content in seeds ranges from 0.3% to 2.5% and is twice as high in Coffee Robusta as in Coffee Arabica [3,5]. Ground coffee brews are also rich in phenolic compounds, such as chlorogenic acid, hydroxycinnamic acids, and their derivatives such as caffeic and ferulic acids and alkaloids (mainly caffeine and small amounts of theobromine and theophylline), diterpenoid alcohols (cafestol and kahweol), carbohydrates, lipids, and volatile and heterocyclic compounds [5,15].

Table 1. Health-promoting effect of coffee infusions on the human body.

Area of Impact/Type of Dysfunction	Effect
The nervous system The central nervous system (CNS) - Alzheimer's disease - Parkinson's disease - Depression Peripheral nervous system - Sense organs	An adenosine receptor antagonist—caffeine stimulates the CNS, improves concentration and thought processes [16–19]. Coffee consumption improves the metabolism and uptake of the antiparkinsonian drugs, which reduces the latency to a motor response and reduces the risk of Parkinson's disease [16–18]. Caffeine stimulates the secretion of serotonin and dopamine and, in the proper dose, it can reduce the risk of depression [17]. The soluble and volatile infusion components provide aroma and flavor [17,18].
The gastrointestinal system	Caffeine stimulates gastric acid secretion by activating bitter taste receptors, what decreases the pH of the gastric juice. Low pH improves the solubility of weakly alkaline drugs as they form soluble salts [16].
Obesity and type II diabetes (metabolic disorders)	Chlorogenic acid and trigonelline significantly reduce blood glucose and insulin levels [17–19]. Cafestol increases insulin sensitivity in muscle cells [17–19]. Chlorogenic acid intensifies the adipose tissue decomposition, and caffeine inhibits the absorption of fatty acids in the intestinal lumen [17–19]. Infusions are characterized by a low calorific value [17].
The cardiovascular system	Antioxidants improve the bioavailability of nitric oxide in the vascular system and enhance the vascular endothelium [17–19].
Carcinogenesis	Components contained in coffee repair and protect DNA against oxidative damage, show anti-inflammatory activity, increase apoptosis of cancer cells, and cause tumor suppression [17–20].

Table 1. *Cont.*

Area of Impact/Type of Dysfunction	Effect
Large intestine	Coffee increases intestinal peristalsis, excretion of bile acids with the feces, and modifies the composition of the intestinal microbiota [19].
Breast cancer	Phytohormones in coffee increase the concentration of globulin, which binds sex hormones and reduces the absorption of testosterone and affects the level of luteal estrogens [17,20].
Ovarian cancer	Chlorogenic, caffeic acids, and caffeine show antiproliferative properties in ovarian cancer cells. Cytochrome P450 isozymes involved in caffeine metabolism may contribute to the development of ovarian cancer or reduce the risk of its occurrence [17,19].
Endometrial cancer (EC)	This effect of coffee is associated with the correlation between the prevalence of obesity and EC and with the increased sensitivity of cellular receptors to insulin [19].

There are many reports on the coffee brewing process, but most of them are focused on the assessment of selected parameters, such as the impact of the intensity of the roasting process, the thickness of the grinding, or the method of brewing. The present study aimed to evaluate several parameters of the coffee brewing process, such as the method of making infusions (cold and hot brew), water temperature (cold, below or above 90 °C), and brewing time (9 and 24 h as well as 4 and 10 min). The details of the various brewing methods are presented in Table 2. For this purpose, unroasted and roasted Arabica coffee beans, imported from various countries (Brazil, Colombia, India, Peru, and Rwanda), belonging to the world's largest suppliers of this raw material, were analyzed. The influence of these factors on the in vitro antioxidant activity of infusions as well as on the content of polyphenols, flavonoids, and caffeine was analyzed. The results show that the bean's origin, roasting process, and brewing technique had a significant effect on the tested properties. The factors such as the difference in brewing time and water temperature (below and above 90 °C) had less impact. The obtained results could extend our knowledge on the brewing process of the most frequently consumed beverage in the world to verify parameters affected the content of health-promoting biologically active compounds, especially antioxidants.

Table 2. Description of the brewing methods.

Signature	Description of the Brewing Methods
Cold brew	
CB, 9 h	The ground grains were poured over with boiled and cooled tap water at 23–25 °C and stored at +4 °C for 9 h.
CB, 24 h	The ground grains were poured over with boiled and cooled tap water at 23–25 °C and stored at +4 °C for 24 h.
Hot brew	
86 °C, 4′	The ground grains were poured over with boiled tap water at 84–86 °C and brewing for 4 min.
86 °C, 10′	The ground grains were poured over with boiled tap water at 84–86 °C and brewing for 10 min.
95 °C, 4′	The ground grains were poured over with boiled tap water at 93–95 °C and brewing for 4 min.
95 °C, 10′	The ground grains were poured over with boiled tap water at 93–95 °C and brewing for 10 min.

2. Results and Discussion

2.1. In Vitro Antioxidant Activity of Coffee Infusion

Figure 1 presents free radical scavenging activities (RSA [%]) of infusions prepared using various brewing methods from unroasted (green) and roasted (brown) coffee beans from different countries, assessed by the DPPH and ABTS techniques. The brew's abilities to reduce ferric ions evaluated by the FRAP and PFRAP methods as well as to reduce cupric ions determined with CUPRAC method are presented in Figure 2.

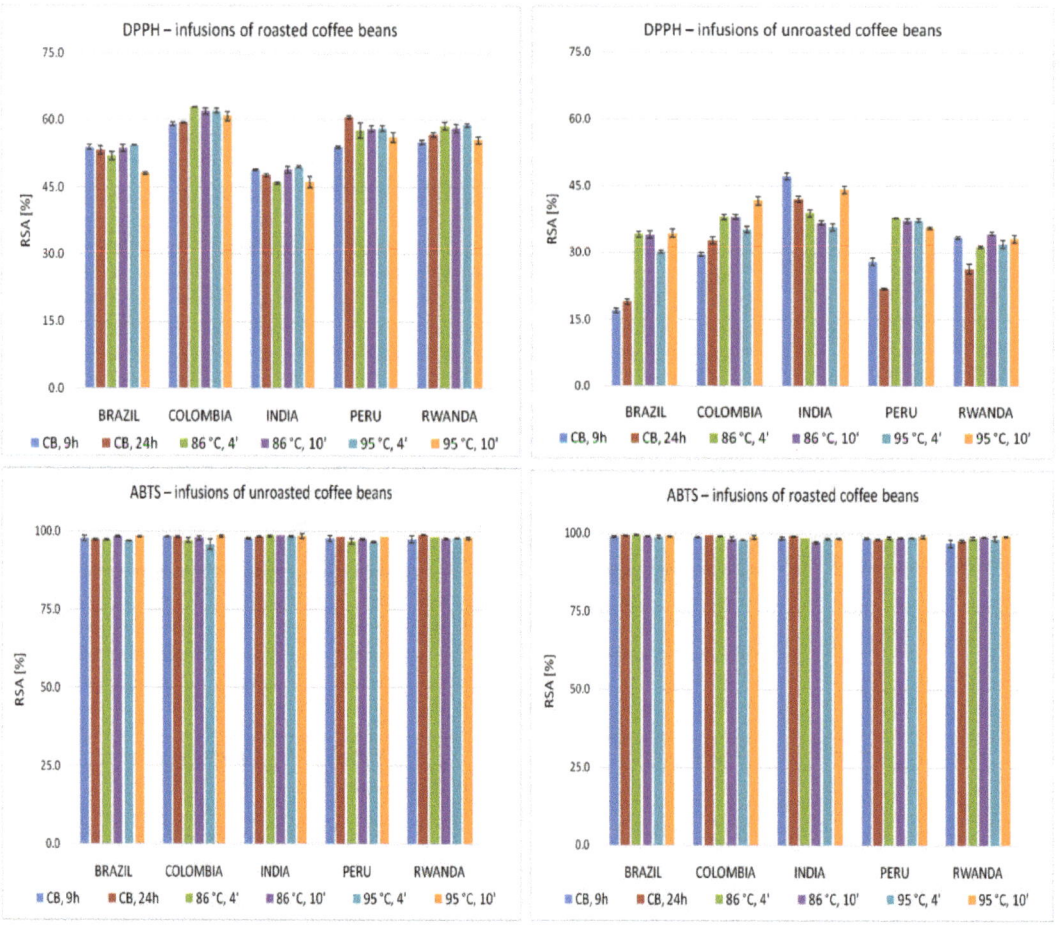

Figure 1. Radical scavenging activity (RSA [%]) of coffee infusions evaluated using DPPH and ABTS methods. Vertical lines represent standard deviation (SD). Details regarding brewing methods are summarized in Table 2.

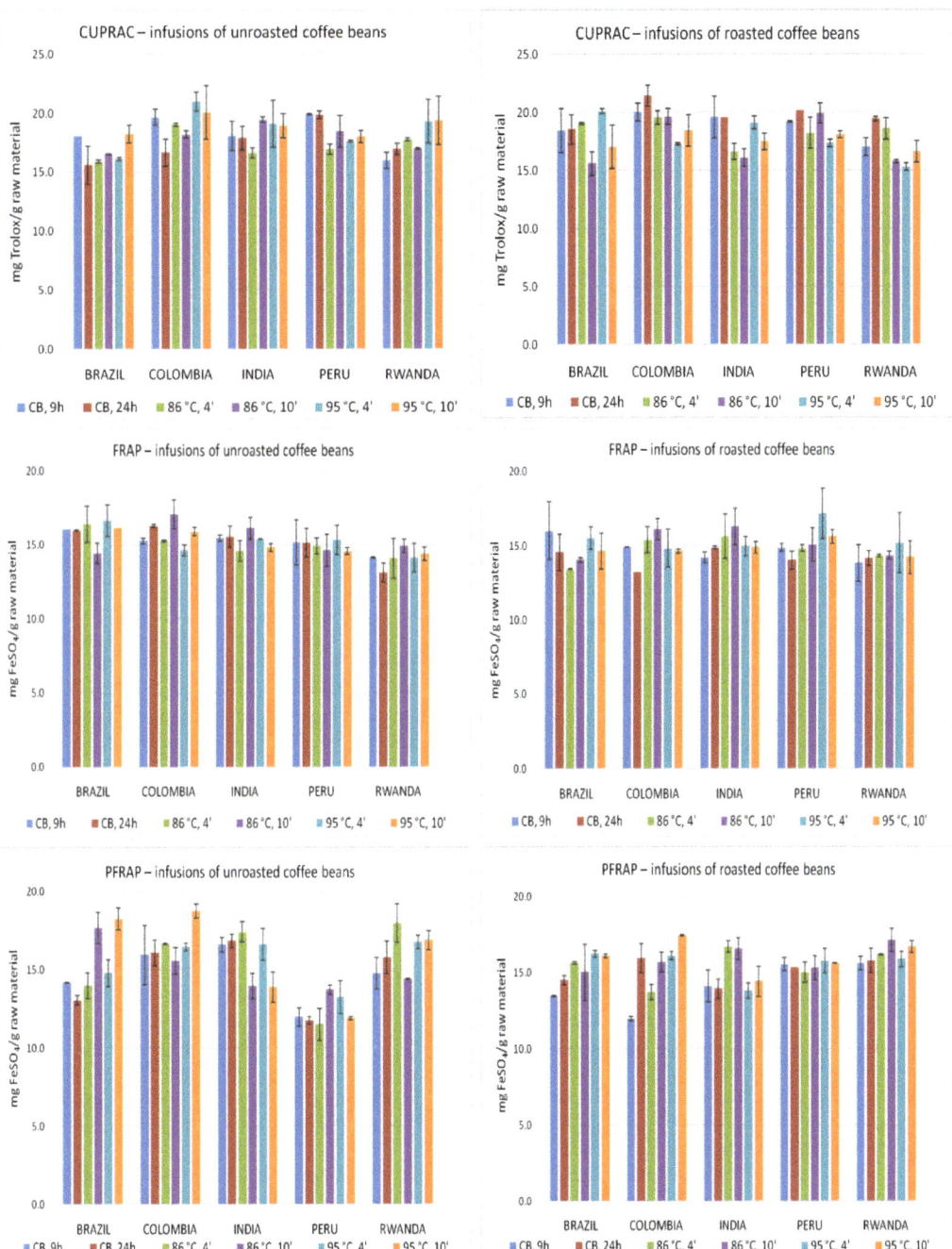

Figure 2. The ability of coffee infusions to reduce cupric and ferric ions determined by CUPRAC, FRAP, and PFRAP methods. Vertical lines represent standard deviation (SD). Details regarding brewing methods are summarized in Table 2.

The infusions prepared from roasted beans were characterized by a higher antioxidant potential expressed as RSA [%] evaluated by DPPH technique (Figure 1), as compared to infusions from unroasted beans. The highest activity evaluated using DPPH method was found for the Colombian roasted coffee beans infusion (86 °C, 4 min), whereas the lowest for the Brazilian green coffee beans infusion brewed using the cold brew method for 9 h. The highest RSA [%] in the roasted coffee beans infusions group prepared using different brewing methods was most often observed for extracts from Colombian beans, whereas the lowest was for Indian bean brews. In the case of unroasted beans, the highest activity of infusions was found for Indian coffee, whereas the lowest was for infusions prepared from Brazil and Rwanda coffee beans. Prolongation of roasted beans brewing time generally increased the activity of cold brew infusions but reduced the activity of infusions brewed at a temperature above 90 °C. In the case of unroasted beans, the increase of activity due to the extension of the brewing time was observed only for coffee brewed at a temperature above 90 °C. All the results obtained by DPPH method could suggest that the hot brew method led to obtain infusions with higher antioxidant activity.

The infusions analyzed using ABTS method (Figure 1) were characterized by very high activities, ranging from 95.76% RSA (green beans from Colombia, brewed at 95 °C for 4 min) to 99.43% RSA (infusion of roasted coffee from Brazil—86 °C, 4 min). As a rule, the roasted coffee bean infusions were characterized by a higher antioxidant potential than analogously prepared extracts from unroasted beans. The highest activities of the infusions prepared from roasted coffee beans were observed most often for Brazilian beans, while in the group of extracts from green coffee beans, for the brews from Indian and Colombian beans. In the group of unroasted beans extracts, it was also found that infusions of Peru beans are frequently characterized by slightly lower activity assessed by ABTS method. However, prolongation of brewing time led to enhance of the antioxidant activity, especially for extracts prepared from unroasted beans. This tendency was also found for infusions prepared with the cold brew method and at a temperature above 90 °C. Therefore, infusions prepared using the cold and hot brew techniques showed a very high free radical scavenging potential evaluated using the ABTS technique; however, it is rather difficult to unequivocally evaluate the effect of brewing temperature on antioxidant activity of brews.

The reduction potential of the infusions was evaluated using the FRAP, PFRAP, and the CUPRAC methods (Figure 2). The highest activity determined by the FRAP method was found for roasted beans from Peru (95 °C, 4 min), while the lowest for the unroasted beans infusion from Rwanda beans (CB, 24 h). Moreover, it was found that activity of extracts from unroasted beans was often higher as compared to infusions prepared from roasted beans. This tendency was especially observed for infusions prepared using the cold brew method. In the case of roasted beans, the highest activity was often observed for coffee beans from India and Peru, and the lowest for beans from Colombia and Rwanda. Moreover, the highest activity evaluated by FRAP method was found for unroasted Brazil and Colombia beans, whereas the lowest for Rwanda coffee. Evaluation of the brewing time effect of roasted and unroasted beans showed that in the case of the cold method and during application water of above 90 °C, a shorter brewing time seemed to be more effective. In the case of the hot brew method using water at a temperature of ~85 °C, brewing for 10 min seems to be more effective. The impact of brewing method on the infusion's potential showed that the hot brewing technique led to obtain infusions with a higher reduction activity.

The highest reduction activity of iron ions assessed by the PFRAP method (Figure 2) was observed for unroasted Colombian coffee beans infusion (95 °C, 10 min), whereas the lowest for unroasted beans from Peru (CB, 24 h). Based on the analysis of the results obtained for roasted and unroasted coffee beans, it is rather difficult to clearly define the group showed higher activity. However, the highest potential for roasted beans was found for infusions brewed at 86 °C, whereas for unroasted beans at 95 °C. Moreover, in the group of unroasted and roasted beans infusions, the highest activities were obtained most often for extracts from Rwanda beans. Additionally, also roasted Indian coffee beans brews were highly active. The lowest potential showed the infusions prepared from Peru coffee, both roasted and unroasted. In contrary to roasted, unroasted Indian coffee bean infusion had generally quite low antioxidant potential. The analysis of brewing time has established no beneficial effect of its prolongation on the tested potential of the extracts. The results suggested that in the case of hot brew (brown beans), 10 min process is generally more effective, while in the case of unroasted beans (85 °C)—4 min. Similar to the FRAP method, the analysis of the impact of the brewing method showed that hot coffee brewing techniques led to infusions with a greater reduction in the activity of ferric ions evaluated using PFRAP technique.

Application of CUPRAC method (Figure 2) to determine cupric ion reduction capacity suggest that Colombian roasted coffee extract (CB, 24 h) was characterized by the highest activity, whereas the lowest was found for the infusion prepared using the same method from Colombian unroasted beans. Comparison of the activities of roasted and unroasted coffee bean infusions leads to the conclusion that after application either the cold brewing method or 86 °C (4 min) roasted coffee bean infusions are more active, in contrary to the other brewing methods, where the green bean extracts were characterized by higher potential. Moreover, the highest ability to reduce cupric ions was found most often for Colombian coffee extracts (both roasted and unroasted), while the lowest for Rwanda roasted and Brazil unroasted coffee beans. Shorter brewing time was more effective to prepare infusions from brown and green beans using water below 90 °C and the cold brew method for unroasted beans. In the other brewing methods, prolongation of brewing time up to 24 h in cold method and up to 10 min in hot method seems to be more efficient.

The analysis of the effect of roasting coffee beans on the antioxidant activity of infusions showed that as a rule antioxidant potential of roasted coffee beans was higher, as compared to unroasted beans. Priftis et al. [21] evaluated the antioxidant activity of 13 varieties of coffee (roasted and unroasted) and confirmed that both types of coffee showed the high ability to scavenge free radicals. The impact of roasting on the activity of the obtained infusions depended on the variety of beans. This phenomenon may be related to the different chemical composition of beans. Moreover, the burning time also influenced the antioxidant activity of the obtained extracts. Dybkowska et al. [22] analyzed the antioxidant properties of coffee brews prepared from beans cultivated in Brazil, Ethiopia, Colombia, and India. The beans with various roasting degrees were analyzed—light, medium, and dark. They noticed that the process of roasting coffee beans increased the antioxidant potential of the obtained infusions. This phenomenon is directly related to the formation of melanoidins as a result of the Maillard reaction in coffee beans upon roasting. Melanoidins influence the antioxidant activity of coffee and its sensory properties. Their content in coffee depends, among others, on the intensity of the roasting process—the higher the roasting temperature, the higher content of these compounds, but lower their molecular weight. Ribeiro et al. [23] confirmed a higher content of melanoidins in roasted coffee bean infusions than in unroasted. In their study, higher antioxidant activity evaluated using FRAP and ABTS methods was found for roasted bean infusions as compared with infusions prepared from green coffee beans. Hečimović et al. [24] also confirmed our observations, that both factors—coffee variety and the roasting degree—affect the antioxidant activity. In their study, similarly to ours, infusions prepared from unroasted beans showed a lower potential than extracts from roasted beans.

The country of the coffee bean's cultivation could also affect the antioxidant activity of infusions. High antioxidant potential was found quite often for coffee from Colombia and India, while infusions from beans from Peru and Rwanda were characterized by lower activity. Oszmiański et al. [25,26], based on the apple analysis, concluded that the factors such as year of harvest, growth period, storage conditions, geographic location and genetic variation, the effect of the region, agricultural practices, and cultivation method could have an impact on the plant biochemical profile including antioxidant potential. It is assumed that the roasting degree of beans could have a significant impact, apart from the individual composition of particular varieties. The beans from Colombia and India were burned medium-light to medium. Coffee from Peru was the most roasted of all the tested varieties, in contrary to the least roasted from Rwanda. The observations are confirmed by the suggestion of Priftis et al. [21] that the roasting degree of coffee beans should be optimized for high antioxidant activity. Dybkowska et al. [22] also suggest that for nutritional reasons, consumption of coffee with a short or medium degree of burnout is the most beneficial for human health.

The analysis of the brewing method suggests that the hot technique could have a positive effect to obtain infusions with a higher antioxidant potential than the cold method. Rao and Fuller [27] showed that antioxidant activity of hot-brewed infusions was higher as compared to cold-brewed infusions. They suggested that this phenomenon could be related to the hot water extraction of additional bioactive compounds, including those with antioxidant potential. It may be related to the higher content of caffeoylquinic and chlorogenic acid isomers in hot-brewed coffee than in cold-brewed infusions. Rao et al. [28] also suggested that hot water can more easily wet the oily surface of coffee beans, to enhance the efficiency of extraction of active compounds, including those with antioxidant potential. Coffee brewing using hot or cold water could affect the different solubilities of compounds with higher molecular weight, mainly melanoidins.

Temperature of the water to be used to prepare infusions (hot brew method) is another parameter to be taken into consideration. The antioxidant activity of infusions brewing with water at a temperature of above 90 °C was higher. There are many reports on the effect of the roasting degree or the method of brewing coffee on the antioxidant activity of infusions. However, there is less information on the influence of small differences in water temperature on the activity of the obtained infusions. Castiglioni et al. [29] investigated the effect of water temperature (70 °C, 90 °C, and cold) on the antioxidant activity of white and green tea from China and Malawi. They found a maximum efficiency using water at temperature of 90 °C and cold brewing method. Pramudya and Seo [30] studied the effect of the temperature of serving coffee (5 °C, 25 °C, 65 °C) on the sensor attributes and emotional responses of the coffee brews. The respondents most often described the taste of coffee served at 65 °C as "roasted flavor", while the taste of the brew served at 5 °C as "pungent aroma", "metallic flavor", and "skunky flavor". They also perceived similar observations when serving green tea at different temperatures. The authors found that the respondents valued more positive sensory features of infusions served at higher than at lower temperature.

However, it is difficult to clearly evaluate how prolongation of the brewing time could affect the antioxidant activity of the infusions. Górecki and Hallmann [31] compared the antioxidant activity of infusions brewing for 3 and 6 min. They obtained slightly higher results for infusions prepared during a 6 min process. However, these differences were not significant. Moreover, the authors also suggest that other factors, such as the roasting degree of beans, could affect the antioxidant potential of the infusions.

2.2. Total Polyphenols and Flavonoids Content

The total polyphenols and flavonoids content in the studied infusions are presented in Figure 3. The highest polyphenols content was found in the Rwanda roasted coffee beans infusion, brewed using the cold brew method for 9 h, whereas the lowest in unroasted Colombian coffee extract prepared during a 4-min brewing (86 °C). Generally, a higher content of polyphenols was found in roasted coffee bean infusions, particularly in those prepared using hot water. The cold brewing method was effective to obtain infusions with high content of polyphenols from unroasted coffee beans. In brews from roasted beans, the highest polyphenol content was found in the Rwanda coffee extracts, while the lowest in Colombian and Indian infusions. In unroasted bean infusions, the highest concentration of polyphenols was found most often in Indian coffee bean brews, while the lowest in Colombian. In the case of roasted beans, the extension of brewing time to 10 min in the hot brewing method usually increased the polyphenols content. However, no similar relationships were observed in the case of green coffee. The obtained results suggest that cold brewing increases the concentration of total polyphenols in infusions, as compared to traditional hot brewing.

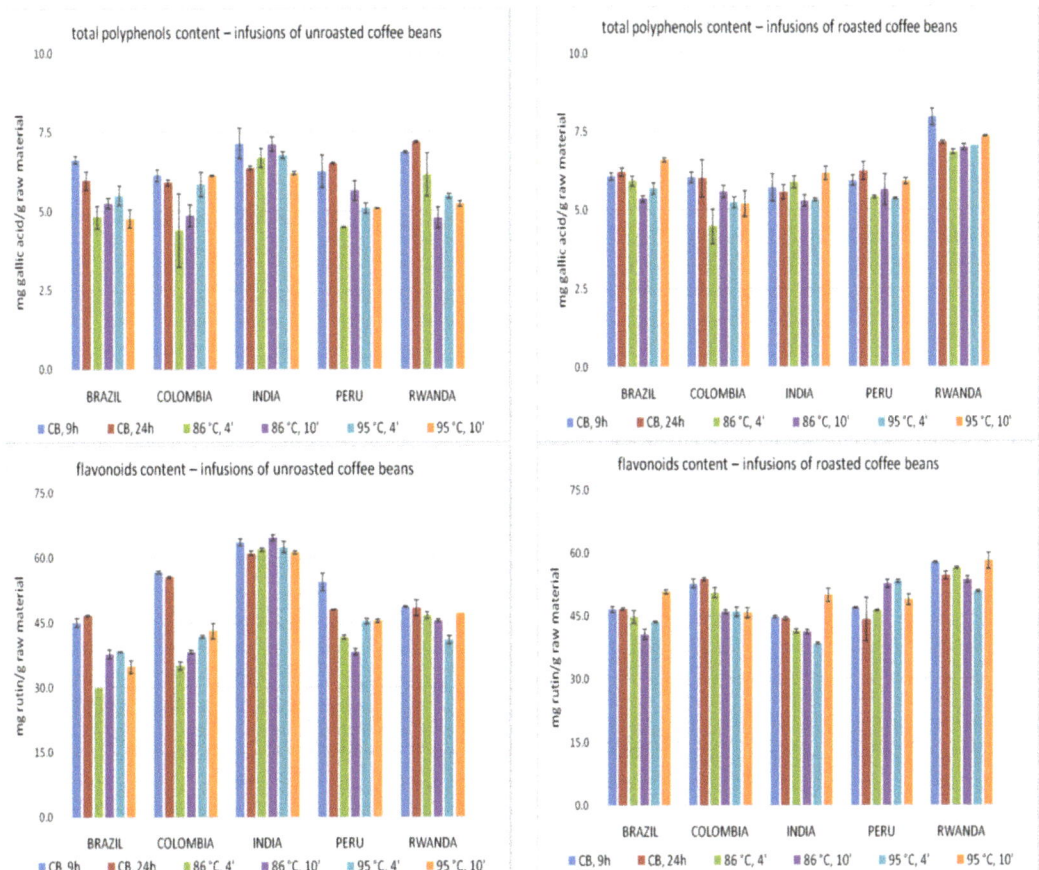

Figure 3. The total polyphenols and flavonoids content in coffee infusions. Vertical lines represent standard deviation (SD). Details regarding brewing methods are summarized in Table 2.

The highest content of flavonoids (Figure 3) was found in the unroasted Indian coffee infusion (85 °C, 10 min), while the lowest in unroasted Brazilian coffee (85 °C, 4 min). In the group of infusions prepared with hot water, a higher content of flavonoids was found in extracts from roasted beans, while in the cold brew method, from unroasted beans. In unroasted bean infusions, the brews prepared from Indian coffee showed the highest flavonoid content, while Brazil beans the lowest concentration of these group of compounds. Among infusions obtained from roasted beans, the highest content of flavonoids was found for samples obtained from Rwanda beans, whereas the lowest for Indian coffee infusions. It is difficult to clearly assess the effect of time extension on the content of flavonoids in the tested brews. In cold brewing, the infusions prepared during the 9-h process are generally characterized by a higher content of the flavonoids. A shorter brewing time also seems to be rather optimal for brewing roasted coffee with water below 90 °C. Extending the brewing time to 10 min seemed to be more effective in the case of roasted beans brewing with water at 95 °C and green coffee with water below 90 °C. The obtained results suggest that in most cases the cold brewing contributes to obtain infusions with a higher content of flavonoids than hot brewing. Similar results were observed for total polyphenols content.

Similar to the antioxidant activity, it was found that roasted bean infusions contained more polyphenols, including flavonoids, than unroasted. The highest content of these compounds was found in Rwanda coffee characterized by the lowest roasting degree. Dybkowska et al. [22] showed a decrease in the content of polyphenols in 100% Arabica beans infusions and blend coffee of Arabica and Robusta beans because of the roasting process. The thermolabile nature of these compounds contributes to their degradation after prolonged exposure to high temperature. The authors also emphasize that the loss of polyphenols is unfavorable due to the health-promoting effect of these compounds on the human body. Król et al. [32] also indicate a decrease of polyphenols content in the brews because of the extension of the roasting beans process.

The brewing method could also affect the polyphenols and flavonoids content. Cold brewing infusions of unroasted beans lead to higher content of these compounds, while the hot brewing technique seems to be more effective for roasted beans. Fibrianto et al. [33] compared the effect of the hot and cold brewing method on the polyphenols content in infusions prepared from roasted Arabica beans. Similar to our results, they also found a higher content of these compounds in extracts obtained using hot water.

The evaluation of the effect of water temperature in the hot brewing method showed that a higher content of polyphenols and flavonoids was observed in slightly more infusions prepared with water at 95 °C rather than at 86 °C. Merecz et al. [34] investigated the effect of the brewing method (hot water, percolator, and coffee machine) on the content of polyphenols and flavonoids in brews. In their study, the roasted and unroasted Arabica and Robusta beans were evaluated. However, their results cannot clearly confirm the influence of the brewing method on the content of these compounds in infusions. The concentration of polyphenols and flavonoids depended on the type of coffee (species, roasted/unroasted, and country of the bean's origins), as well as on the number of the brewings (1 to 3). In the case of roasted beans, the most effective method seemed to be application of a percolator (flooding the ground beans with cold water and then placed over a heat source). The content of polyphenols and flavonoids in unroasted beans was lower than in roasted. In the case of green coffee, the content of these compounds was higher in infusions prepared in a percolator and using hot water as compared to the brews from a coffee machine. Results of our study also lead to the conclusion that the type of coffee used (degree of roasting, country of origin, brewing method) had an impact on the content of biologically active compounds, including polyphenols and flavonoids in contrary to the slight differences in temperature of the water used to prepare the infusions. Merecz et al. [34] also emphasized that factors such as storage method and the degree of grinding beans could affect the profile of biologically active compounds in coffee infusions.

Furthermore, infusion time could affect the polyphenols content. In our study, it was found that extending of the brewing time, both in the cold (up to 24 h) and hot methods (up to 10 min), generally had a positive effect on the content of these compounds. In contrary, this tendency was not observed for the content of flavonoids, because in some cases, shorter brewing time seemed to be more optimal. Slightly different observations were made by Górecki and Hallmann [31]. They found that extending brewing time from 3 to 6 min contributed to a slight increase of flavonoids content and to a slight decrease of total phenols in coffee brews. However, these authors analyzed only the extracts prepared using the hot brewing technique. On the other hand, Cordoba et al. [11] confirmed our observation: extending the brewing time from 14 to 22 h (cold brewing method) increased the polyphenol content in coffee infusions.

2.3. Caffeine Content in Coffee Infusion

The caffeine content in studied infusions is presented in Table 3, whereas the chromatogram presenting the analysis of the selected infusion (unroasted beans from Peru—86 °C, 4 min) in Figure 4. The highest caffeine content determined by HPLC method was found in the Indian roasted bean infusion (CB, 24 h), while the lowest in the Peru unroasted beans brews (95 °C, 4 min). The higher caffeine concentration was found rather in brown bean infusions than in green coffee beans. The cold method was more effective to prepare infusions with a higher caffeine content than the traditional hot brewing technique. However, infusions brewed with water at 95 °C for 4 min were characterized by the lowest caffeine content. The obtained results suggest that the relatively high content of caffeine (over 60 mg/100 mL in 5% (w/w) infusion) was found in brews prepared from Indian coffee. The lowest caffeine content was generally found in coffee from Peru and Rwanda, especially in brews obtained from unroasted beans.

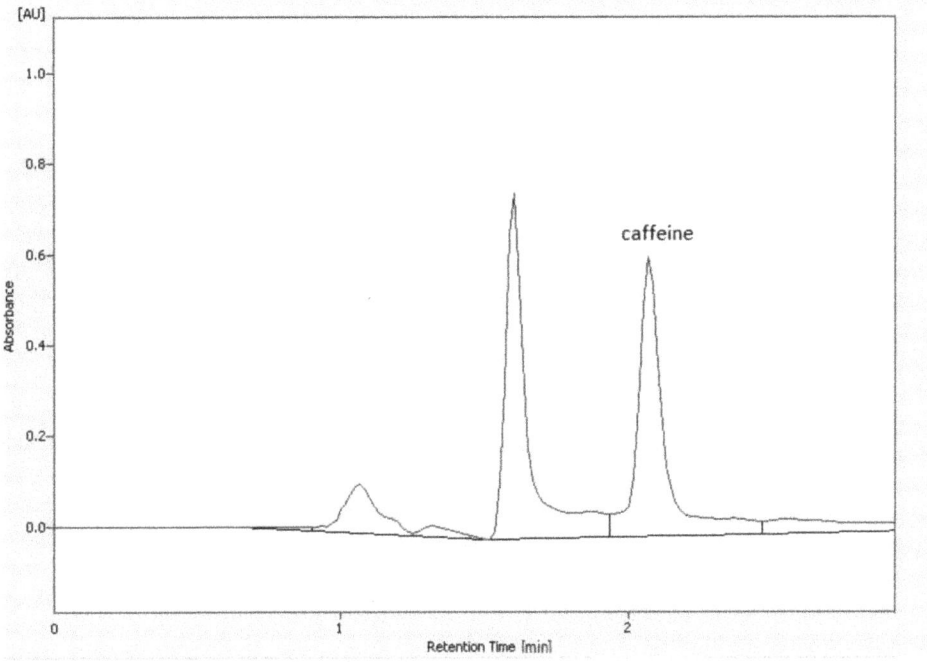

Figure 4. Chromatogram of the determination of caffeine in the infusion of unroasted beans from Peru (temperature of water—84–86 °C, brewing time—4 min).

Similar to the antioxidant activity as well as to the content of total polyphenols and flavonoids, higher caffeine concentration was usually found in roasted coffee infusions than in brews of green coffee beans. The highest caffeine content was observed in Indian coffee infusions, while the lowest concentrations were observed in coffee beans grown in Peru and Rwanda. Similar results, i.e., higher caffeine content in roasted than unroasted beans, were also obtained by Mubarak [14] and Motor and Beyen [35]. The influence of the roasting degree on the caffeine content is emphasized by Górecki and Hallmann [31]. They observed a significant decrease in caffeine content after long-term roasting of the beans. Moreover, they compared the content of this alkaloid in beans from conventional and organic crops. Conventional crops samples were characterized by a higher caffeine content, probably due to the use of nitrogen fertilizers that lead to increase the percentage of caffeine in coffee beans. Moreover, according to Gebeyehu and Bikila [36], the growing conditions of coffee trees could also modify the caffeine content in beans.

Table 3. The mean (±SD) caffeine content in studied infusions. Details regarding brewing methods are summarized in Table 2.

Brewing Method	mg/100 mL of Coffee Infusion	
	Unroasted Bean Infusion	Roasted Bean Infusion
Brazil		
CB, 9 h	54.13 ± 1.35	48.87 ± 0.08
CB, 24 h	51.18 ± 0.59	67.72 ± 2.36
86 °C, 4'	34.50 ± 0.52	46.00 ± 0.11
86 °C, 10'	42.68 ± 0.33	47.53 ± 0.18
95 °C, 4'	43.22 ± 0.46	53.07 ± 0.39
95 °C, 10'	29.90 ± 0.32	49.08 ± 0.63
Colombia		
CB, 9 h	62.30 ± 0.55	50.61 ± 0.17
CB, 24 h	60.11 ± 0.17	57.04 ± 0.82
86 °C, 4'	36.02 ± 0.03	52.78 ± 0.57
86 °C, 10'	37.64 ± 0.20	48.65 ± 0.24
95 °C, 4'	34.26 ± 0.12	56.77 ± 0.25
95 °C, 10'	32.15 ± 0.07	45.15 ± 0.28
India		
CB, 9 h	65.53 ± 0.09	66.60 ± 0.36
CB, 24 h	65.61 ± 0.16	78.30 ± 0.34
86 °C, 4'	51.32 ± 0.08	53.38 ± 0.09
86 °C, 10'	61.58 ± 0.27	61.22 ± 0.17
95 °C, 4'	49.78 ± 0.13	62.12 ± 0.72
95 °C, 10'	52.93 ± 0.21	57.80 ± 0.56
Peru		
CB, 9 h	38.97 ± 0.22	59.27 ± 0.20
CB, 24 h	41.88 ± 0.10	59.62 ± 0.15
86 °C, 4'	27.79 ± 0.15	44.73 ± 0.34
86 °C, 10'	27.23 ± 0.07	57.27 ± 0.23
95 °C, 4'	18.15 ± 0.30	53.98 ± 0.20
95 °C, 10'	28.68 ± 0.18	51.80 ± 0.35
Rwanda		
CB, 9 h	39.26 ± 0.14	50.08 ± 0.20
CB, 24 h	49.01 ± 0.45	54.01 ± 0.07
86 °C, 4'	27.80 ± 0.13	49.38 ± 0.14
86 °C, 10'	29.75 ± 0.43	52.77 ± 0.20
95 °C, 4'	25.72 ± 0.22	49.25 ± 0.43
95 °C, 10'	47.32 ± 0.47	50.63 ± 0.30

The evaluation of the effect of the brewing method showed that cold brew infusions usually are characterized by a high caffeine content. Moreover, it can be assumed that longer brewing time favor the preparation of infusions with a higher content of this alkaloid. Similar results were obtained by Fuller and Rao [37]. They found that cold-brew infusions were characterized by a higher caffeine content as compared to extracts prepared using the hot method. The authors suggest that the higher caffeine content in cold infusions may be caused, among others, by extending the brewing time. In their study, the time was extended from 6 min (hot brew) to even 24 h (cold brew). Such a procedure could increase the intragranular diffusion and decrease the concentration of extractable coffee compounds in the hot brew, as compared to the cold brew. Moreover, the extraction from the surface and near-surface matrix occurs more rapidly than the diffusion of compounds through the intragranular pore network to the grain surface. In another study, Rao et al. [28] compared, among others, the content of bioactive compounds in infusions prepared using cold and hot methods, from coffee beans with varying roasting degrees. They found that the roasting process led to several chemical and physical changes in the bean matrix. Depending on the water temperature using to prepare the infusion, the above-mentioned changes affected most likely the ability, speed, and permeation efficiency of the various compounds. In their study, the water temperature affected the caffeine content in the brews. As in the case of our research, cold brew infusions seemed to be more effective to obtain higher caffeine content than hot water infusions. The high caffeine content in cold drip infusions was also demonstrated by Córdoba et al. [38].

Moreover, the water temperature could affect the caffeine content. Infusions prepared using the hot brew method with water temperature not exceeding 90 °C were a little more often characterized by a higher content of this alkaloid. Caprioli et al. [39] analyzed the Arabica and Robusta beans infusions prepared in two espresso machines used different pressure and temperature to brew coffee—at a temperature of 88–92 °C at a pressure of 9 bar and a temperature of 92–98 °C at a pressure of 7 bar. The caffeine content in Arabica bean infusions was higher in brews prepared at a higher temperature and lower pressure, while for Robusta coffee at lower temperature and higher pressure. In another study, Caprioli et al. [40] confirmed our observations: it is rather difficult to find consistent comparative data in the literature on the influence of coffee brewing parameters on the concentration of biologically active compounds in brews. The reason for this may be as a rule the application of a non-standard brewing method, characterized by different parameters such as the coffee-water ratio, the degree of beans roasting as well as differences in the units of the presented results. These factors can make it difficult to compare the data from different studies.

The analysis of the impact of brewing time on the caffeine content suggests that for the tested coffee varieties in our study, a longer brewing time seems to be more optimal. Similar results were obtained by Fuller and Rao [37]. In their study, the extending of brewing time from 400 to 1440 min increased the caffeine content in coffee infusions. The influence of the brewing method on the content of biologically active compounds, including caffeine, is also mentioned by Zaguła et al. [41]. The authors analyzed the influence of the application of a variable magnetic field on the caffeine content in black and green tea infusions. They suggested that a magnetic field assisted extraction could enhance the effectiveness of extracting the active substances from tea leaves to the infusion. Moreover, the authors emphasized that properly selected techniques designed to facilitate water-based extraction, using ultrasounds, magnetic fields, or microwaves may lead to technological advancements in the extraction of bioactive compounds from plant material.

2.4. Tannins Content and pH of Coffee Infusions

In our study, all the analyzed infusions contained tannins. The tannins in roasted coffee beans infusions were also found by Choi and Koh [42]. Patay et al. [43] also confirmed the content of these compounds in ripe and unripe seeds and pericarp of coffee beans.

The pH of all tested infusions was slightly acidic (Table 4). The pH of the unroasted bean infusions ranged from 5.16 (beans from Rwanda, cold-brewed for 9 h) to 6.58 (beans from Peru, brewed for 4 min with water at 95 °C). The pH of roasted bean infusions was more acidic, from 4.99 (Rwanda coffee, cold-brewed for 9 h) to 5.71 (Indian beans, cold-brewed for 24 h). Fibrianto et al. [33] analyzed the pH of infusions depending on the degree of roasting beans (light, medium, and dark). As the degree of roasting increased, the pH of the infusions was more alkaline. Slightly roasted bean infusions were more acidic.

Table 4. pH of coffee infusions. Details regarding brewing methods are summarized in Table 2.

pH of Coffee Infusion					
infusion of unroasted beans	Brazil	Colombia	India	Peru	Rwanda
CB, 9 h	6.04	5.75	6.00	5.17	5.16
CB, 24 h	5.92	6.11	6.24	6.17	6.44
86 °C, 4′	6.11	6.48	6.40	6.47	6.35
86 °C, 10′	6.06	6.28	6.20	5.94	6.50
95 °C, 4′	6.26	6.13	6.26	6.58	6.50
95 °C, 10′	6.16	6.32	6.29	6.23	6.35
infusion of roasted beans	Brazil	Colombia	India	Peru	Rwanda
CB, 9 h	5.25	5.07	5.62	5.12	4.99
CB, 24 h	5.31	5.07	5.71	5.19	5.21
86 °C, 4′	5.15	5.07	5.50	5.05	5.17
86 °C, 10′	5.14	5.03	5.48	5.07	5.14
95 °C, 4′	5.19	5.06	5.53	5.11	5.12
95 °C, 10′	5.20	5.07	5.50	5.02	5.10

The analysis of the influence of the brewing method on the pH of the obtained infusions showed that in the case of unroasted beans, cold brewing leads to extracts with a lower pH, while the hot method, with a higher pH. The opposite relationship was noticed in the group of roasted bean infusions, as application of the hot-brew method generally led to more acidic infusions than with the cold-brew method. The exception was coffee from Rwanda (CB, 9 h) with the lowest pH. Rao and Fuller [27] compared the pH of infusions of roasted beans from different countries, prepared using the hot- and cold-brew methods. In most cases, cold infusions were characterized by a more alkaline reaction. These observations were confirmed in our study. Rao and Fuller [27] also noted that coffee vendors often suggested that infusions prepared using cold- and hot-brew methods were characterized by different taste profiles due to different acidity levels. Therefore, it is believed that consumption of cold-brewed coffee, due to its lower acidity, could cause fewer gastrointestinal symptoms, sometimes observed after consuming coffee infusions. Rao and Fuller [27] clearly distinguish the pH assessment of infusions and their total titratable acidity. pH refers to the concentration of aqueous hydrogen ions, providing a metric for the quantity of deprotonated acid molecules in a tested sample, whereas the total titratable acidity is a measure of all acidic protons in a sample, including non-dissociated protons. Based on the obtained results, authors concluded that coffee infusions prepared using cold and hot brewing technique are similar, taking into account the total concentration of deprotonated acid compounds; however, they differ in the concentration and possibly the complexity of protonated acids at the pH of extraction. No correlation between perceived acidity in the flavor of coffee brews and pH was observed by Gloess et al. [44] and Andueza et al. [45]. Furthermore, Gloess et al. [44] found no correlation between the pH and the titratable acidity of the coffee brews. The authors explain that many of the acids presented in the coffee infusion may not be completely deprotonated at pH measurement of this infusions and as a consequence does not affect its pH, but could be measured during titration with alkali.

The evaluation of the impact of water temperature in the hot brew method on the pH showed that infusions prepared with water at 95 °C were often characterized by a more alkaline reaction. Salamanca et al. [46] evaluated the effect of the type of coffee (natural and washed Arabica as well as natural Robusta) and the extraction temperature profile (88–93 °C, 90 °C, 93–88 °C) on the pH of the infusion. The pH varied depending on the type of coffee, as well as the temperature of brewing. In the case of Arabica beans, the infusions prepared at 93–88 °C were more acidic, while those obtained in a constant temperature of 90 °C were more alkaline. In the case of the Robusta variety, the most acidic infusions were those brewed at 88–93 °C, while the alkaline were prepared at 93–88 °C. Regardless of the water temperature, as in our study, all prepared infusions were acidic, and pH ranging from 5.01 ± 0.82 to 5.74 ± 0.04.

The analysis of the influence of the brewing time on the pH of the obtained infusions showed that in the case of the cold brew method, the extracts obtained during a longer brewing time (24 h) had a higher pH, whereas, in the hot brewing technique, the infusions obtained during a shorter brewing time (4 min) had a more alkaline pH. Fuller and Rao [37] analyzed the pH of infusions prepared using the cold brew method for 400 and 1440 min. They observed more alkaline reactions for extracts prepared during a shorter brewing time.

The comparison of the pH of the infusions depending on the country of origin of the beans has shown that in the case of unroasted beans, the most alkaline are usually the infusions from Rwanda coffee, while the most acidic—the beans grown in Brazil. In the case of roasted beans, the most alkaline pH, regardless of the water temperature and infusion time, was found for infusions of beans imported from India, while acidic for extracts obtained from beans grown in Colombia and Peru. Rao and Fuller [27] also compared the pH of infusions made from roasted beans grown in different countries (Brazil, Ethiopia, Myanmar, Colombia, and Mexico). In the case of the hot-brew method, the infusion made from Brazilian beans was the most alkaline, whereas the most acidic was made from the coffee grown in Ethiopia. In the case of cold brewing, the most alkaline was the infusion of beans grown in Myanmar, and the most acidic, also the extracts of Ethiopian beans. In another study of Fuller and Rao [37], it was noted that pH of infusions depended not only on the hot or cold method, but also on the degree of roasting and grinding the beans. The most acidic reaction was found for medium-coarse coffee, while the most alkaline for dark roast and medium coarse ground coffee (dark-medium).

2.5. Statistical Analysis

The statistically significant Pearson correlation coefficients were obtained between methods: DPPH vs. ABTS ($r = 0.489$; $p < 0.0001$), FRAP vs. F-C ($r = 0.314$; $p < 0.02$), ABTS vs. flavonoids content ($r = 0.270$; $p < 0.04$) as well as F-C vs. flavonoids content ($r = 0.688$; $p < 0.0001$). Correlations between the caffeine content and the results of antioxidant activity as well as the total polyphenols and flavonoids content, were also assessed. Statistically significant correlation coefficients were obtained between the caffeine content and antioxidant activity evaluated with DPPH ($r = 0.390$; $p < 0.003$) and ABTS ($r = 0.453$; $p < 0.001$) methods. Moreover, a significant correlation was found for caffeine vs. total polyphenols ($r = 0.355$; $p < 0.006$) and for caffeine vs. flavonoids content ($r = 0.445$; $p < 0.001$). The statistical significance of differences between the results obtained for infusions prepared using various brewing parameters was also assessed. The differences between the antioxidant activity of infusions prepared from roasted and unroasted beans were statistically significant ($z = 4.871$; $p < 0.0001$). Caffeine content in infusions of green and brown beans also differed significantly ($z = 4.206$; $p < 0.0001$). The above-mentioned differences, between the concentration of polyphenols and flavonoids, were statistically insignificant. The assessment of differences between the coffee brewing temperature (CB vs. 84–86 °C and CB vs. 93–95 °C) showed that in the case of antioxidant activity, the differences were statistically significant between the cold-brew method and 93–95 °C ($z = 2.274$; $p < 0.03$). The content of polyphenols and flavonoids differed significantly between the cold-brew method and 84–86 °C as well as cold brew method and 93–95 °C ($z = 4.436$ and $z = 3.212$, respectively;

$p < 0.01$). Furthermore, the caffeine content differed depending on the brewing method (CB vs. 84–86 °C—$z = 3.808$; $p < 0.001$ as well as CB vs. 93–95 °C—$z = 2.688$; $p < 0.01$). The differences between the brewing temperatures in the hot brew method (84–86 °C vs. 93–95 °C) were not statistically significant taking into account antioxidant activity, polyphenols and flavonoids content, as well as caffeine concentration in the analyzed infusions. The evaluation of differences between shorter and longer brewing time in individual brewing techniques (9 h vs. 24 h and 4 min vs. 10 min) showed that only the differences between caffeine content in cold brew infusions (9 h vs. 24 h), were statistically significant ($z = 1.988$; $p < 0.05$). The statistically significance of differences between the antioxidant activity, the content of caffeine, polyphenols, and flavonoids in infusions from beans (both roasted and unroasted) cultivated in different countries was also assessed. In the case of antioxidant activity, the differences were statistically significant between coffees imported from Brazil and Colombia ($z = 3.806$; $p < 0.001$), Colombia and Peru ($z = 3.622$; $p < 0.001$), as well as Colombia and Rwanda ($z = 4.167$; $p < 0.001$). The content of polyphenols and flavonoids differed significantly between infusions obtained from beans cultivated in Brazil vs. Colombia ($z = 2.057$; $p < 0.04$), Brazil vs. Rwanda ($z = 4.171$; $p < 0.001$), Colombia vs. Rwanda ($z = 2.743$; $p < 0.01$) as well as Peru vs. Rwanda ($z = 2.600$; $p < 0.01$). Caffeine content differed significantly between infusions brewed with coffee beans from Brazil and India, Colombia and India, India and Peru as well as India and Rwanda ($z = 3.059$; $p < 0.01$).

3. Materials and Methods

3.1. Chemicals

Acetic acid (99.5%), aluminum chloride hexahydrate, copper(II) chloride dihydrate, disodium hydrogen phosphate dihydrate, 96% ethanol, 36% hydrochloric acid, iron(III) chloride hexahydrate, methanol, phosphoric acid, potassium persulfate, potassium dihydrogen phosphate, potassium hexacyanoferrate(III), sodium acetate anhydrous, sodium carbonate anhydrous, sodium hydroxide, sodium nitrite, and trichloroacetic acid were purchased from Chempur, Poland. Neocuproine was delivered by J&K Scientific, Germany. Folin–Ciocalteu reagent, acetonitrile, iron(II) sulfate heptahydrate, gallic acid were supplied by Merck, Germany, whereas rutin trihydrate by Roth, Germany. ABTS (2,2'-azino-bis(3-ethylbenzothiazoline-6-sulfonic acid), DPPH (2,2-diphenyl-1-picrylhydrazyl), TPTZ (2,4,6-tris(2-pyridyl)-s-triazine), Trolox (6-hydroxy-2,5,7,8-tetramethylchromane-2-carboxylic acid), caffeine were purchased from Sigma-Aldrich, USA. All the chemicals were of analytical grade.

3.2. Preparation of Coffee Brews

Unroasted and roasted Arabica coffee beans from Brazil, Colombia, India, Peru, and Rwanda were used to prepare the infusions. The region of coffee from individual countries and the degree of roasting are summarized in Table 5. Coffee beans were ground using electric grinder (CTC Clatronic KSW 3306, Germany), immediately before sample preparation. The roasted beans were ground for 15 s, while unroasted, due to the greater hardness, for 70 s, until the coffee was finely ground. The ground beans were poured over with boiled tap water at different temperatures (hot-brew and cold-brew method) and subjected to different brewing times. The details of the various brewing methods are presented in Table 2. The completed brews were filtered through filter papers. Prepared 5% (w/w) infusions were filtered through Whatman's filter papers no. 4. All the extracts were stored at +4 °C until the analysis.

Table 5. The origin of the analyzed coffee beans.

Country of the Beans Origins	Region	Roasting Degree
Brazil (Cerrado)	Cerrado Mineiro	medium
Colombia (Medellin)	Antioquia/Medellin	medium light
India (Monsooned Malabar)	Karnataka, Western Ghats	medium
Peru (Cepro Yanesha)	Villa Rica, Oxapampa, Pasco	medium dark
Rwanda (Sake)	Ngoma District, Eastern Province	light

3.3. Evaluation of Antioxidant Activity

The antioxidant activity of infusions was evaluated by several in vitro methods. The ability to scavenge free radicals (RSA [%]) was assessed by the DPPH and ABTS methods. Moreover, the ability of samples to reduce ferric and cupric ions was evaluated using FRAP (ferric reducing antioxidant power), PFRAP (potassium ferricyanide reducing power), and CUPRAC (cupric ion reducing antioxidant capacity) methods. The evaluation of antioxidant activity by DPPH, ABTS, and FRAP methods was performed as described by Muzykiewicz et al. [47]. To evaluate ferric reducing capacity of infusions, the FRAP method, as described by Apak et al. [48], and the PFRAP technique (with slight modifications), according to Jayaprakasha et al. [49], were used. The incubation time was reduced to 10 min and absorbance was measured at 734 nm. The spectrophotometric measurements were performed in 1 cm cuvettes using Hitachi U-5100 spectrophotometer (Japan). In DPPH and ABTS methods the activity was expressed as RSA [%], whereas in CUPRAC technique as Trolox equivalents (TEAC)—mg Trolox/g RM (raw material). The reducing power evaluated using FRAP and PFRAP method was presented as $FeSO_4$ equivalents—mg $FeSO_4$/g RM. Three samples were prepared from each extract and the results are presented as an arithmetic mean ± standard deviation (SD).

3.4. Evaluation of Total Polyphenols and Flavonoids Content

The total polyphenols content (Folin–Ciocalteu method) was evaluated as described by Muzykiewicz et al. [47], whereas the flavonoids according to Saeed et al. [50]. The spectrophotometric measurements were performed in 1 cm cuvettes using Hitachi U-5100 spectrophotometer (Japan). The total polyphenols content was expressed as gallic acid (GA) equivalents (GAE)—mg GA/g RM, whereas flavonoids content as rutin equivalents—mg rutin/g RM. Three samples were prepared from each extract and the results are presented as an arithmetic mean ± standard deviation (SD).

3.5. Evaluation of Tannins Content and pH of Infusions

Tannins content in infusions was analyzed according to Saeed et al. [50]. The few drops of 0.1% $FeCl_3$ were added to the coffee infusion. The appearance of a blue color indicated the presence of tannins in the coffee infusion. The pH of brews was measured using Thermo Electron Orion Benchtop 410A pH meter (USA).

3.6. HPLC Analysis

The concentration of caffeine in all coffee infusions was determined by high-performance liquid chromatography (HPLC-UV, Knauer, Germany). The tested compound was separated on a 125 × 4 mm column containing Hyperisil ODS (C_{18}), particle size 5 µm. The mobile phase consisted of 0.5 M H_3PO_4 (pH 2.5), acetonitrile and MeOH in the ratio 180:20:10 ($v/v/v$), flow rate was 1 mL/min 20 µL of the analyzed sample was injected on the column. The determinations were carried out at 272 nm. The correlation coefficient of the calibration curve was r = 0.999 (y = 370683x + 32.205, retention time—2.05 min). Each sample was analyzed in triplicate, and the results are presented as arithmetic mean ± standard deviation (SD).

3.7. Statistical Analysis

The Pearson's linear correlation between the antioxidant activity (DPPH, ABTS, FRAP, PFRAP, CUPRAC methods), polyphenols, flavonoids as well as caffeine content was determined. The significance of differences between the results of antioxidant activity, the content of polyphenols, flavonoids, and caffeine, obtained for infusions prepared using various parameters (method, time and temperature of brewing), considering the roasting and origin of beans was determined with Wilcoxon signed rank-test (parameter z). $p < 0.05$ was considered to be statistically significant. All the calculations were done with Statistica 13.3PL Software (StatSoft, Poland).

4. Conclusions

The results of the study showed that the selection of beans and brewing methods could have a significant effect on antioxidant activity, polyphenols, flavonoids, and caffeine content, as well as the pH of the infusions prepared from Arabica coffee beans. In general, a higher antioxidant activity and content of the above-mentioned biologically active compounds were obtained in the infusions prepared from roasted beans, as compared to the unroasted coffee beans. The origin of the beans and the brewing technique (hot or cold brew) also influenced the tested properties. Cold-brew infusions were generally characterized by a higher caffeine and total polyphenols (including flavonoids) content in the case of unroasted beans. The hot brewing method led to obtain extracts with higher antioxidant activity and the content of phenolic compounds in the case of roasted beans. In this study, the coffee beans were imported from different countries and were characterized by different degree of roasting, which also had a significant impact on the characteristics of infusions. It seems that factors such as brewing time (9 h vs. 24 h as well as 4 min vs. 10 min) and water temperature (below and above 90 °C) had a less significant impact on the tested properties. All infusions were slightly acidic and contained tannins. The results suggest that origin of coffee beans and brewing parameters seem to be responsible for the tested properties of infusions, therefore of their preparation should be optimized to obtain infusions with the most favorable content of biologically active compounds.

Author Contributions: Conceptualization, A.M.-S., A.N. and D.W.; methodology, A.M.-S., A.N., D.W. and A.K.; validation, A.M.-S., A.N. and A.K.; formal analysis, A.M.-S. and A.N.; investigation, A.M.-S., A.N. and D.W.; resources, A.M.-S. and D.W.; writing—original draft preparation, A.M.-S., D.W. and A.N.; writing—review and editing, A.M.-S. and A.K.; visualization, A.M.-S.; supervision, A.K.; project administration, A.M.-S.; All authors have read and agreed to the published version of the manuscript.

Funding: This research received no external funding. The APC was funded by Pomeranian Medical University in Szczecin.

Institutional Review Board Statement: Not applicable.

Informed Consent Statement: Not applicable.

Data Availability Statement: The data presented in this study are available in this article.

Acknowledgments: We express our gratitude to Adam Sołtysiak from the coffee roastery "To Kawa" in Szczecin (http://tokawa.pl/, accessed on 15 June 2021), for providing the coffee samples used in the study.

Conflicts of Interest: The authors declare no conflict of interest. The funders had no role in the design of the study; in the collection, analyses, or interpretation of data; in the writing of the manuscript; or in the decision to publish the results.

References

1. Dos Santos, A.; Marques, L.; Gonçalves, C.; Marcucci, M. Botanical aspects, caffeine content and antioxidant activity of Coffea arabica. *Am. J. Plant. Sci.* **2019**, *10*, 1013–1021. [CrossRef]
2. Goodin, M.; Dos Reis Figueira, A. Good to the last drop: The emergence of coffee ringspot virus. *PLoS Pathog.* **2019**, *15*, 1–6. [CrossRef]

3. Matysek-Nawrocka, M.; Cyrankiewicz, P. Biological active substances derived from tea, coffee and cocoa and their application in cosmetics. *Post. Fitoter.* **2016**, *17*, 139–144.
4. Krishnan, S. Sustainable coffee production. *ORE Environ. Sci.* **2017**, 1–34. [CrossRef]
5. Kohlmünzer, S. *Pharmacognosy*, 5th ed.; Wyd. Lek. PZWL: Warsaw, Poland, 2013; pp. 475–476.
6. Murata, M. Browning and pigmentation in food through the Maillard reaction. *Glycoconj J.* **2021**, *38*, 283–292. [CrossRef] [PubMed]
7. Janda, K.; Jakubczyk, K.; Baranowska-Bosiacka, I.; Kapczuk, P.; Kochman, J.; Rebacz-Maron, E.; Gutowska, I. Mineral composition and antioxidant potential of coffee beverages depending on the brewing method. *Foods* **2020**, *9*, 121. [CrossRef]
8. Cordoba, N.; Fernandez-Alduenda, M.; Moreno, F.L.; Ruiz, Y. Coffee extraction: A review of parameters and their influence on the physicochemical characteristics and flavour of coffee brews. *Trends Food Sci. Technol.* **2020**, *96*, 45–60. [CrossRef]
9. Kim, S.Y.; Kang, B.S. A colorimetric sensor array-based classification of coffees. *Sens. Actuators B Chem.* **2018**, *275*, 277–283. [CrossRef]
10. Gonzales, E.C.I.; Lloren, K.G.M.; Al-shdifat, J.S.; Valdez, L.B.; Gines, K.R.; Garcia, E.V. Effect of pressure on the particle size distribution of espresso coffee. *KIMIKA* **2018**, *29*, 30–35. [CrossRef]
11. Cordoba, N.; Pataquiva, L.; Osorio, C.; Leonardo Moreno, F.; Yolanda Ruiz, R. Effect of grinding, extraction time and type of coffee on the physicochemical and flavour characteristics of cold brew coffee. *Sci. Rep.* **2019**, *9*, 1–6. [CrossRef]
12. Angeloni, G.; Guerrini, L.; Masella, P.; Innocenti, M.; Bellumori, M.; Parenti, A. Characterization and comparison of cold brew and cold drip coffee extraction methods. *J. Sci. Food Agric.* **2018**, *99*, 391–399. [CrossRef]
13. Amanpour, A.; Selli, S. Differentiation of volatile profiles and odor activity values of Turkish coffee and French press coffee. *J. Food Process. Preserv.* **2016**, *40*, 1116–1124. [CrossRef]
14. Mubarak, A.; Croft, K.D.; Bondonno, C.B.; Din, N.S. Comparison of liberica and arabica coffee: Chlorogenic acid, caffeine, total phenolic and DPPH radical scavenging activity. *Asian J. Agric. Biol.* **2019**, *7*, 130–136.
15. Affonso, R.; Voytena, A.; Fanan, S.; Pitz, H.; Coelho, D.; Horstmann, A.; Pereira, A.; Uarrota, V.; Hellmann, M.; Ravela, L.; et al. Phytochemical composition, antioxidant activity, and the effect of the aqueous extract of Coffee (*Coffea arabica* L.) Bean residual press cake on the skin wound healing. *Oxid. Med. Cell Longev.* **2016**. [CrossRef]
16. Belayneh, A.; Molla, F. The Effect of Coffee on Pharmacokinetic Properties of Drugs: A Review. *BioMed. Res. Int.* **2020**, *20*, 1–11. [CrossRef]
17. Pelczyńska, M.; Bogdański, P. Health-promoting properties of coffee. *Varia Med.* **2019**, *3*, 311–317.
18. Gemechu, F.G. Embracing nutritional qualities, biological activities and technological properties of coffee by products in functional food formulation. *Trends Food Sci. Technol.* **2020**, *104*, 235–261. [CrossRef]
19. Witkowska, A.; Mirończuk-Chodakowska, I.; Terlikowska, K.; Kulesza, K.; Zujko, M. Coffee and its biologically active components: Is there a connection to breast, endometrial, and ovarian cancer?—A review. *Pol. J. Food Nutr. Sci.* **2020**, *70*, 207–222. [CrossRef]
20. Aguiar, J.; Estevinho, B.N.; Santos, L. Microencapsulation of natural antioxidants for food application—The specific case of coffee antioxidants—A review. *Trends Food Sci. Technol.* **2016**, *58*, 21–39. [CrossRef]
21. Priftis, A.; Stagos, D.; Konstantinopoulos, K.; Tsitsimpikou, C.; Spandidos, D.A.; Tsatsakis, A.M.; Tzatzarakis, M.N.; Kouretas, D. Comparison of antioxidant activity between green and roasted coffee beans using molecular methods. *Mol. Med. Rep.* **2015**, *12*, 7293–7302. [CrossRef] [PubMed]
22. Dybkowska, E.; Sadowska, A.; Rakowska, R.; Dębowska, M.; Świderski, F.; Świąder, K. Assessing polyphenols content and antioxidant activity in coffee beans according to origin and the degree of roasting. *Rocz. Panstw. Zakl. Hig.* **2017**, *68*, 347–353. [PubMed]
23. Ribeiro, E.; de Souza Rocha, T.; Prudencio, S.H. Potential of green and roasted coffee beans and spent coffee grounds to provide bioactive peptides. *Food Chem.* **2021**, *348*, 1–12. [CrossRef] [PubMed]
24. Hečimović, I.; Belščak-Cvitanović, A.; Horžić, D.; Komes, D. Comparative study of polyphenols and caffeine in different coffee varieties affected by the degree of roasting. *Food Chem.* **2011**, *129*, 991–1000. [CrossRef]
25. Oszmiański, J.; Lachowicz, S.; Gławdel, E.; Cebulak, T.; Ochmian, I. Determination of phytochemical composition and antioxidant capacity of 22 old apple cultivars grown in Poland. *Eur. Food Res. Technol.* **2018**, *244*, 647–662. [CrossRef]
26. Oszmiański, J.; Lachowicz, S.; Gamsjäger, H. Phytochemical analysis by liquid chromatography of ten old apple varieties grown in Austria and their antioxidative activity. *Eur. Food Res. Technol.* **2020**, *246*, 437–448. [CrossRef]
27. Rao, N.Z.; Fuller, M. Acidity and antioxidant activity of cold brew coffee. *Sci. Rep.* **2018**, *8*, 1–9. [CrossRef]
28. Rao, N.Z.; Fuller, M.; Grim, M.D. Physiochemical characteristics of hot and cold brew coffee chemistry: The effects of roast level and brewing temperature on compound extraction. *Foods* **2020**, *9*, 902. [CrossRef]
29. Castiglioni, S.; Damiani, E.; Astolfi, P.; Carloni, P. Influence of steeping conditions (time, temperature, and particle size) on antioxidant properties and sensory attributes of some white and green teas. *Int. J. Food Sci. Nutr.* **2015**, *66*, 491–497. [CrossRef]
30. Pramudya, R.C.; Seo, H.S. Influences of product temperature on emotional responses to, and sensory attributes of, coffee and green tea beverages. *Front. Psychol.* **2018**, *8*, 1–16. [CrossRef]
31. Górecki, M.; Hallmann, E. The antioxidant content of coffee and its in vitro activity as an effect of its production method and roasting and brewing time. *Antioxidants* **2020**, *9*, 308. [CrossRef]
32. Król, K.; Gantner, M.; Tatarak, A.; Hallmann, E. The content of polyphenols in coffee beans as roasting, origin and storage effect. *Eur. Food Res. Technol.* **2020**, *246*, 33–39. [CrossRef]

33. Fibrianto, K.; Umam, K.; Wulandari, E.S. Effect of roasting profiles and brewing methods on the characteristics of bali kintamani coffee. *Adv. Eng. Res.* **2018**, *172*, 194–197.
34. Merecz, A.; Marusińska, A.; Karwowski, B.T. The content of biologically active substances and antioxidant activity in coffee depending on brewing method. *Pol. J. Natur. Sci.* **2018**, *33*, 267–284.
35. Motora, K.G.; Beyene, T.T. Determination of caffeine in raw and roasted coffee beans of ilu abba bora zone, South West Ethiopia. *Indo Am. J. Pharm. Res.* **2017**, *7*, 463–470.
36. Gebeyehu, B.T.; Bikila, S.L. Determination of caffeine content and antioxidant activity of coffee. *Am. J. Appl. Chem.* **2015**, *3*, 69–76. [CrossRef]
37. Fuller, M.; Rao, N.Z. The effect of time, roasting temperature, and grind size on caffeine and chlorogenic acid concentrations in cold brew coffee. *Sci. Rep.* **2017**, *7*, 1–9. [CrossRef]
38. Córdoba, N.; Moreno, F.L.; Coralia, O.; Velaśqueaz, S.; Ruiz, Y. Chemical and sensory evaluation of cold brew coffees using different roasting profiles and brewing methods. *Food Res. Int.* **2021**, *141*, 110141. [CrossRef]
39. Caprioli, G.; Cortese, M.; Maggi, F.; Minnetti, C.; Odello, L.; Sagratini, G.; Vittori, S. Quantification of caffeine, trigonelline and nicotinic acid in espresso coffee: The influence of espresso machines and coffee cultivars. *Int. J. Food Sci. Nutr.* **2014**, *65*, 465–469. [CrossRef]
40. Caprioli, G.; Cortese, M.; Sagratini, G.; Vittori, S. The influence of different types of preparation (espresso and brew) on coffee aroma and main bioactive constituents. *Int. J. Food Sci. Nutr.* **2015**, *66*, 505–513. [CrossRef]
41. Zaguła, G.; Bajcar, M.; Saletnik, B.; Czernicka, M.; Puchalski, C.; Kapusta, I.; Oszmiański, J. Comparison of the effectiveness of water-based extraction of substances from dry tea leaves with the use of magnetic field assisted extraction techniques. *Molecules* **2017**, *22*, 1656. [CrossRef]
42. Choi, B.; Koh, E. Spent coffee as a rich source of antioxidative compounds. *Food Sci. Biotechnol.* **2017**, *26*, 921–927. [CrossRef] [PubMed]
43. Patay, É.B.; Sali, N.; Kőszegi, T.; Csepregi, R.; Balázs, V.L.; Németh, T.S.; Németh, T.; Papp, N. Antioxidant potential, tannin and polyphenol contents of seed and pericarp of three Coffea species. *Asian Pac. J. Trop Med.* **2016**, *9*, 366–371. [CrossRef]
44. Gloess, A.N.; Schönbächler, B.; Klopprogge, B.; D'Ambrosio, L.; Chatelain, K.; Bongartz, A.; Strittmatter, A.; Rast, M.; Yeretzian, C. Comparison of nine common coffee extraction methods: Instrumental and sensory analysis. *Eur. Food Res. Technol.* **2013**, *236*, 607–627. [CrossRef]
45. Andueza, S.; Vila, M.A.; Paz de Peña, M.; Cid, C. Influence of coffee/water ratio on the final quality of espresso coffee. *J. Sci. Food Agric.* **2007**, *87*, 586–592. [CrossRef]
46. Salamanca, C.A.; Fiol, N.; González, C.; Saez, M.; Villaescusa, I. Extraction of espresso coffee by using gradient of temperature. Effect on physicochemical and sensorial characteristics of espresso. *Food Chem.* **2017**, *214*, 622–630. [CrossRef]
47. Muzykiewicz, A.; Zielonka-Brzezicka, J.; Klimowicz, A. The antioxidant potential of flesh, albedo and flavedo extracts from different varieties of grapefruits. *Acta Sci. Pol. Technol. Aliment.* **2019**, *18*, 453–462. [CrossRef]
48. Apak, R.; Güçlü, K.; Özyürek, M.; Karademir, S.E. Novel total antioxidant capacity index for dietary polyphenols and vitamins C and E, using their cupric ion reducing capability in the presence of neocuproine: CUPRAC method. *J. Agric. Food Chem.* **2004**, *52*, 7970–7981. [CrossRef] [PubMed]
49. Jayaprakasha, G.K.; Singh, R.P.; Sakariah, K.K. Antioxidant activity of grape seed (*Vitis vinifera*) extracts on peroxidation models in vitro. *Food Chem.* **2001**, *73*, 285–290. [CrossRef]
50. Saeed, N.; Khan, M.R.; Shabbir, M. Antioxidant activity, total phenolic and total flavonoid contents of whole plant extracts *Torilis leptophylla* L. *BMC Complement. Altern. Med.* **2012**, *12*, 1–12. [CrossRef]

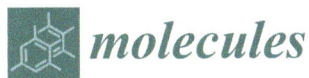

Article

Development of a High-Fibre Multigrain Bar Technology with the Addition of Curly Kale

Hanna Kowalska [1,*], Jolanta Kowalska [1], Anna Ignaczak [1,*], Ewelina Masiarz [1,*], Ewa Domian [1], Sabina Galus [1], Agnieszka Ciurzyńska [1], Agnieszka Salamon [2], Agnieszka Zając [1] and Agata Marzec [1]

[1] Department of Food Engineering and Process Management, Institute of Food Sciences, Warsaw University of Life Sciences, 159c Nowoursynowska St., 02-776 Warsaw, Poland; jolanta_kowalska@sggw.edu.pl (J.K.); ewa_domian@sggw.edu.pl (E.D.); sabina_galus@sggw.edu.pl (S.G.); agnieszka_ciurzynska@sggw.edu.pl (A.C.); agnieszkazajac230@gmail.com (A.Z.); agata_marzec@sggw.edu.pl (A.M.)

[2] Institute of Agriculture and Food Biotechnology—State Research Institute, 36 Rakowiecka St., 02-532 Warsaw, Poland; agnieszka.salamon@ibprs.pl

* Correspondence: hanna_kowalska@sggw.edu.pl (H.K.); annaignaczak475@gmail.com (A.I.); ewelina_masiarz@sggw.edu.pl (E.M.); Tel.: +48-225937565 (H.K.)

Citation: Kowalska, H.; Kowalska, J.; Ignaczak, A.; Masiarz, E.; Domian, E.; Galus, S.; Ciurzyńska, A.; Salamon, A.; Zając, A.; Marzec, A. Development of a High-Fibre Multigrain Bar Technology with the Addition of Curly Kale. *Molecules* **2021**, *26*, 3939. https://doi.org/10.3390/molecules26133939

Academic Editors: Jan Oszmianski, Sabina Lachowicz and Francesco Cacciola

Received: 20 May 2021
Accepted: 24 June 2021
Published: 28 June 2021

Publisher's Note: MDPI stays neutral with regard to jurisdictional claims in published maps and institutional affiliations.

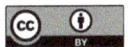

Copyright: © 2021 by the authors. Licensee MDPI, Basel, Switzerland. This article is an open access article distributed under the terms and conditions of the Creative Commons Attribution (CC BY) license (https://creativecommons.org/licenses/by/4.0/).

Abstract: The aim of this study was to find the effect of kale and dietary fibre (DF) on the physicochemical properties, nutritional value and sensory quality of multigrain bars. A recipe of multigrain bars was prepared with the addition of fresh kale (20% and 30%) and DF preparations (apple, blackcurrant, chokeberry and hibiscus). The bars were baked at 180 °C for 20 min. These snack bars, based on pumpkin seeds, sunflower seeds, flaxseed and wholegrain oatmeal, are a high-calorie product (302–367 kcal/100 g). However, the composition of the bars encourages consumption. In addition to the ability to quickly satisfy hunger, such bars are rich in many natural ingredients that are considered pro-health (high fibre content (9.1–11.6 g/100 g), protein (11.2–14.3 g/100 g), fat (17.0–21.1 g/100 g, including unsaturated fatty acids), carbohydrates (20.5–24.0 g/100 g), as well as vitamins, minerals and a large number of substances from the antioxidant group. The addition of kale caused a significant increase of water content, but reduction in the value of all texture parameters (TPA profiles) as well as calorific values. The content of polyphenols was strongly and positively correlated with the antioxidant activity ($r = 0.92$). In the bars with 30% addition of kale (422 mg GA/100 g d.m.), the content of polyphenols was significantly higher than based ones (334 mg GA/100 g d.m.). Bars with the addition of the DF were characterized by a higher antioxidant activity, and the content of carotenoids, chlorophyll A and B and polyphenols. High sensory quality was demonstrated for all (from 4.8 to 7.1 on a 10-point scale). The addition of fibre preparations was also related to technological aspects and allows to create attractive bars without additional chemicals.

Keywords: snack; baking; carotenoids content; chlorophyll content; total polyphenols content; calorific value; sensory properties

1. Introduction

Consumers are increasingly turning to snack foods. This trend may be due to the fast pace of people's lives, which results in a lack of time to prepare and eat traditional meals. In addition, they are paying attention to what they eat because they are more aware of the effects of food on their health. Cereal products, fruits and vegetables occupy an important place in the daily diet because they contain many valuable ingredients such complex carbohydrates, including dietary fibre (DF), vitamins, antioxidant compounds and minerals that can be considered pro-health. However, their consumption is still too low. Producers, to meet the requirements of consumers, introduce new, innovative products to the market such as cereal-based products with the addition of fruit or vegetables. Replacing traditional high-calorie snacks with products with a high content of bio-ingredients may have a beneficial effect on health. It can prevent many diseases, such as diabetes, arteriosclerosis, or high blood pressure.

Fresh and processed vegetables are a source of valuable nutrients. A greater degree of consumer attention should be focused on cruciferous vegetables, which are little appreciated. Kale is not a popular vegetable in the diet of consumers because of its taste, flavour and characteristic texture. Cruciferous vegetables are good sources of fibre, polyphenols, and glucosinolates. It is rich in biologically active substances with antioxidant, bactericidal and fungicidal properties [1]. This vegetable contains polyphenols, including flavonoids, which by inhibiting the activity of phosphodiesterase and cyclooxygenases can reduce platelet aggregation; therefore, it is recommended in atherosclerotic diseases. Glucosinolates may reduce the risk of cancer development [2]. Sulforaphane has the strongest anticancer properties. It shows an inhibitory effect on angiogenesis and the formation of metastases [3]. Kale is characterized by a high content of vitamins, such as in edible parts: C (120 mg/100 g), A (0.9 mg/100 g), B1 (0.1 mg/100 g), B2 (0.2 mg/100 g), B6 (1.6 mg/100 g), and E (1.7 mg/100 g), and also contains folic acid and niacin. In addition, it contains a large number of essential micro and macro elements, including, in edible parts: calcium (157 mg/100 g), potassium (530 mg/100 g) and iron (1.7 mg/100 g) [4,5]. Carotenoids, but also quercetin and camferol, are responsible for its strong antioxidant capacity [6]. The multitude of active compounds in kale translates into the health benefits of its consumption. Many studies have shown that frequent kale consumption reduces the incidence of cancer in various parts of the digestive tract, lung cancer and others. Son et al. [7], in view of the nutritional needs of patients with impaired renal function, attempted the production of kale with reduced potassium content without compromising the yield and quality. The potassium deficiency in kale was eaten up by an increase in total glucosinolate content, which is an indicator of the anticancer activity of cruciferous vegetables. Chlorophyll, contained in the raw material, has an antiseptic and immunizing effect [8,9]. The fresh leaves are suitable for direct consumption, and they can be added to salads or boiled as an ingredient of soups or fried. Michalak et al. [10] presented the possibility of using kale fermentation by autochthonous lactic acid bacteria in the creation of bioactive derivatives of phenolic compounds that may have anticancer properties. In recent years, it has also become a fashionable addition to juices or smoothies [11]. In the USA, powdered kale is used to make dietary supplements. On the local market, there are capsules with kale powder as an ingredient.

Dietary fibre is a heterogeneous mixture of carbohydrate polymers found in plant raw materials. It refers to a large number of substances that exhibit a wide variety of physicochemical properties, with a general division into water-soluble and insoluble compounds. However, the way of processing, e.g., cereals, reduces its content in products. There is a need to make DF preparations that can be added to enrich various products. In addition, DF has important health and technological functions in food production. The raw materials for the production of DF preparations are industrial fruit and vegetable waste (apple pomace, blackcurrant pomace, waste from the processing of carrots, tomatoes) as well as bran, corn cobs, chaff and straw, and legumes (mainly soybeans and peas) [12]. The soluble fraction includes pectin, ß-glucans, gums, mucilage, and a wide range of indigestible oligosaccharides (including inulin). The insoluble fraction includes: lignin, cellulose, and hemicellulose. Each of the two types of fractions has different physiological effects. Soluble DF is less common in food than insoluble DF, but it has a significant impact on digestive and absorbent processes [12–14]. Fruit and vegetable DF has a much higher proportion of soluble DF, while cereal DF contains more insoluble cellulose and hemicellulose [15].

The addition of DF to bakery products, such as cereal snacks or multigrain snack bars, is justified both in terms of health and technology. Consuming products with DF helps to prevent many civilization diseases, such as: obesity, type 2 diabetes, ischemic heart disease, gallstone disease, constipation, and flatulence. It also reduces the risk of developing certain cancers. Its use in food production results from its ability to bind water, gel formation, emulating and stabilizing properties, and fat mimetic properties, therefore it is primarily a structure-forming component and filler and affects the sensory quality of food [12,16]. The European Food Safety Authority (EFSA) allows the nutrition claims "source of fibre" and "high fibre" on food packaging with a content of at least 3% (1.5 g/100 kcal) or at least 6% fibre, respectively (3 g/100 kcal) [17–19]. Food has an increased level of fibre when it is at least 25% higher than similar foods. Products that contain health claims for dietary fibre must also meet requirements for adequately low fat, including saturated fat and low cholesterol [20]. Products containing a large amount of DF can be classified as functional and/or health-promoting food. In the technology of producing granular bars, DF allows for a better, more compact combination of ingredients and obtaining the appropriate structure of the product, mainly due to water absorption and mechanical durability. When deciding to use a DF blend in the product, it should be taken into account that their effect on texture may vary depending on the product formulation.

The aim of the research was to evaluate the use of kale and fibre preparations as an added value to multigrain bars. The scope of the study was the effect of kale and dietary fibre (DF) on the physicochemical proper-ties, nutritional value and sensory quality of multigrain bars.

2. Results

2.1. Development of the Recipe Composition and Production Technology of Multigrain Bars

At the stage of preliminary research, the recipe composition of the base bars was developed using baking. To improve the attractiveness of such a snack in terms of sensory and health, the recipe has been enriched with kale and DF preparations. Table 1 presents the chemical characteristics of fresh kale and multigrain bars with the addition of fresh and dried (microwave-blanched) kale.

Table 1. Chemical characteristics of kale and multigrain bars with the addition of fresh and dried kale (microwave-blanched).

Chemical Characteristics	Fresh Kale	Base Bar — Baking	Bar + Kale 30%	Bar + Dried Kale 10%
Humidity, g/100 g	87.1	27	39.2	30.5
Total protein (N × 6.25), g/100 g	3.3	14.3	12.2	13.9
Total protein (N × 6.25), g/100 g d.m.	25.9	19.6	20.1	20
Fat (no hydrolysis), g/100 g	0.4	21.2	17	19.2
Fat (no hydrolysis), g/100 g d.m.	3.2	29	28	27.7
Total ash, g/100 g	1.1	1.9	1.9	2.3
Total ash, g/100 g d.m.	8.3	2.6	3.2	3.3
Total dietary fibre, g/100 g	5.1	11.6	9.1	11.4
Total dietary fibre, g/100 g d.m.	39.5	15.8	15	16.4
including: soluble fibre fraction, g/100 g	0.3	2.5	2	2.2
soluble fibre fraction, g/100 g d.m.	2.4	3.4	3.3	3.1
insoluble fibre fraction, g/100 g	4.8	9.1	7.1	9.2
insoluble fibre fraction, g/100 g d.m.	37	12.4	11.7	13.3
Total carbohydrates, g/100 g	3	24	20.5	22.6
Total carbohydrates, g/100 g d.m.	23.3	32.9	33.8	32.5
including: sugars, g/100 g	2.6	12.9	10.6	12.5
sugars, g/100 g d.m.	19.9	17.7	17.5	18
Energy value, kcal/100 g	39	367	302	342
Energy value, kJ/100 g	164	1528	1259	1424

The raw material composition allowed to obtain a product with a DF content of 11.5%. Unrefined cereal products are characterized by a high content of DF, especially the insoluble fraction, similar to vegetables. Whole-grain oat flakes and flaxseed could play a significant role in the resulting DF content. The addition of kale did not have a significant effect on the differentiation of the bar composition in terms of DF content, but it caused a partial reduction in the caloric content of the bars (Table 1). The snacks obtained in this way can be a valuable source of both DF fractions, as well as fat (pumpkin and sunflower seeds) and protein. Due to their high calorific value, they can be a tasty and valuable snack that can replace one of the main meals.

Korus [21] analysed the composition of fresh vegetables. She showed a slightly higher content of proteins (about 4.3 g/100 g), emphasizing the beneficial composition of amino acids, including exogenous ones. Korus [5] showed that the pre-treatment of kale leaves reduced the content of minerals and vitamins by 26–52% (blanching) and 29–75% (cooking). The highest content of minerals, B vitamins and tocopherols was recorded in the frozen kale leaves after blanching. After 12 months of storage of frozen leaves, they contained 24–74% of macronutrients, 40–71% of micronutrients, 45–71% of vitamin B_1, 27–47% of vitamin B_2 and 69–85% of total tocopherols. In the study by Olsen et al. [22], green and red kale extracts have undergone a treatment including blanching, freezing and heat treatment by boiling in a bag. In both kale varieties, processing significantly decreased total phenolics, antioxidant capacity, and the content and distribution of flavonols, anthocyanins, hydroxycinnamic acids, glucosinolates, and vitamin C. Both extracts continued to inhibit colon cancer cell proliferation, but fresh kale extract had a much stronger effect. According to Korus [21], vegetables are low in fat, high in carbohydrates and DF and minerals, as well as vitamins and other important ingredients like antioxidants. Cruciferous vegetables deserve special attention. The author [21] showed that among all vegetables, this vegetable contains the most easily digestible calcium and protein and an exceptionally high amount of iron. Kale is also a significant source of DF, vitamins C and E (more than spinach and lettuce), provitamin A and antioxidants (more active than garlic, spinach, Brussels sprouts and broccoli).

Based on literature [5,21,22] data showing that kale processing reduces the content of many components, and because the content of individual ingredients was quite similar in both types of bars with fresh and dried kale (Table 1), the bars with 20 and 30% addition of fresh kale and DF preparations were used for a more detailed assessment of the physico-chemical properties. This was to make bars with lower calories and to facilitate the preparation of ingredients. Depending on the method of drying the kale, it could take up to several hours.

2.2. Water Activity and Its Content in Multigrain Bars

The water activity (Aw) in the bars was in the range of 0.857–0.953 (Table 2). This level of Aw classifies bars in the group of moist foods (in the range of 0.90–1.00) and with average Aw (in the range of 0.55–0.90), and thus in the food in which some microorganisms can develop (no microbiological stability). With the increase in the proportion of kale in the composition, the water activity increased. The base bars, i.e., bars without kale, were characterized by the lowest water activity (0.857). The type of added DF preparation had a significant effect on the water activity of the obtained bars (Table 2). Among the bars with 20% addition of kale, these with apple and chokeberry DF (0.943–0.944) were characterized by higher Aw, while bars with hibiscus DF (0.914) has significantly lower Aw.

The analysis of water content in the tested bars showed a significant effect of the type of added DF preparation and the amount of added kale on this parameter (Table 2). This varied widely, from approximately 17.3 to 41.1%. The water content in the control bars (without the addition of kale) differed significantly from the water content in the samples with the addition of kale. Increasing the proportion of kale from 20 to 30% resulted in a significant increase in the water content in the bars.

Table 2. The effect of kale and fibre preparation on water content, water activity (Aw), and compression force (Fmax) and work (W) in multigrain bars.

Type of Bars	Water Activity [-]	Water Content [%]	Compression Work [mJ]
Control (based)	0.857 ± 0.000 [A]	17.34 ± 1.13 [A]	604.3 ± 33.6
DF-apple-K20	0.944 ± 0.001 [cB]	29.86 ± 0.87 [abB]	383.5 ± 64.3
DF-apple-K30	0.953 ± 0.003 [C]	41.12 ± 2.63 [C]	271.4 ± 21.2
DF-blackcurrant-K20	0.931 ± 0.001 [b]	27.48 ± 2.27 [a]	360.3 ± 45.2
DF-chokeberry-K20	0.943 ± 0.000 [c]	27.54 ± 2.57 [a]	438.3 ± 41.4
P-hibiscus-K20	0.916 ± 0.001 [a]	35.39 ± 0.23 [b]	268.6 ± 95.8
One-way analysis of variance (ANOVA)			
Factors		p-value	
Kale addition (A,B,C)	0.0001 *	0.0020 *	0.0000 *
Type of fibre (a,b,c)	0.0001 *	0.0310 *	0.0138 *

*—means significant difference at a confidence level of 0.05; a, b, c and A, B, C—homogeneous groups, the same letters mean no statistically significant differences between the analysed values of indicators; the codes are described in Table 4.

2.3. The Effect of the Addition of Kale and Fibre Preparation on the Texture of the Multigrain Bars

2.3.1. Compression Test

The texture of the bars was tested on the basis of the compression test and the work required was calculated. The control bars showed the highest compression work (604.3 mJ), about 2 times higher than the other bars (Table 2). A significant effect of increasing the amount of kale on the value of this indicator was demonstrated; for bars with 20 and 30% addition of kale, the work/deformation energy of the samples was about 383.5 and 271.4 mJ, respectively. Higher humidity decreased the hardness and the work needed for the deformation in the compression test was lower. The type of DF had a significant effect on the hardness of the bars. The bars with the addition of DF-Chokeberry were distinguished by significantly greater hardness (Fmax = 438.3 mJ), and P-Hibiscus by significant softness (268.6 mJ). This type of DF turned out to be less useful in the production of bars already at the stage of preparation before baking.

2.3.2. Texture Profile Analysis (TPA) Test

The addition of kale had a statistically significant effect on all parameters of the texture profile (Table 3), but no significant differences were observed in the amount of kale addition. The DF preparations had a significant effect on the parameters of the texture profile, only in the case of elasticity, no such effect was observed (Table 3).

The values of the hardness parameter for the tested bars ranged from 89 to 299 N. The control bars (298.2 N) had the highest hardness value, significantly lower values were achieved in bars with 20 (121.5 N) and 30% (94.6 N) kale addition. Therefore, it can be concluded that the kale bars were more brittle or soft than the base bars. However, the amount of kale added did not significantly affect the hardness of the bars. The results of this parameter were significantly influenced by the type of DF preparation used. The bars with the addition of apple and hibiscus DF had significantly lower hardness values than the bars with the addition of blackcurrant and chokeberry DF.

Elasticity discriminants of the tested bars changed, as did the hardness of bars with and without kale. The addition of kale decreased the value of this parameter. The base bars (without the addition of kale) had an elasticity of 0.54, the bars with 20% addition of kale 0.40, and the bar with 30% addition of 0.383. For bars with the addition of various DF preparations, the values of elasticity were at a similar level (0.40–0.48 N).

Table 3. The effect of kale and fibre preparation on the texture profile of multigrain bars. The bar codes are explained in Table 4.

Type of Bars	Hardness [N]	Elasticity [-]	Cohesiveness [-]	Guminess [N]	Chewing [N]
Control	298.2 ± 25.4 [B]	0.54 ± 0.03 [B]	0.48 ±0.064 [B]	145.0 ± 29.0 [B]	77.0 ± 15.7 [B]
DF-Apple-K20	121.5 ± 16.0 [aA]	0.40 ± 0.03 [A]	0.26 ± 0.021 [aA]	32.2 ± 4.7 [aA]	12.9 ± 1.9 [aA]
DF-Apple-K30	94.6 ± 21.3 [A]	0.38 ± 0.06 [A]	0.40 ± 0.070 [A]	38.4 ± 15.4 [A]	14.4 ± 2.5 [A]
DF-Blackcurrant-K20	171.9 ± 21.4 [b]	0.46 ± 0.02	0.43 ± 0.063 [bc]	75.7 ± 18.8 [b]	35.1 ± 9.5 [b]
DF-Chokeberry-K20	184.4 ± 25.4 [b]	0.48 ± 0.03	0.48 ± 0.021 [c]	88.8 ± 13.6 [b]	44.9 ± 5.8 [b]
P-Hibiscus-K20	89.5 ± 24.8 [a]	0.42 ± 0.02	0.37 ± 0.031 [b]	33.0 ± 9.052 [a]	13.8 ± 3.1 [a]
Factors	\multicolumn{5}{c}{One-way analysis of variance (ANOVA) p-value}				
Kale addition (A,B,C)	0.0000 *	0.0013 *	0.0013 *	0.0000 *	0.0000 *
Type of fibre (a,b,c)	0.0002 *	0.1201	0.0000 *	0.0000 *	0.0000 *

*—means significant difference at a confidence level of 0.05; a, b, c and A, B, C—homogeneous groups, the same letters mean no statistically significant differences between the analysed values of indicators; the codes are described in Table 4.

The addition of kale significantly influenced the cohesiveness. The bars without the addition (base) were characterized by higher cohesiveness than the bars with the addition of kale. The type of DF preparation also had a significant effect. The bars with the addition of apple DF and 20% kale had the lowest cohesiveness values (0.26), the bars with the addition of hibiscus powder (0.37), blackcurrant DF (0.43) and chokeberry DF (0.48) were characterized by higher values.

Guminess significantly depended on the addition of kale. The base bars (without addition) had higher values (145.0 N) than the bars with the addition of kale. The greater addition of kale did not cause any significant changes in the guminess of the bars. The effect of the various DF preparations was also significant. The bars with apple and hibiscus DF were characterized by low values of guminess (about 32 N), while the value of this parameter for bars with the addition of blackcurrant DF (75.7 N) and samples with the addition of chokeberry DF (88.8 N) was significantly higher.

The chewiness of the bars decreased significantly (to about 6 times) in the bars with the addition of kale compared to the control bars, from 77.0 to 12.9 N for bars with 20% additive and 14.4 N with 30% additive. Moreover, bars with apple DF (12.9 N) and hibiscus (13.8 N) were characterized by low chewiness values, significantly higher values were obtained for bars with blackcurrant and chokeberry DF addition.

2.4. The Effect of the Addition of Kale and Fibre Preparation on the Color of the Multigrain Bars

The addition of kale in the amount of 20 and 30% did not significantly affect the brightness of the colour of the bars (Figure 1a). On the other hand, the type of added DF preparation significantly influenced the brightness of the colour of bars. The addition of blackcurrant, chokeberry and hibiscus DF caused a significant darkening of the colour bars. The bars with the addition of apple DF showed up to about 16% higher values of the L* parameter. This dependence may be due to the colour of the DF preparations, apple DF is a light beige powder, while the remaining DF are dark red powders. Dark red discoloration of the preparations may be due to the presence of anthocyanin pigments.

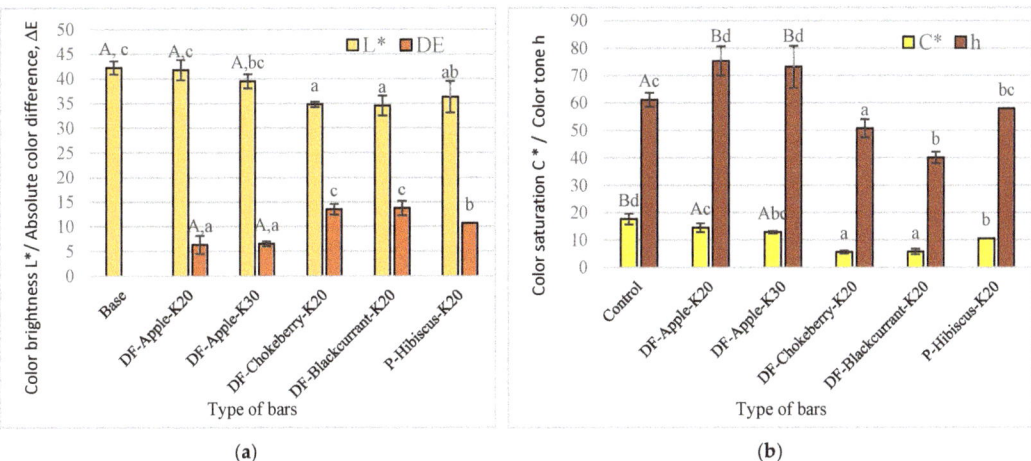

Figure 1. The influence of kale and fibre preparation addition on the colour parameters of multigrain bars: (**a**) Colour brightness L* and absolute colour difference ΔE, (**b**) colour saturation C* and colour tone h. Designation: a, b, c, d—homogeneous groups, the influence of: fibre preparations and A, B—kale at α = 0.05. The bar codes are explained in Table 4.

Table 4. The recipe of multigrain bars based on the weight of all ingredients, with the addition of kale and fibre preparation or powder of dried hibiscus flower.

Ingredient	Content [%]	Code bars
Whole grain oatmeal (Kupiec, Poland)	20	
Flaxeed (Kresto, Russia)	20	
Sunflower seeds (Bakaland, Poland)	20	
Pumpkin seeds (Bakaland, Poland)	20	
Fresh kale (VitalFresh, Poland)	20 or 30	K20 or K30
Honey (Huzar, Poland)	10	
Water (tap water)	25	
m-40 * apple fibre;	10	DF-Apple
m-40 * chokeberry fibre;	10	DF-Chokeberry
m-40 * blackcurrant fibre	10	DF-Blackcurrant
Dried hibiscus flower—powder (GreenField, Poland)	10	P-Hibiscus

* Coarse fibre, particle size approx. 40 μm.

To evaluate the effect of the addition of kale and DF preparation on the colour changes of the bars, the absolute colour difference ΔE was calculated, and the colour of the control bars was set as a standard. The colour of the bars was clearly differentiated, because the absolute colour difference ranged from 6.3–13.7 (Figures 1a and 2), from the colour of the bars with apple DF to those with blackcurrant and chokeberry DF.

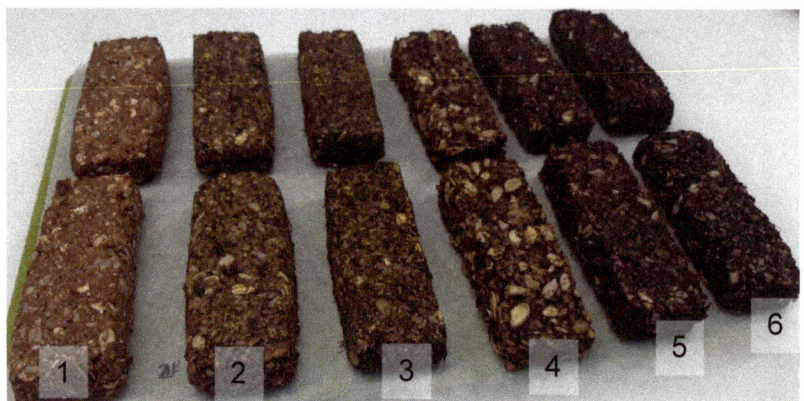

Figure 2. Pictures of baked bars, respectively: 1—base (Control), 2—with apple fibre and 20% kale, 3—with apple fibre and 30% kale, 4—with hibiscus fibre and 20% kale, 5—with fibre from blackcurrant and 20% kale, 6—with chokeberry fibre and 20% kale.

The higher colour saturation is perceived by consumers as the more "alive", while the lower the colour saturation, the more muffled it is, the closer to grey [23]. The values of the C* parameter in the bars tested ranged from 5 to 18% (Figure 1b). The base bars (approx. 17.5%) had higher values of the C* parameter, while the lower values of the bars with the addition of blackcurrant DF and chokeberry (approx. 5.5%). The addition of kale to the recipe significantly influenced the saturation of the colour of the bars, bars without the addition of kale had significantly higher values of the C* parameter than bars with the addition of 20 or 30% kale. The type of DF preparation used also significantly influenced the colour saturation. Bars with the addition of chokeberry and currant DF were characterized by the lowest values, significantly higher values were found for bars with the addition of hibiscus, while the most "vivid" colour was characterized by the bars with the addition of apple DF.

The colour hue of h bars was also analysed, which informs how much a given colour differs from white [23]. All tested bars had the h parameter in the range of 40–75°, which corresponds to the range of colours from red to yellow. Low h values were characteristic for bars with the addition of chokeberry DF (approx. 40°), higher bars with the addition of blackcurrant DF (approx. 50°) and bars with the addition of hibiscus (approx. 57°). The bars with the addition of apple DF had the highest colour shade values. The type of DF preparation used had a significant effect on the colour shade. The amount of kale addition used in the bar recipe was not significant. On the other hand, the addition of kale (20 and 30%) resulted in significantly higher h values than in bars without this additive.

2.5. The Effect of the Addition of Kale and Fibre on the Antioxidant Content of Multigrain Bars

The addition of kale significantly (Figure 3a) increased the antioxidant activity from 23.6 mM Trol/g d.m. for base bars without kale addition to 29.3 mM Trol/g d.m. for bars with 30% addition of kale. Bars with a 20% addition of kale and chokeberry DF (43.2 mM Trol/g d.m.) were characterized by high antioxidant activity, the value in these bars was nearly two times higher than in the based bars. It can be assumed that the DF preparation had a significant effect on this index.

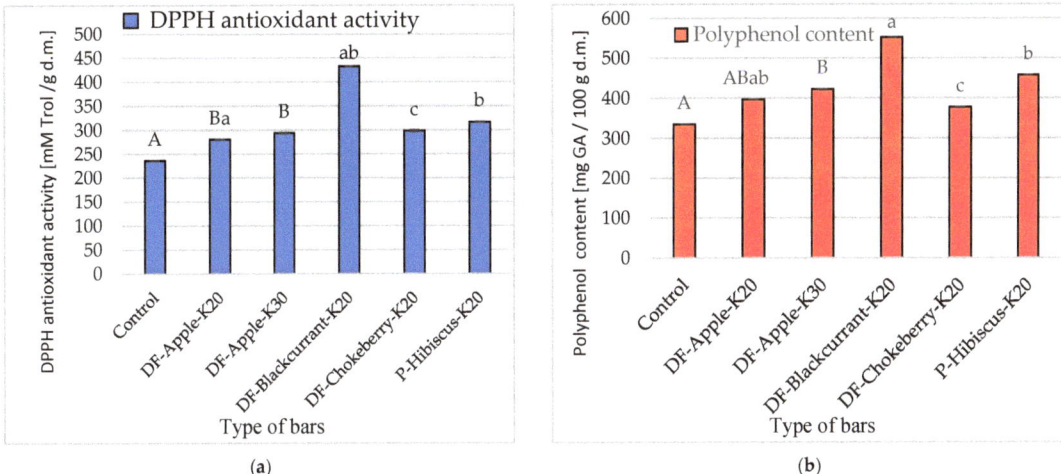

Figure 3. The influence of the kale (factor I) and fibre preparations (factor II) addition in multigrain bars on the: (**a**)—DPPH antioxidant activity [mM Trol/ g d.m.] and (**b**)—polyphenol content [mg GA/100 g d.m.]. Designations: A, B—homogeneous groups (factor I), and a, b, c—(factor II) at α = 0.05. The bar codes are explained in Table 4.

In the study by Korus [21], the antioxidant activity of kale was at the level of 14.7–23.7 µM Trol/g, so lower than in the bars tested. In terms of dry matter content, the results would be more similar. Moreover, the values of this indicator depend on many factors related to both the preparation of the product and the method of determination [24]. Due to the large number of different compounds influencing the antioxidant activity (soluble in water or organic solvents), the obtained results may depend on the method of preparation of the extract. The bars enriched with chokeberry DF had the highest value of polyphenol content (Figure 3b), i.e., about 552.5 mg GA/100 g d.m., significantly lower bars with the addition of hibiscus powder, about 457.5 mg GA/100 g d.m. For bars with the addition of blackcurrant DF and bars with the addition of apple DF, this value was in the range 377–396 mg GA/100 g d.m.

Korus [21] showed a high content of polyphenols in kale, at the level of 256–531 mg/100 g of fresh weight. Such a large range is influenced by the variety, growing conditions and maturity. This vegetable is therefore a very valuable source of these compounds, which are largely preserved in the bars.

Green vegetables are rich in chlorophyll and often contain carotenoids, the colour of which is not always discernible due to the predominant chlorophyll. In fresh kale tested by Korus [21], the total content of chlorophyll was 81–165 mg/100 g and carotenoids 16.8–34.2 mg/100 g. The control bars were characterized by a low content of chlorophyll (approx. 5.0 mg/100 g d.m.) and carotenoids (0.14 mg/100 g d.m.), and the addition of kale caused a 3–5 fold increase in chlorophyll content and 23–34 fold in carotenoids content (Figure 4a,b). This content increased with the increase in the percentage share of kale in the recipe. The DF preparations did not cause significant changes in the chlorophyll content in the bars. On the other hand, the content of carotenoids was significantly different, depending on the type of DF in the bar recipe (Figure 4b). The bars with the addition of blackcurrant DF contained significantly less (approx. 2.4 mg/100 g d.m.) carotenoids than the bars with the addition of chokeberry DF (approx. 4.1 mg/100 g d.m.).

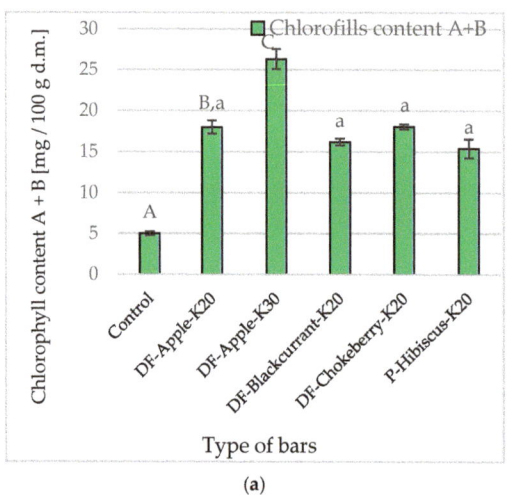
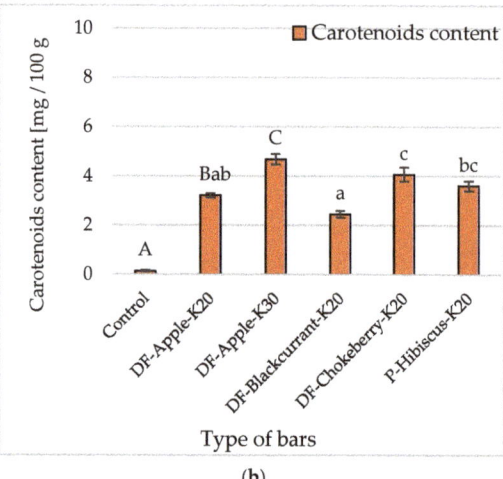

Figure 4. The influence of the kale (factor I) and fibre preparations (factor II) addition in multigrain bars on the: (**a**)—chlorophyll content A + B [mg/100 g d.m.] and (**b**)—carotenoids content [mg/100 g d.m.]. Designations: A, B, C—homogeneous groups (factor I), and a, b, c—(factor II) at $\alpha = 0.05$. The bar codes are explained in Table 4.

2.6. The Effect of the Addition of Kale and Fibre on the Sensory Quality of the Multigrain Bars

The bars were positively assessed by potential consumers (Figure 5). Within the five sensory discriminants on a 10-point scale, apart from the overall quality of the chokeberry DF bars, all bars scored higher than 5.0, but not higher than 7.3 points. Most of the lower scores were given to bars with the addition of chokeberry DF (from 4.8 to 6.4 points). Most of the higher ratings were given to bars with P-Hibiscus, especially for texture and overall quality.

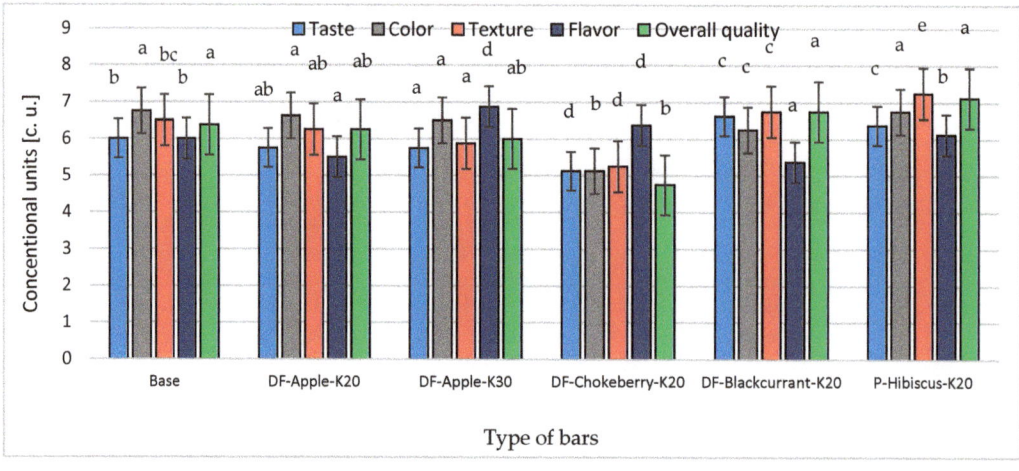

Figure 5. The effect of kale and fibre preparation or powder of dried hibiscus flower addition on sensory properties of multigrain bars. Designations: a, b, c, d, e—homogeneous groups (the influence of type of bars) at $\alpha = 0.05$. The bar codes are explained in Table 4.

3. Discussion

Currently, the daily intake of DF by most consumers is too low. This is due to the high degree of processing of many products. DF is supplied mainly from cereals and cereal products, seeds of legumes and fruits and vegetables. These products differ not only in their DF content, but also in the type of DF compounds. They are found in vegetables and cereals are grouped into water-soluble (pectins, gums) and water-insoluble (cellulose, lignin, some of the hemicellulose) [25]. All bars contained fibre at the level above 9% (Table 1), which allows them to be classified as products with a high fibre content. Bars tested by Márquez-Villacorta and Vásquez [26] with a composition of 4.12% oat bran; 10.04% of pineapple peel powder and 17.18% of quinoa flakes contained more DF (13.28%) and protein (11.37%), and the overall acceptance score was slightly higher (7.47 points). Epidemiological studies suggest that regular consumption of fruits and vegetables containing both DF and natural antioxidant compounds may reduce the risk of many chronic diseases [27,28]. The current diet also focuses on the caloric content of food. Vatankhah et al. [29] investigated the suitability of stevioside, a natural low calorie sweetener, as a replacement for sucrose in Iranian sweet bread. They showed that the replacement of sucrose in the amount of 50%, the physical, chemical and sensory properties of the bread were similar to the base product, but the calorific value was reduced by 11%. Ibrahim et al. [30] assessed the possibilities of using date fruit in the bar recipe and replacing honey with date paste. With regard to the use of date paste up to 70%, bars with a share of 50% were characterized by the highest overall acceptability.

Due to their sensory value, wide availability and convenience, snacks are popular and frequently consumed products [31]. Consumers like snacks very much, but also pay increasingly attention to what they eat and are aware of the issue of healthy eating. The current market trends force the food industry to introduce such products that can be part of a healthy and balanced diet, but also tasty and encouraging consumption [32].

Depending on the composition, various methods are used for the production of snacks, which can generally be divided into the so-called "cold" and "hot", respectively, without and with the use of increased temperature. The use of baking has benefits in terms of quality and product safety without the use of chemicals. During baking, starch gelatinization, browning reactions, changes in structure, surface properties and other mechanical behaviour of the bakery products occur [29], and the formation of their characteristic sensory properties. Based on the composition of the bars, they may be classified as snack bakery products. An additional advantage of choosing this method of producing bars was obtaining relatively soft products, such as bread. In order to increase the content of natural ingredients in multi-grain (wholegrain oatmeal, sunflower seeds, pumpkin seeds, flaxseed) bars, kale and DF were added to increase the high health-promoting potential of the bars, without chemicals. The taste of fresh kale does not encourage consumption, so an attempt was made to mask it. As a result, in the sensory evaluation, the addition of kale was less significant than the type of fibre. The addition of chokeberry to the fibre preparation was the least acceptable for most indications (4.8–5.2 points), but its flavour was distinguished (6.4 points).

The water activity (Aw) in the bars was high (0.857–0.953), but when analysing bars with the addition of 20% kale, all Aw were below 0.95. No pathogenic microorganisms develop in such a product. Many bakery products are characterized by higher water activity [33]. The shelf life of the bars is short. To retain all the value of the snacks and extend their freshness, for example, modified atmosphere packaging should be used. Water is an essential ingredient in many foods. Affects a number of processes and reactions that can reflect the quality and stability of food during storage. Whether certain reactions will occur is primarily determined by the state of the water, which is characterized by its activity [34]. From the point of view of water activity, food can be divided into [35] wet with water activity in the range of 0.90–1.00, medium water content—water activity in the range of 0.55–0.90 and low water content—water activity in the range 0.00–0.55.

In general, a stable food is considered the one with a water activity in the range of 0.07–0.35. However, the development of microorganisms is almost completely limited already at the water activity below 0.60 [36].

With the increase in the share of kale in the recipe, the water content in the bars increased. This was due to the increase in the water content in the bar recipe, which was caused by the addition of kale containing about 85% water [6]. This form of kale addition was justified by the possibility of enriching the bars. However, from the technological point of view, the addition of kale in the amount of 20% was sufficient. The type of DF preparation significantly influenced the water content in the tested bars (Table 2). The water content in bars with the addition of currant and chokeberry DF was the lowest (about 27%), while the bars with the addition of hibiscus preparation (about 35%) had a significantly higher water content. This may indicate the different sorption properties of the DF preparations used. According to Miastowski et al. [36], water binding is one of the most important features of DF preparation. However, their large diversity in terms of the presence of DF compounds, depending on the source of origin, has a large impact on the degree of water binding in bars. This property also depends on the degree of micronization and the particle size composition. Therefore, the use of various preparations resulted in different values of water activity. This is advantageous in the manufacture of bars that should have the desired texture.

The water content has influenced the mechanical properties of bars. The correlation coefficient for the water content and compression force was about -0.92 ($p = 0.0098$), and for the compression work -0.94 ($p = 0.0053$). This proves a strong negative correlation between these properties and the water content.

The TPA test is used to test the texture of food based on indicators that reflect the consumer's perception of the chewing experience [37]. For multigrain bars about 2 cm thick, softness is required and those up to about 1 cm thick can be crunchy. In the case of thin ones, especially those with increased carbohydrate content, one should aim to obtain a glassy (amorphous) state. The structure of the bars is influenced by the method of their production, especially the temperature value. In the research by Nikmaram et al. [38], the optimal conditions for the production of extrudates depended on the amount of sesame seeds added and the temperature of the process. The addition of kale and DF preparations had a statistically significant effect on the parameters of the texture profile. The higher content of sesame seed, incorporated into corn expanded extrudates, increased the hardness of the extrudates, possibly due to the content of fat, protein and fibre [38]. Similarly relationships Kowalczewski and Ivanišová [39] showed that the addition of fruit to the muffin recipe had a significant impact on the parameters of the texture profile. According to Wójtowicz and Baltyn [40], the hardness of snacks should be as low as possible, as it proves the fragility of these products. In the study by Kubiak and Dolik [41], the result for apples was 62.02 N, Wójtowicz and Balatyn [40], potato pancakes were characterized by a hardness in the range of 102–106 N, while in Heo et al. [42] muffins enriched with DF were characterized by a hardness of 412–491 N. In the research by Kubiak and Dolik [41], the bread was characterized by elasticity at the level of 0.94. The tested bars were characterized by almost two times lower elasticity. This may indicate their compact structure.

In a properly functioning organism, it is necessary to ensure a balance in so-called redox processes. If reactive oxygen species are not effectively quenched, it may lead to oxidative stress [39]. To prevent the formation and protect the body against reactive oxygen species, one should eat food rich in antioxidant compounds [43]. Polyphenols are compounds synthesized by plants. Several thousand compounds belong to the group of phenol compounds, but they all have one thing in common, which is the antioxidant properties. The content of polyphenols was strongly and positively correlated with the antioxidant activity ($r = 0.92$). The use of kale addition caused changes in the content of polyphenolic compounds (Figure 3b). In the case of 30% addition of kale (422 mg GA /100 g d.m.), the content of polyphenols was significantly higher than for bars without addition (334.6 mg GA/100 g d.m.). The amount of polyphenolic compounds largely depended on the DF preparation used. The bars enriched with chokeberry DF had the highest value, i.e., about 552 mg GA/100 g d.m. In the study by Nawirska et al. [44], chokeberry pomace was also characterized by the highest polyphenol content among the tested fruits, and significantly lower values were obtained for blackcurrant. Biegańska-Marecik et al. [45] showed that kale has one of the highest values of antioxidant activity. The addition of frozen and freeze-dried kale on beverages based on apple juice resulted in a two- and three-fold increase in antioxidant activity, respectively. Murugesan et al. [1] showed that the antioxidant capacity of kale leaf ethanol extract was 62.9% (DPPH*), and GC-MS chromatographic analysis included profiles of more than 17 major phytochemicals in the extract. Additionally, Satheesh et al. [46] reported that there has been a growing trend in recent times to include more green leafy vegetables in the human diet, and kale has great potential for use in a variety of food and nutritional applications. Kale has been shown to have the nutritional and anti-nutritional components of kale, with research showing its multiple health benefits.

The anthocyanin pigments present in the bars had a positive effect on the antioxidant activity, but they could cause colour changes of the product. Colour is a parameter that has a large impact on the perception of food by consumers, as it can reflect the quality of food products. According to Kowalczewski and Ivanišová [39], these changes may not be accepted by consumers for some products. Moreover, in the case of bars, it can be noticed that the addition of chokeberry DF preparation, which had a positive effect on the content of polyphenols, translated into high oxidative activity and caused colour changes (Figure 1a,b). In addition, the bars were darker because the L* values were lower (Figure 1a). However, no significant differences were observed in consumer assessments regarding the colour of the bars (Figure 5).

Carotenoids and chlorophylls are plant pigments that give colour to vegetables and fruits, they are located in chloroplasts. Carotenoids are responsible for the red, orange and yellow colours. They are considered one of the strongest antioxidants and are credited with the ability to extinguish free radicals. They are also precursors of vitamin A. Chlorophylls are credited with bacteriostatic and anti-inflammatory properties, supporting the removal of carcinogenic toxins and with antioxidant properties. They give plants and products a characteristic green colour [47].

According to Karwowska et al. [47], fresh kale is characterized by the content of chlorophyll A and B at the level of 904.5 mg/100 g d.m. Kale added to the recipe increased the content of chlorophyll in the bars. This content increased with the increase in the percentage share of kale in the recipe. The addition of kale in the amount of 20 and 30% resulted in a 3.6 and 5.3-fold increase in their chlorophyll content, respectively, in comparison with the control samples (approx. 5.0 mg/100 g d.m.). The DF preparations of blackcurrant, chokeberry and hibiscus did not cause significant changes in the chlorophyll content in the bars. However, in the bars with the addition of chokeberry and hibiscus DF, the content of chlorophyll was lower by 10–14% than for those with chokeberry DF.

The addition of kale enriched bars with carotenoids. As in the case of chlorophyll, the addition of kale caused a greater increase in the carotenoid content. The bars with 20% additive (3.2 mg/100 g d.m.) contained about 23 times more dye than the base bars (0.136 mg/100 g d.m.). Bars with more kale contained the most carotenoids (4.7 mg/100 g d.m.). According to Karwowska et al. [47], it contains carotenoids in the amount of about 175 mg/100 g d.m. The effect of the DF preparation used on the content of dyes was also observed. The bars with the addition of blackcurrent DF contained significantly less carotenoids than the bars with the addition of chokeberry DF. Aronia contains 140–230 mg of carotenoids per 100 g of d.m., while blackcurrant only 20–40 mg/100 g of d.m. [48]. This translated into the final content of these dyes in the baked bars.

4. Materials and Methods

4.1. Material

The materials for the research were multi-grain bars with the addition of fresh kale prepared according to the established recipe (Table 4). The type of DF added and the percentage of fresh kale (*Brassica oleracea* L. var. *acephala*) added was variable in the recipe. The raw materials were purchased in a large-area store, while the DF preparations were obtained directly from the producer (GreenField, Poland).

4.2. Experimental Procedure

4.2.1. Preparation of BARS

The dry ingredients were ground in a grinder (Bosch MKM6000) for 20 s. Ground flaxseed was poured over with hot water to gel. The kale was ground in a Thermomix TM 31 device (Vorwerk Ltd., Wroclaw, Poland) for 10 s, speed of rotation—level 7. Then, all ingredients were combined and mixed for about 2 min. After receiving the mass, it was placed in rectangular form with dimensions of 100 × 40 × 20 mm. The formed bars were baked or dried in three different variants.

4.2.2. Baking

Baking was carried out in an electric Piccolo oven (Winkler Wachtel Ltd., Wroclaw, Poland) for 25 min. The temperature of the lower and upper chamber of the furnace was 180 °C.

4.3. Analytical Methods

4.3.1. Determination of Dry Matter Content

The dry matter content of the bars was determined by drying in a laboratory dryer (WAMED SUP-65 WG, Warsaw, Poland) at 130 °C for 1 h. The vessels with/without samples were weighed on an analytical balance (ME54E/M, Metler, Warsaw, Poland) with an accuracy of 0.001 g. The measurement was performed in duplicate.

4.3.2. Determination of Water Activity

Water activity was determined with an AQUALAB CX-2 device (Decagon Devices Inc. Pullman, WA, USA). Measurements were carried out at the temperature of 23 ± 1 °C. The measurement was performed in duplicate, the final result was the mean of the measurements.

4.3.3. Colour Parameters

The colour of the bars was measured with the Konica Minolta CR-300 colorimeter (standard observer CIE 2°, illuminat D65, measuring gap 8 mm) in the CIE Lab system. The measurement was performed in 5 replications. The mean of the measurements was taken as the result.

4.3.4. Examination of Bars Structure

Compression Test

The mechanical properties were tested in a TA-HD plus texturometer (Stable Micro Systems, Godalming, UK). The compression test was performed with a 75 mm diameter head. Bars with dimensions of 25 × 40 × 20 mm were used for the measurement. The head speed was 1 mm/s. The samples were compressed to 50% of their height. The measurement was performed in 10 replications. The compression test was performed for the bars 4 h after the end of drying or baking. On the basis of the test, the compression work calculated as the product of the half of the area under the deformation curve and the head travel speed were determined.

Texture Profile Analysis (TPA) Test

The texture profile test was performed with a TA-HD plus texturometer (Stable Micro Systems, Godalming, UK). The measurement was performed 4 h after the end of drying or baking. Bars with dimensions of $25 \times 40 \times 20$ mm were used for the measurement. The tested samples were compressed twice to about 50% of the original height. The head speed was 1 mm/s. The measurement was performed in 10 replications. On the basis of the test, the mechanical determinants of texture, such as hardness, elasticity, cohesiveness, gumminess, and chewiness, were determined as follows:

- Hardness—the maximum value of the force used during the test [N];
- Elasticity—the ratio of the compression time in the second cycle to the compression time in the first test cycle;
- Cohesiveness (compressibility)—the ratio of the compression work in the second cycle to the compression work in the first cycle;
- Gumminess—the product of hardness and cohesiveness [N];
- Chewiness—product of gumminess and elasticity [N].

4.3.5. Chemical Determinations

Chemical determinations were carried out in an accredited laboratory at the Institute of Agriculture and Food Biotechnology—State Research Institute in Warsaw, Poland. All determinations were performed at least in duplicate.

Nutritional Value

Determination of the nutritional value, i.e., protein, fat, ash, DF and carbohydrates, was carried out in the accredited laboratory of the Institute of Agricultural and Food Biotechnology—National Research Institute in Warsaw Poland. All determinations were performed at least twice.

Determination of Protein Content

Total nitrogen content was determined by the reference titration method (Kjeldahl) and converted into total protein content, taking into account the nitrogen to protein conversion factor 6.25 according to PN-EN ISO 20483: 2014 standard.

The principle of the method consists in converting organic nitrogen compounds contained in a dry sample of ammonium sulphate with concentrated sulfuric acid in the presence of a catalyst, basifying the solution, distilling and titrating ammonia bound in boric acid with the addition of indicators with sulfuric acid.

Determination of Fat Content

The fat content was determined in accordance with the PN-A-79011-4: 1998 standard. The principle of the method is based on the extraction of fat from a dry sample under predefined conditions using petroleum ether by means of a Soxhlet apparatus, and then weighing the residue of the sample after complete evaporation of the solvent.

Determination of Ash Content

The ash content was determined by the gravimetric method after the samples were incinerated according to the PN-EN ISO 2171: 2010 standard. The principle of the method is based on incineration of the dry sample (pre-dried) at the temperature of 900 °C and determination of the inorganic residues after ashing by weight.

Determination of Total Dietary Fibre Content

The total dietary DF content, including the soluble and insoluble fractions was determined by the gravimetric method after prior enzymatic hydrolysis of the samples using the Megazyme Total Dietary Fibre Kit (Bray, Bray Business Park, Co. Wicklow, A98 YV29, Ireland).

Calculation of Carbohydrates Content, Including Sugars

The carbohydrate content (CC) in g/100 g d.m. was calculated from the formula:

$$CC = 100 - (H + A + F + P + DF) \quad (1)$$

where:

H—humidity of the sample, [g/100 g d.m];
A—ash content of the sample, [g/100 g d.m];
F—fat content of the sample, [g/100 g d.m];
P—protein content of the sample, [g/100 g d.m];
DF—dietary fibre content of the sample, [g/100 g d.m].

Determination of the content of individual sugars, including: fructose, glucose, disaccharides (sum of sucrose and maltose) was performed using high performance liquid chromatography (HPLC) with refractometric detection of sugars contained in the aqueous solution obtained from the sample. The result of the sugar content was given as the sum of individual sugars [g/100 g d.m.].

Calculation of Energy Value

The energy value (EV) of the product (bars) was calculated on the basis of the energy content of protein (1 g = 4 kcal or 17 kJ), carbohydrates (1 g = 4 kcal or 17 kJ), fat (1 g = 9 kcal or 37 kJ) and dietary fibre (1 g = 2 kcal or 8 kJ) contained in them. The energy value in kcal/100 g and kJ/100 g of product was calculated [49]:

$$EV \; [kcal/100 \; g] = (P + CC) \cdot 4 + F \cdot 9 + DF \cdot 2 \quad (2)$$

$$EV \; [kJ/100 \; g] = (P + CC) \cdot 7 + F \cdot 37 + DF \cdot 8 \quad (3)$$

where:

P—protein content of the sample [g/100 g];
CC—carbohydrates content of the sample [g/100 g];
F—fat content of the sample [g/100 g];
DF—dietary fibre content of the sample [g/100 g].

Determination of DPPH Radical Scavenging Activity

The antioxidant activity (AA) was determined using the spectrophotometric method with the DPPH radical based on the method of Urbańska at el. [50] and Wong at el. [51]. For the preparation of samples, 2.4 mL of DPPH methanolic radical solution (60 µM) was used and 100 µL of acetone extract of the samples (the extract was prepared in the same way as for the determination of carotenoids/chlorophylls) was added. The samples were mixed and incubated at room temperature for 30 min in the dark. After this time, the absorbance was measured at the wavelength λ = 515 nm against the blank. The acetone solution and DPPH solution were collected for the control sample. The blank was a sample containing of methanol and of 80% acetone.

The antioxidant activity (quenching/scavenging capacity) of the DPPH radical (% inhibition) was calculated:

$$\%inhibition = \frac{A_0 - A_1}{A_0} \cdot 100 \quad (4)$$

where:

A_1—absorbance of the DPPH radical with acetone extract from the sample;
A_0—absorbance of the DPPH radical with acetone (control sample).

When the calculated inhibition was greater than the 95% value, the sample was diluted with 80% (v/v) acetone solution so that the absorbance value was linear over the range of the analysed concentrations.

The antioxidant activity (AA) based on the DPPH free radical scavenging ability of the extract was expressed as mM Trolox per 1 g of dry matter (d.m.) of the sample.

Determination of Total Polyphenol Content by the Folin–Ciocaletau Method

The total polyphenol content was determined by spectrophotometric method with the use of the Folin–Ciocaleteu reagent, which consisted of a coloured reaction of polyphenolic compounds with this reagent [50]. To the test tube was added 15% sodium carbonate (0.5 mL), distilled water (8.9 mL), acetone extract of the sample (0.5 mL; the extract was obtained in the same way as for the determination of carotenoids/chlorophylls, chapter 3.3.6), and 100 µL of Folin–Ciocalteu reagent. The sample was then mixed and incubated for 45 min in the dark (room temperature). After this time, the absorbance was measured at the wavelength λ = 765 nm against the blank. When the measured absorbance of the sample was greater than 0.650 value, the sample was diluted with 80% (v/v) acetone solution. The determination was performed in duplicate. The content of total polyphenols was expressed as mg of gallic acid (GA) per 100 g dry matter (d.m.) of the sample.

Determination of Carotenoids and Chlorophyll A and B Content

Determination of carotenoids and chlorophyll content in the bar samples was performed using the BECKMAN DU-530 spectrophotometer (Beckman, UK). The samples were milled with a Sencor grinder to obtain the extract. An 80% (v/v) acetone solution (25 mL) was added to the weighed sample (about 1.0 g). The samples were homogenized for 30 s at a speed of 13,500 rpm in an ULTRA-TURRAX T25 basic homogenizer (IKA-WERKE, Germany). Then, the obtained homogenate was centrifuged in a laboratory centrifuge MPW 375 (MPW-Med-Instruments, Poland) for 3 min at a speed of 10,000 rpm. The measurements were made for chlorophyll A at wavelengths λ = 663 nm, for chlorophyll B λ = 647 nm, and at λ = 470 nm for carotenoids with the blank, which was an 80% (v/v) acetone solution. When the measured absorbance of the sample was greater than 0.900 in value, the sample was diluted with an 80% (v/v) acetone solution. The determination was performed in duplicate. The content of carotenoid pigments, chlorophyll A and B in the acetone extract was calculated from the equations [52]:

$$C_C = \frac{1000 \cdot A_{470} - 1.82 \cdot C_A - 85.02 \cdot C_B}{198} \tag{5}$$

$$C_A = 12.25 \cdot A_{663} - 2.79 \cdot A_{647} \tag{6}$$

$$C_B = 21.50 \cdot A_{647} - 5.10 \cdot A_{663} \tag{7}$$

$$C_{A+B} = 7.15 \cdot A_{663} + 18.71 \cdot A_{467} \tag{8}$$

where:

C_C—content of carotenoids in acetone extract [µg/mL];
C_A—content of chlorophyll A in acetone extract [µg/mL];
C_B—content of chlorophyll B in the acetone extract [µg/mL];
C_{A+B}—content of chlorophyll (total A + B) in the acetone extract [µg/mL];
A_{663}—absorbance of acetone extract measured at wavelength λ = 663 nm;
A_{647}—absorbance of acetone extract measured at a wavelength of λ = 647 nm;
A_{470}—absorbance of acetone extract measured at wavelength λ = 470 nm.

The content of chlorophyll or carotenoid dyes in the sample was calculated in mg per 100 g dry matter (d.m.). All determinations were performed at least in duplicate.

Sensory Evaluation

The sensory evaluation was performed by a team of 30 unqualified people, aged 18 to 45, using a 10-point scale. The evaluators were instructed on how to evaluate the selected discriminants such as taste, colour, smell, texture, and overall desirability (Table 5).

Table 5. Quality features to be assessed and their characteristics.

Sensory Discriminants	Definition	Boundary Terms
Colour	Bar colour (colouring)	10 points—desirable, even 0 points—undesirable, uneven surface colouring
Smell	Intensity of perceived smell	10 points—characteristic for cereal snacks, mild 0 points—imperceptible, atypical
Texture	Fragility and porosity	10 points—desirable, brittle, porous 0 points—undesirable, non-brittle, non-porous, too cohesive
Taste	Taste felt after biting and chewing	10 points—characteristics of cereal snacks 0 points—imperceptible, alien
General suitability	General impression of the quality of the bars	10 points—very desirable 0 points—unacceptable

4.4. Statistical Analysis

The statistical analysis of the obtained results was performed with the use of Microsoft Excel and STATISTICA 13 PL programs. To determine the effect of the amount of curly kale and the addition of DF on the selected indicators, a one- or two-factor analysis of variance and Tukey's HSD test were performed to determine homogeneous groups (post hoc test). Pearson's correlation was also performed to investigate the relationship between the selected indicators.

5. Conclusions

The addition of kale and DF preparations had a beneficial effect on the physicochemical, sensory and pro-healthy properties of snacks. In the production of bars, DF also played a technological role, enabling the appropriate consistency of the mix before baking and the texture of the final products. Multigrain raw materials are characterized by a high content of DF. Multigrain bars with the addition of kale and DF preparations can be a valuable source of both DF fractions, antioxidant compounds, as well as fat, protein, vitamins and minerals. They can be an offer of snacks for people struggling with health problems, as well as for healthy people who are looking for tasty and valuable products.

Author Contributions: Conceptualization, H.K., A.Z. and A.I.; methodology, H.K., A.S. and J.K.; software, H.K. and A.I.; validation, H.K., J.K., E.D., S.G., A.C. and A.S.; formal analysis, H.K., J.K., S.G. and A.M.; investigation, A.Z. and E.M.; resources, A.Z.; data curation, H.K. and E.M.; writing—original draft preparation, H.K., A.C. and A.I.; writing—review and editing, J.K., A.M., E.D., A.I. and E.M.; visualization, E.M.; supervision, H.K.; funding acquisition, H.K. All authors have read and agreed to the published version of the manuscript.

Funding: This research was financed under the Warsaw University of Life Sciences (WULS) Support System (decision No. SMPB 7/2020).

Institutional Review Board Statement: Not applicable.

Informed Consent Statement: Not applicable.

Data Availability Statement: Not applicable.

Conflicts of Interest: The authors declare no conflict of interest.

Sample Availability: Samples are available from the corresponding author.

References

1. Murugesan, K.; Mulugeta, K.; Hailu, E.; Tamene, W.; Yadav, S.A. Insights for integrative medicinal potentials of Ethiopian Kale (*Brassica carinata*): Investigation of antibacterial, antioxidant potential and phytocompounds composition of its leaves. *Chin. Herb. Med.* **2021**, *13*, 250–254. [CrossRef]
2. Sun, B.; Liu, N.; Zhao, Y.; Yan, H.; Wang, Q. Variation of glucosinolates in three edible parts of Chinese kale (*Brassica alboglabra* Bailey) varieties. *Food Chem.* **2011**, *124*, 941–947. [CrossRef]
3. Asakage, M.; Tsuno, N.H.; Kitayama, J.; Tsuchiya, T.; Yoneyama, S.; Yamada, J.; Okaji, Y.; Kaisaki, S.; Osada, T.; Takahashi, K.; et al. Sulforaphane induces inhibition of human umbilical vein endothelial cells proliferation by apoptosis. *Angiogenesis* **2006**, *9*, 83–91. [CrossRef] [PubMed]
4. Flaczyk, E.; Przeor, M.; Kobus-Cisowska, J.; Biegańska-Marecik, R. Assessment of the sensory quality of new kale dishes (*Brassica Oleracea*). *Bromatol. Toxicol. Chem.* **2014**, *47*, 392–396.
5. Korus, A. Changes in the content of minerals, B-group vitamins and tocopherols in processed kale leaves. *J. Food Compos. Anal.* **2020**, *89*, 103464. [CrossRef]
6. Bąk-Sypień, I.I.; Karmańska, A.; Kubiak, K.; Karwowski, B.T. Antioxidant activity of fresh and thermal processed green and red cultivares of curly kale (*Brassica oleracea* L.). *Bromatol. Toxicol. Chem.* **2017**, *50*, 246–251. (In Polish)
7. Son, Y.-J.; Park, J.-E.; Kim, J.; Yoo, G.; Lee, T.-S.; Nho, C.W. Production of low potassium kale with increased glucosinolate content from vertical farming as a novel dietary option for renal dysfunction patients. *Food Chem.* **2021**, *339*, 128092. [CrossRef]
8. Rose, P.; Huang, Q.; Ong, C.N.; Whiteman, M. Broccoli and watercress suppress matrix metalloproteinase-9 activity and invasiveness of human MDA-MB-231 breast cancer cells. *Toxicol. Appl. Pharmacol.* **2005**, *209*, 105–113. [CrossRef]
9. Szwejda-Grzybowska, J. Anticarcinogenic components of cruciferous vegetables and their importance in the prevention of neoplastic diseases. *Bromatol. Toxicol. Chem.* **2011**, *4*, 1039–1046. (In Polish)
10. Michalak, M.; Szwajgier, D.; Paduch, R.; Kukula-Koch, W.; Waśko, A.; Polak-Berecka, M. Fermented curly kale as a new source of gentisic and salicylic acids with antitumor potential. *J. Funct. Foods* **2020**, *67*, 103866. [CrossRef]
11. Mazzeo, T.; N'Dri, D.; Chiavaro, E.; Visconti, A.; Fogliano, V.; Pellegrini, N. Effect of two cooking procedures on phytochemical compounds, total antioxidant capacity and colour of selected frozen vegetables. *Food Chem.* **2011**, *128*, 627–633. [CrossRef]
12. Godula, K.; Czerniejewska-Surma, K.; Dmytrów, I.; Plust, D.; Surma, O. Possible applications of dietary fibre in functional food production. *Food Sci. Technol. Qual.* **2019**, *2*, 5–17. [CrossRef]
13. Rana, V.; Bachheti, R.K.; Chand, T.; Barman, A. Dietary fibre and human health. *Int. J. Food Saf. Nutr. Public Health* **2011**, *4*, 101. [CrossRef]
14. Yangilar, F. The application of dietary fibre in food industry: Structural features, effects on health and definitione, obtaining and analysis of dietary fibre: A review. *J. Food Nutr. Res.* **2013**, *1*, 13–23. [CrossRef]
15. Figuerola, F.; Hurtado, M.L.; Estévez, A.M.; Chiffelle, I.; Asenjo, F. Fibre concentrates from apple pomace and citrus peel as potential fibre sources for food enrichment. *Food Chem.* **2005**, *91*, 395–401. [CrossRef]
16. Górecka, D.; Anioła, J.; Dziedzic, K.; Ławniczak, P. Impact of particle size reduction degree of micronized high-fibre preparations on their selected functional properties. *Food Sci. Technol. Qual.* **2008**, *3*, 89–95. (In Polish)
17. Wojtasik, A.; Pietraś, E.; Kunachowicz, H. Dietary fiber. In *Nutrition Standards for the Polish Population and Their Application*; Jarosz, M., Rychlik, E., Charzewska, J., Eds.; Food and Nutrition Institute: Warsaw, Poland, 2020; pp. 148–170. Available online: https://www.pzh.gov.pl/wp-content/uploads/2020/12/Normy_zywienia_2020web-1.pdf (accessed on 17 June 2021). (In Polish)
18. Regulation (EC) No 1924/2006 of the European Parliament and of the Council of 20 December 2006 on Nutrition and Health Claims Made on Foods. 2006R1924—EN—13.12.2014—004.001. ANNEX: Nutrition Claims and Conditions Applying to Them. Available online: https://eur-lex.europa.eu/legal-content/en/ALL/?uri=CELEX%3A32006R1924 (accessed on 31 January 2021).
19. Commission Regulation (EU) No 1047/2012 of 8 November 2012 Amending Regulation (EC) No 1924/2006 with Regard to the List of Nutrition Claims. Available online: https://eur-lex.europa.eu/legal-content/EN/TXT/?uri=celex%3A32012R1047 (accessed on 17 June 2021).
20. Sharma, S.K.; Bansal, S.; Mangal, M.; Dixit, A.K.; Gupta, R.K.; Mangal, A.K. Utilization of food processing by products as dietary, functional, and novel fiber: A Review. *Crit. Rev. Food Sci. Nutr.* **2016**, *56*, 1647–1661. [CrossRef] [PubMed]
21. Korus, A. Kale (*Brassica oleracea* L. var. acephala DC.): A valuable Brassica vegetable. Part I. Origin, cultivation and utilization. *Fermentation Fruits Veg. Ind.* **2015**, *59*, 11–12. (In Polish)
22. Olsen, H.; Grimmer, S.; Aaby, K.; Saha, S.; Borge, G.I.A. Antiproliferative Effects of Fresh and Thermal Processed Green and Red Cultivars of Curly Kale (*Brassica oleracea* L. convar. acephala var. sabellica). *J. Agric. Food Chem.* **2012**, *60*, 7375–7383. [CrossRef]
23. Stokman, H.; Gevers, T.; Koenderink, J. Color Measurement by Imaging Spectrometry. *Comput. Vis. Image Underst.* **2000**, *79*, 236–249. [CrossRef]
24. Tiveron, A.P.; Melo, P.S.; Bergamaschi, K.B.; Vieira, T.M.F.D.S.; Regitano-D'Arce, M.A.B.; De Alencar, S.M. Antioxidant Activity of Brazilian Vegetables and Its Relation with Phenolic Composition. *Int. J. Mol. Sci.* **2012**, *13*, 8943–8957. [CrossRef]
25. Nawirska, A.; Kwaśniewska, M. Dietary fibre fractions from fruit and vegetable processing waste. *Food Chem.* **2005**, *91*, 221–225. [CrossRef]
26. Márquez-Villacorta, L.F.; Vásquez, C.C.P. Evaluación de características de calidad en barras de cereales con alto contenido de fibra y proteína. *Biotecnol. Sect. Agropecu. Agroind.* **2018**, *16*, 69–78. [CrossRef]

27. Sun-Waterhouse, D.; Teoh, A.; Massarotto, C.; Wibisono, R.; Wadhwa, S. Comparative analysis of fruit-based functional snack bars. *Food Chem.* **2010**, *119*, 1369–1379. [CrossRef]
28. Charron, C.S.; Novotny, J.A.; Jeffery, E.H.; Kramer, M.; Ross, S.A.; Seifried, H.E. Consumption of baby kale increased cytochrome P450 1A2 (CYP1A2) activity and influenced bilirubin metabolism in a randomized clinical trial. *J. Funct. Foods* **2020**, *64*, 103624. [CrossRef]
29. Vatankhah, M.; Garavand, F.; Mohammadi, B.; Elhamirad, A.H. Quality attributes of reduced-sugar Iranian traditional sweet bread containing stevioside. *J. Food Meas. Charact.* **2017**, *11*, 1233–1239. [CrossRef]
30. Ibrahim, S.; Fidan, H.; Aljaloud, S.; Stankov, S.; Ivanov, G. Application of Date (*Phoenix dactylifera* L.) Fruit in the Composition of a Novel Snack Bar. *Foods* **2021**, *10*, 918. [CrossRef] [PubMed]
31. Kowalska, H.; Marzec, A.; Kowalska, J.; Samborska, K.; Tywonek, M.; Lenart, A. Development of apple chips technology. *Heat Mass Transf.* **2018**, *54*, 3573–3586. [CrossRef]
32. Błońska, A.; Marzec, A.; Błaszczyk, A. Instrumental Evaluation of Acoustic and Mechanical Texture Properties of Short-Dough Biscuits with Different Content of Fat and Inulin. *J. Texture Stud.* **2014**, *45*, 226–234. [CrossRef]
33. Pałacha, Z.; Makarewicz, M. Water activity of selected groups of food products. *Technol. Prog. Food Process.* **2011**, *2*, 24–29. (In Polish)
34. Pałacha, Z.; Mazur, P. Analysis of water activity in selected fruit products. *Technol. Prog. Food Process.* **2019**, *1*, 18–22. (In Polish)
35. Reid, D.S. Water Activity: Fundamentals and Relationships. In *Water Activity in Foods: Fundamentals and Applications*; Barbosa-Cánovas, G.V., Fontana, A.J., Jr., Schmidt, S.J., Labuza, T.P., Eds.; John Wiley and Sons: Hoboken, NJ, USA, 2020; pp. 13–26. [CrossRef]
36. Miastowski, K.; Bakoniuk, R.; Czaplicka, M.; Obidziński, S. Charakterystyka wiązania wody przez błonnik kakaowy. *Technol. Prog. Food Process.* **2015**, *1*, 15–19. (In Polish)
37. Kubiak, M.S.; Dolik, K. Instrumental texture profile analysis test. *J. Eng. Sci. Technol.* **2013**, *3*, 23–28. (In Polish)
38. Nikmaram, N.; Garavand, F.; Elhamirad, A.H.; Beiraghi-Toosi, S.; Goli-Movahhed, G. Production of high quality expanded corn extrudates containing sesame seed using response surface methodology. *Qual. Assur. Saf. Crop. Foods* **2015**, *7*, 713–720. [CrossRef]
39. Kowalczewski, P.; Ivanišová, E. Effect of the addition of dried berries on the characteristics of gluten-free muffins. *Postępy Nauk. Technol. Przem. Rolno—Spoz.* **2018**, *73*, 61–71. (In Polish)
40. Wójtowicz, A.; Baltyn, P. Assessment of selected quality features of popular potato snacks. *Food Sci. Technol. Qual.* **2006**, *2*, 112–123. (In Polish)
41. Kubiak, M.S.; Dolik, K. Instrumental texture profile analysis test. *LAB Lab. Appar. Res.* **2017**, *22*, 23–28.
42. Heo, Y.; Kim, M.-J.; Lee, J.-W.; Moon, B. Muffins enriched with dietary fiber from kimchi by-product: Baking properties, physical-chemical properties, and consumer acceptance. *Food Sci. Nutr.* **2019**, *7*, 1778–1785. [CrossRef]
43. Goetzke, B.; Nitzko, S.; Spiller, A. Consumption of organic and functional food. A matter of well-being and health? *Appetite* **2014**, *77*, 96–105. [CrossRef]
44. Nawirska, A.; Sokół-Łętowska, A.; Kucharska, A.Z. Antioxidant characteristics of pomace from different fruits. *Food Sci. Technol. Qual.* **2007**, *4*, 120–125. (In Polish)
45. Biegańska-Marecik, R.; Radziejewska-Kubzdela, E.; Marecik, R. Characterization of phenolics, glucosinolates and antioxidant activity of beverages based on apple juice with addition of frozen and freeze-dried curly kale leaves (*Brassica oleracea* L. var. acephala L.). *Food Chem.* **2017**, *230*, 271–280. [CrossRef]
46. Satheesh, N.; Fanta, S.W. Kale: Review on nutritional composition, bio-active compounds, anti-nutritional factors, health beneficial properties and value-added products. *Cogent Food Agric.* **2020**, *6*, 1811048. [CrossRef]
47. Karwowska, K.; Skotnicka, M.; Pieszko, M. Bioactive substances in the „green" dietary supplements. *Bromatol. Toxicol. Chem.* **2020**, *53*, 129–136. (In Polish)
48. Sikora, J.; Markowicz, M.; Makiciuk-Olasik, E. The role and healing properties of black chokeberry in the prevention of civilization diseases. *Bromatol. Toxicol. Chem.* **2009**, *42*, 10–17. (In Polish)
49. Regulation of the European Parliament and of the Council (EU) No. 1169/2011 of 25 October 2011. Official Journal of the EU L 304 of 22.11.2011. Available online: https://eur-lex.europa.eu/legal-content/EN/TXT/PDF/?uri=CELEX:32011R1169&from=EN (accessed on 17 June 2021).
50. Urbańska, B.; Szafrański, T.; Kowalska, H.; Kowalska, J. Study of Polyphenol Content and Antioxidant Properties of Various Mix of Chocolate Milk Masses with Different Protein Content. *Antioxidants* **2020**, *9*, 299. [CrossRef]
51. Wong, S.P.; Leong, L.P.; Koh, J.H.W. Antioxidant activities of aqueous extracts of selected plants. *Food Chem.* **2006**, *99*, 775–783. [CrossRef]
52. Lichtenthaler, H.K.; Buschmann, C. Chlorophylls and Carotenoids: Measurement and Characterization by UV-VIS Spectroscopy. *Curr. Protoc. Food Anal. Chem.* **2001**, *1*, F4.3.1–F4.3.8. [CrossRef]

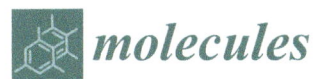

Article

The Qualitative and Quantitative Compositions of Phenolic Compounds in Fruits of Lithuanian Heirloom Apple Cultivars

Aurita Butkevičiūtė [1,*], Mindaugas Liaudanskas [1,2], Darius Kviklys [2,3], Dalia Gelvonauskienė [2] and Valdimaras Janulis [1]

1. Department of Pharmacognosy, Lithuanian University of Health Sciences, Sukileliu av. 13, LT-50162 Kaunas, Lithuania; Mindaugas.Liaudanskas@lsmu.lt (M.L.); farmakog@lsmuni.lt (V.J.)
2. Institute of Horticulture, Lithuanian Research Centre for Agriculture and Forestry, Kauno str. 30, LT-54333 Babtai, Kaunas District, Lithuania; Darius.Kviklys@lammc.lt (D.K.); Dalia.Gelvonauskiene@lammc.lt (D.G.)
3. Norwegian Institute of Bioeconomy Research-NIBIO Ullensvang, Postboks str. 11, NO-1431 Ås Lofthus, Norway
* Correspondence: Aurita.Butkeviciute@lsmu.lt; Tel.: +37-037-621-56190

Academic Editors: Jan Oszmianski and Sabina Lachowicz
Received: 22 October 2020; Accepted: 10 November 2020; Published: 11 November 2020

Abstract: As the interest in heirloom cultivars of apple trees, their fruit, and processed products is growing worldwide, studies of the qualitative and quantitative composition of biological compounds are important for the evaluation of the quality and nutritional properties of the apples. Studies on the variations in the chemical composition of phenolic compounds characterized by a versatile biological effect are important when researching the genetic heritage of the heirloom cultivars in order to increase the cultivation of such cultivars in orchards. A variation in the qualitative and quantitative composition of phenolic compounds was found in apple samples of cultivars included in the Lithuanian collection of genetic resources. By the high-performance liquid chromatography (HPLC) method flavan-3-ols (procyanidin B1, procyanidin B2, procyanidin C2, (+)-catechin and (−)-epicatechin), flavonols (rutin, hyperoside, quercitrin, isoquercitrin, reynoutrin and avicularin), chlorogenic acids and phloridzin were identified and quantified in fruit samples of heirloom apple cultivars grown in Lithuania. The highest sum of the identified phenolic compounds (3.82 ± 0.53 mg/g) was found in apple fruit samples of the 'Koštelė' cultivar

Keywords: apple; phenolic compounds; genetic resources; HPLC-DAD

1. Introduction

Apple trees are among the old cultivated fruit trees in the world [1]. Domestic apple trees (*Malus domestica* Borkh.) were starting to be grown 4000–10,000 years ago in the orchards of Central Asia [2]. Until the end of the 19th century, domestic apple trees were grown in the orchards of manors and monasteries [3,4]. Later on, local farmers started growing apple trees of the traditional cultivars in their orchards. During this period, a number of traditional apple cultivars of genetic resource heritage were bred in Lithuania, including 'Lietuvos pepinas', 'Montvilinis', 'Popierinis', 'Rudeninis dryžuotasis', 'Žemaičių grietininis', etc. [3]. It is expedient to preserve these apple cultivars, as their value has not been assessed yet.

The results of studies on the qualitative and quantitative composition of the fruit samples of apple cultivars grown in industrial orchards have been presented in scientific literature, but research data on the chemical composition of the fruit of heirloom apple cultivars grown in genetic heritage collections are fragmented [5]. The qualitative and quantitative composition of phenolic compounds in apples grown in Lithuanian industrial orchards has been investigated [5]. Secondary metabolites are phenolic compounds such as flavanols, flavonols, hydroxycinnamic acids, dihydrochalcones and anthocyanins were identified in fruit of the heirloom apple cultivars grown in Portuguese and Polish orchards [6,7]. Fruit samples of heirloom apple cultivars grown in Italian orchards and collections were found to have higher levels of phenolic compounds compared to those found in samples of apples of cultivars grown in industrial orchards [8,9].

Phenolic compounds have a wide range of biological effects: they act as strong antioxidants, scavenging free radicals [9,10], inhibit inflammatory processes [11,12] and the multiplication of bacteria [13] and they also have anti-cancer [14,15] and anti-aging effects [16–18]. The recommended daily diet should include apples, their processed products, and dietary supplements for the prevention of diabetes, asthma, cancer, and neurodegenerative and chronic cardiovascular diseases [11,15,19].

Industrial horticulture has been developing highly intensively during recent decades [1]. New apple cultivars are bred in industrial orchards, taking into account the needs of consumers in different regions of the world [1,20]. The introduction of new apple cultivars by fruit tree breeders reduced the demand for heirloom cultivars of apples grown in orchards [1,21]. Numerous cultivars of apple-specific trait donors have been used to create new apple cultivars grown in industrial orchards. Therefore, the characteristics of fruit trees of these cultivars (adaptability to biotic and abiotic factors, fruit taste, texture of the flesh, etc.) based on genetic factors are "harmonized". Consumers are missing the traditional cultivars due to the variety of their fruit taste, aroma, consistency and suitability for unique national heritage products. Many countries, including Lithuania, have signed the Convention on Biological Diversity [22], the TREATY agreement [23] and the Nagoya Protocol [24] to assess the genetic uniqueness, distinctiveness and risk of extinction of heirloom varieties of garden plants. The signatories of the mentioned documents are committed to collecting, preserving and researching the diversity and economic, biological and medical value of the genetic resources of heirloom varieties of agricultural plants.

Currently, consumers are looking for high-quality products with a known composition and health benefits [25]. Research into the qualitative and quantitative composition of biologically active compounds is important in assessing the quality and nutritional properties of apples. In Lithuania, apple cultivars belonging to the collection of genetic resources are grown in private orchards. In order to study the genetic heritage of heirloom cultivars with the aim of promoting their cultivation in orchards, it is important to carry out detailed studies on the variability of the chemical composition of phenolic compounds with biological effects. Data on qualitative and quantitative chemical composition will provide new scientific knowledge about variability of the qualitative and quantitative composition of biologically active compounds in the fruit of apple trees of heirloom cultivars.

The aim of the study was to investigate variability of the qualitative and quantitative composition of phenolic compounds in the samples of heirloom apple cultivars, to substantiate the cultivation of heirloom cultivars in Lithuanian orchards, and to preserve the genetic heritage of heirloom cultivars.

2. Results and Discussion

2.1. Qualitative and Quantitative Analysis of Phenolic Compounds of Apple of Heirloom Cultivars

Scientific literature provides data on the variability of the chemical composition of phenolic compounds in fruit samples of apple trees grown in industrial orchards [26]. The total amount of phenolic compounds found in fruit samples of apple cultivars 'Aldas', 'Auksis', 'Ligol', and 'Šampion' grown in Lithuanian industrial orchards ranged from 1.64 mg/g to 5.75 mg/g [27,28]. In Lithuania as well as in many other countries, collections and private orchards contain heirloom apple cultivars that form the heritage of genetic resources. Fruit of the heirloom apple cultivars are characterized by a high nutritional value and are of different shapes, colors, sizes and organoleptic properties (crispness, juiciness, and sweetness) [29]. Studies of the chemical composition of the fruit of heirloom apple cultivars are patchy.

The sum of the identified phenolic compounds in the samples of heirloom apple cultivars included in the collection of the Lithuanian heritage of genetic resources varied from 0.15 ± 0.01 mg/g to 3.82 ± 0.53 mg/g (Figure 1). The highest sum of the identified phenolic compounds (3.82 ± 0.53 mg/g) was detected in samples of the 'Koštelė' apple cultivar, which differed statistically significantly from the amount of these compounds detected in apple fruit samples of the other studied cultivars ($p < 0.05$) (Figure 1). The lowest content of the sum of the identified phenolic compounds (0.15 ± 0.01 mg/g) was found in fruit samples of the 'Birutės pepinas' cultivar, and it did not differ statistically significantly from that detected in fruit samples of 'Beržininkų ananasinis', 'Danų karalienė Luiza', 'Montvilinis', 'Panemunės baltasis', 'Pilkasis alyvinis', 'Raudonasis alyvinis' or 'Žemaičių grietininis' apple cultivars (Figure 1).

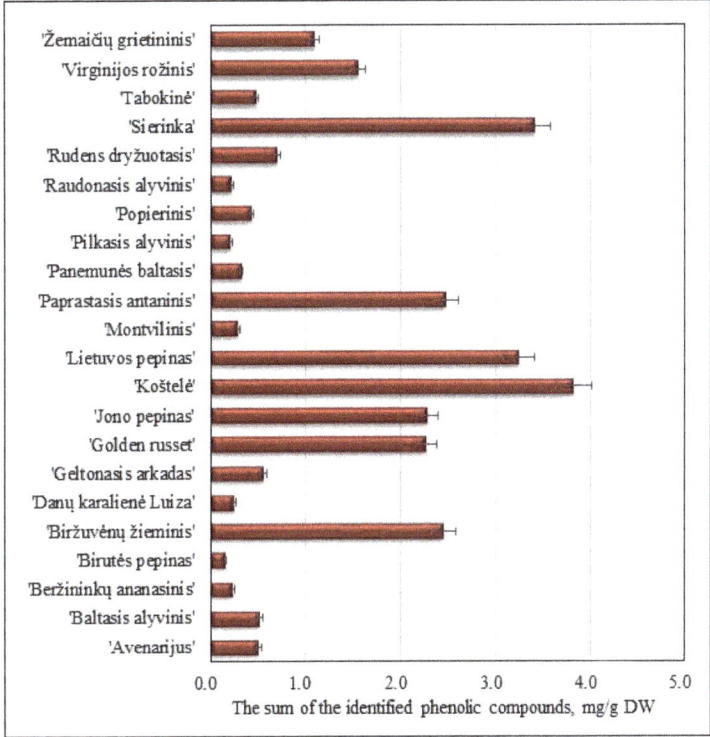

Figure 1. Variability of the sum of the identified phenolic compounds in fruit samples of heirloom apple cultivars.

Studies of the fruit samples of heirloom apple cultivars grown in the orchards of the Marche region of Italy showed that the total amount of phenolic compounds ranged from 0.82 mg/g to 3.60 mg/g [30]. The total amount of phenolic compounds in fruit samples of heirloom apple cultivars grown in Brazilian orchards ranged from 0.46 mg/g to 1.58 mg/g [31]. Meanwhile, the total amount of phenolic compounds in fruit samples of heirloom apple cultivars grown in orchards of the Piedmont region of Italy ranged from 0.45 mg/g to 5.00 mg/g [8]. The sum of the identified phenolic compounds in fruit samples of heirloom apple cultivars grown in Lithuanian orchards was higher than that detected in fruit samples of the heirloom apple cultivars grown in the orchards of the Italian Marche region or Brazil, but lower than that found in fruit samples of the heirloom apple cultivars grown in the orchards of the Italian region of Piedmont.

2.1.1. Variation of the Amount of Flavan-3-ols

Flavan-3-ols (procyanidin B1, procyanidin B2, procyanidin C2, (+)-catechin, and (−)-epicatechin) identified in fruit samples of heirloom apple cultivars grown in Lithuania accounted for 30% of the total amount of the identified and quantified phenolic compounds. The flavan-3-ol content in fruit samples of heirloom apple cultivars ranged from 0.03 ± 0.001 mg/g to 1.40 ± 0.05 mg/g (Figure 2). The flavan-3-ol content in fruit samples of heirloom apple cultivars grown in Croatian orchards was found to vary from 0.02 mg/g to 0.69 mg/g [26]. The flavan-3-ol content in fruit samples of heirloom apple cultivars grown in Italian orchards ranged from 0.02 mg/g to 0.66 mg/g [32]. The flavan-3-ol content in fruit samples of heirloom red-fleshed apple cultivars grown in Spanish orchards was found to range from 0.016 mg/g to 0.022 mg/g, while the flavan-3-ol content in samples of heirloom white-fleshed apples ranged from 0.09 mg/g to 0.20 mg/g [33]. The content of flavan-3-ols in fruit samples of heirloom apple cultivars of the Lithuanian genetic heritage collection was found to be higher than that in fruit samples of heirloom apple cultivars grown in Croatian, Italian, or Spanish orchards.

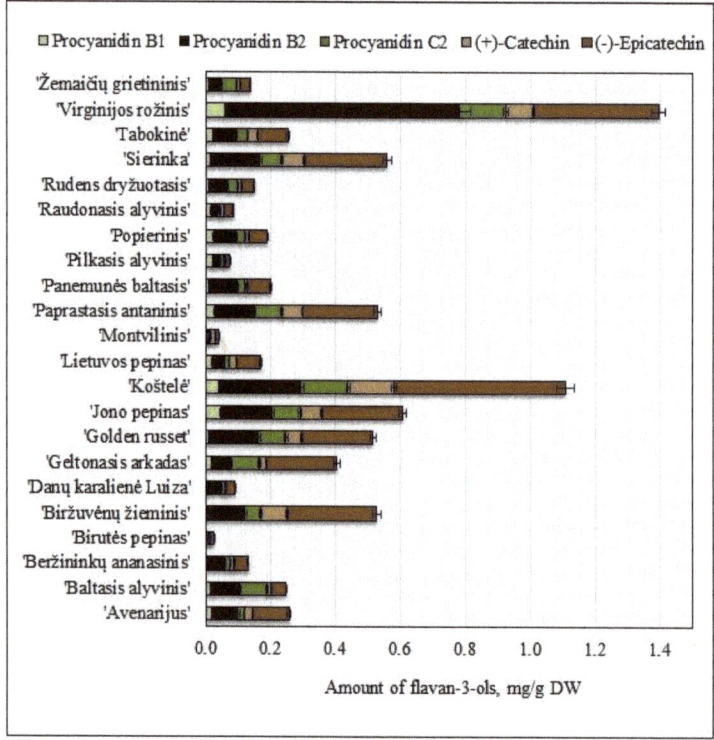

Figure 2. Variability of the amount of flavan-3-ols in fruit samples of heirloom apple cultivars.

The predominant compound of the flavan-3-ol group in fruit samples of heirloom apple cultivars grown in Lithuania was (−)-epicatechin. The highest amount of (−)-epicatechin (0.53 ± 0.01 mg/g) was found in fruit samples of the 'Koštelė' cultivar, and it was statistically significantly ($p < 0.05$) different from the amount of (−)-epicatechin detected in fruit samples of other apple cultivars (Figure 2). The content of (−)-epicatechin in fruit samples of heirloom apple cultivars grown in Polish orchards was found to range from 0.05 mg/g to 2.79 mg/g [34]. The amount of (−)-epicatechin in fruit samples of heirloom apple cultivars grown in Italian orchards ranged from 0.09 mg/g to 0.53 mg/g [8]. The data obtained by Polish and Italian researchers corroborate the results of our research.

The highest amounts of (+)-catechin (0.14 ± 0.01 mg/g) were found in fruit samples of the 'Koštelė' apple cultivar (Figure 2). The analysis of the fruit samples of heirloom apple cultivars showed a statistically significant ($p < 0.05$) difference in (+)-catechin content. The amount of (+)-catechin in fruit samples of heirloom apple cultivars grown in Italian orchards ranged from 0.02 mg/g to 0.05 mg/g [9]. Meanwhile, the amount of (+)-catechin in fruit samples of heirloom apple cultivars grown in Polish orchards ranged from 0.01 mg/g to 0.72 mg/g [35]. Fruit samples of heirloom apple cultivars grown in Lithuanian orchards were found to contain higher amounts of (+)-catechin, compared to that in fruit samples of heirloom apple cultivars grown in Italian orchards, but lower than that found in fruit samples of heirloom apple cultivars grown in Polish orchards. Procyanidins are among the most common flavan-3-ols found in samples of heirloom apple cultivars [8]. The highest amounts of procyanidin B2 (0.72 ± 0.18 mg/g), procyanidin C2 (0.14 ± 0.03 mg/g) and procyanidin B1 (0.06 ± 0.01 mg/g) were found in apple fruit samples of the 'Virginijos rožinis' cultivar ($p < 0.05$) (Figure 2). Procyanidin B2 predominated among the procyanidins identified and quantified in apple samples of heirloom cultivars grown in Lithuania. The amount of procyanidin B2 in fruit samples of heirloom apple cultivars grown in Polish orchards ranged from 0.07 mg/g to 2.00 mg/g [35]. Meanwhile, the amount of procyanidin B2 in fruit samples of heirloom apple cultivars grown in Italian orchards ranged from 0.018 mg/g to 2.09 mg/g [8]. The amount of procyanidin C1 in fruit samples of heirloom apple cultivars grown in Polish orchards ranged from 0.0006 mg/g to 0.97 mg/g [35]. The amount of procyanidin B1 in fruit samples of heirloom apple cultivars grown in Italian orchards ranged from 0.005 mg/g to 0.34 mg/g [8] and from 0.006 mg/g to 0.014 mg/g [32]. The results of studies on the variability of procyanidin content in fruit samples of heirloom apple cultivars from the collection of the Lithuanian heritage of genetic resources are confirmed by the data of research conducted by Polish and Italian scientists.

According to their amount in fruit samples of heirloom apple cultivars grown in Lithuanian orchards, the compounds of the flavan-3-ol group can be arranged in the following order: (−)-epicatechin>procyanidin B2>procyanidin C2>(+)-catechin>procyanidin B1. Studies of the qualitative and quantitative composition of compounds of the flavan-3-ol group are valuable due to the antioxidant properties of this group of compounds [10] and their glucose regulating effects [34].

2.1.2. Variation of the Amount of Flavonols

The following flavonols were identified and quantified in fruit samples of heirloom apple cultivars from the collection of the Lithuanian heritage of genetic resources: rutin, hyperoside, quercitrin, isoquercitrin, reynoutrin, and avicularin. They comprised 13% of all the identified and quantified phenolic compounds. The content of flavonols in fruit samples of heirloom apple cultivars ranged from 0.04 ± 0.001 mg/g to 0.47 ± 0.12 mg/g (Figure 3). Studies of fruit samples of heirloom apple cultivars grown in Croatian orchards showed that flavonol levels ranged from 0.20 mg/g to 1.22 mg/g [26]. Meanwhile, flavonol levels in fruit samples of heirloom apple cultivars grown in Austrian orchards ranged from 0.67 mg/g to 5.66 mg/g [19]. The results of our study are corroborated by research data obtained by Croatian and Polish researchers.

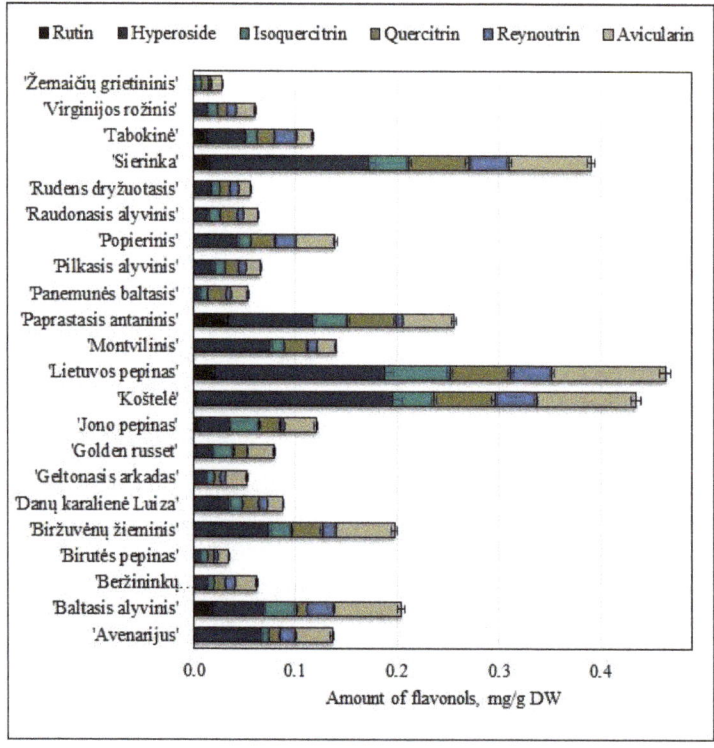

Figure 3. Variability of the amount of flavonols in fruit samples of heirloom apple cultivars.

Hyperoside was the predominant compound of the flavonols group in fruit samples of heirloom apple cultivars grown in Lithuania. The highest amount of hyperoside (0.19 ± 0.01 mg/g) was found in apple fruit samples of the 'Koštelė' cultivar, and it was statistically significantly different from hyperoside content in apple samples of other studied cultivars ($p < 0.05$) (Figure 3). The amount of hyperoside in fruit samples of heirloom apple cultivars grown in Italian orchards ranged from 0.0003 mg/g to 0.002 mg/g [8]. The amount of hyperoside found in fruit samples of heirloom apple cultivars grown in Lithuania was higher than that detected in fruit samples of heirloom apple cultivars grown in Italian orchards. The highest amount of avicularin (0.11 ± 0.01 mg/g) was found in apple fruit samples of the 'Lietuvos pepinas' cultivar (Figure 3). Avicularin content differed statistically significantly between fruit samples of heirloom apple cultivars ($p < 0.05$). The highest amount of quercitrin (0.06 ± 0.002 mg/g) was found in apple fruit samples of the 'Koštelė' cultivar, and it was statistically significantly different from that found in apple samples of other cultivars ($p < 0.05$) (Figure 3). The amount of quercitrin found in fruit samples of heirloom apple cultivars grown in Italian orchards ranged from 0.005 mg/g to 0.043 mg/g [8]. The amount of quercitrin in fruit samples of heirloom apple cultivars grown in Lithuanian orchards was higher, compared to the amount found in fruit samples of heirloom apple cultivars grown in Italian orchards. The highest amounts of isoquercitrin (0.06 ± 0.002 mg/g) and reynoutrin (0.04 ± 0.002 mg/g) were found in apple fruit samples of the 'Lietuvos pepinas' cultivar (Figure 3). The amount of isoquercitrin differed statistically significantly between fruit samples of differed heirloom apple cultivars ($p < 0.05$). There was no statistically significant difference in the amount of reynoutrin between apple fruit samples of the 'Sierinka' and 'Koštelė' cultivars ($p > 0.05$). Among the fruit samples of heirloom apple cultivars grown in Lithuania, the highest amount of rutin (0.04 ± 0.002 mg/g) was found in fruit samples of the 'Paprastasis antaninis' cultivar, and it did not differ statistically significantly from that found in apple samples of 'Pilkasis alyvinis', 'Beržininkų ananasinis', 'Golden russet', 'Jono pepinas', 'Koštelė', 'Sierinka', 'Tabokinė', 'Baltasis alyvinis', or 'Lietuvos pepinas' cultivars ($p > 0.05$) (Figure 3). The amount of rutin found in fruit samples of heirloom apple cultivars belonging to the collection of the Lithuanian heritage of genetic resources was higher compared to the amount of rutin (0.004 mg/g) found in fruit samples of heirloom apple cultivars grown in Italian orchards [9].

According to their amount in fruit samples of heirloom apple cultivars belonging to the collection of the Lithuanian heritage of genetic resources, the compounds of the flavonols group can be arranged in the following order: hyperoside>avicularin>quercitrin>isoquercitrin>reynoutrin>rutin. Studies of the qualitative and quantitative composition of the compounds of the flavonols group are important due to their antioxidant [34], anti-inflammatory [11], and antiallergic properties [36].

2.1.3. Variation of the Amount of Chlorogenic Acid

Phenolcarboxylic acids are an important group of secondary metabolites in apples. It is important to determine the variability of their quantitative composition in fruit samples of heirloom apple cultivars. Chlorogenic acid was the predominant compound, making up 50% of the total amount of the identified and quantified phenolic compounds. The amount of chlorogenic acid in fruit samples of heirloom apple cultivars ranged from 0.01 ± 0.001 mg/g to 2.35 ± 0.03 mg/g (Figure 4).

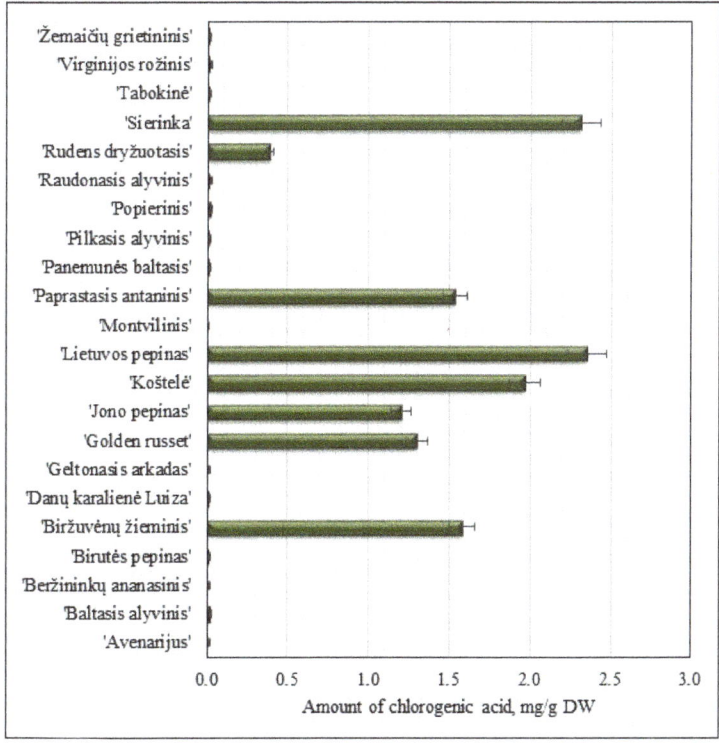

Figure 4. Variability of the amount of chlorogenic acid in fruit samples of heirloom apple cultivars.

The highest amount of chlorogenic acid (2.35 ± 0.03 mg/g) was detected in apple fruit samples of the 'Lietuvos pepinas' cultivar (Figure 4). The content of chlorogenic acid in fruit samples of heirloom apple cultivars differed statistically significantly ($p < 0.05$). The lowest amount of chlorogenic acid (0.01 ± 0.001 mg/g) was found in apple fruit samples of the 'Montvilinis' cultivar (Figure 4). The amount of chlorogenic acid in fruit samples of heirloom apple cultivars grown in orchards in the Tuscan region of Italy was found to vary from 0.12 mg/g to 0.63 mg/g [9]. Meanwhile, the amount of chlorogenic acid in fruit samples of heirloom apple cultivars grown in orchards in the Piedmont region of Italy ranged from 0.13 mg/g to 2.08 mg/g [8]. Fruit samples of heirloom apple cultivars from the collection of the Lithuanian heritage of genetic resources contained higher amounts of chlorogenic acid compared to those found in fruit samples of heirloom apple cultivars grown in Italian orchards.

2.1.4. Variation of the Amount of Phloridzin

Compounds of the dihydrochalcone group are naturally prevalent in the vegetative and generative organs of plants of the apple (*Malus L.*) genus, while in other plant species, they are almost undetectable [33]. Fruit samples of heirloom apple cultivars were found to contain the dihydrochalcone group compound phloridzin, which accounted for 7% of the total amount of the identified and quantified phenolic compounds. The amount of phloridzin in apple samples ranged from 0.02 ± 0.002 mg/g to 0.30 ± 0.005 mg/g (Figure 5).

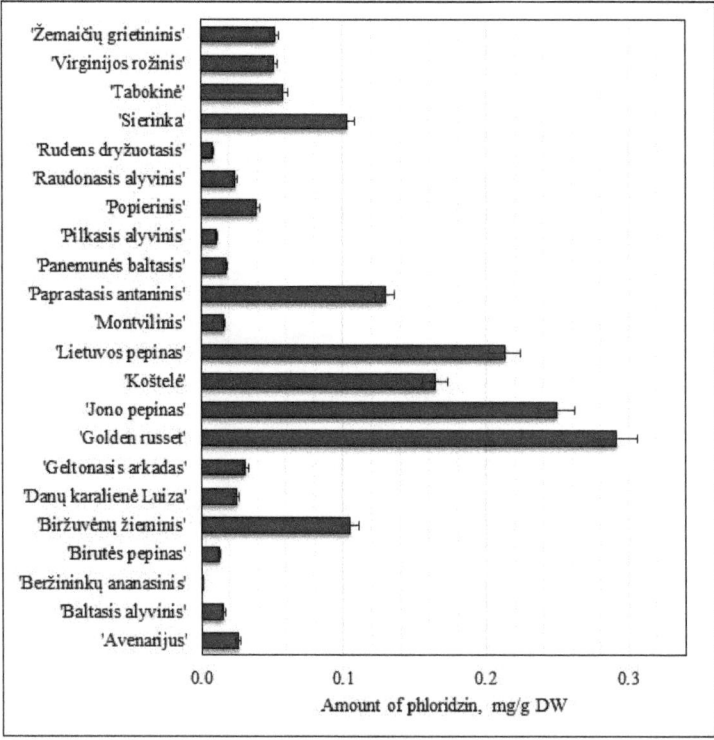

Figure 5. Variability of the amount of phloridzin in fruit samples of heirloom apple cultivars.

The highest content of phloridzin (0.30 ± 0.005 mg/g) was found in apple fruit samples of the 'Golden russet' cultivar (Figure 5), which did not differ statistically significantly only from the amounts found in apple fruit samples of the 'Jono pepinas' cultivar. The lowest amount of phloridzin (0.02 ± 0.002 mg/g) was found in apple fruit samples of the 'Beržininkų ananasinis' cultivar (Figure 5). The amount of phloridzin in fruit samples of heirloom apple cultivars grown in orchards in the Piedmont region of Italy was found to range from 0.001 mg/g to 0.26 mg/g [8]. The amount of phloridzin in fruit samples of heirloom apple cultivars grown in orchards in the Garfagnana region of Italy ranged from 0.01 mg/g to 0.05 mg/g [32]. Fruit samples of heirloom apple cultivars from the collection of the Lithuanian heritage of genetic resources contained higher amounts of phloridzin compared to those found in fruit samples of heirloom apple cultivars grown in Italian orchards.

2.2. Hierarchical Cluster Analysis of Phenolic Compounds of Apple of Heirloom Cultivars

Hierarchical cluster analysis of heirloom apple cultivars was performed, the results of which are presented in Figure 6. Based on the variability of the quantitative composition in apple samples of heirloom cultivars, phenolic compounds were distributed into clusters.

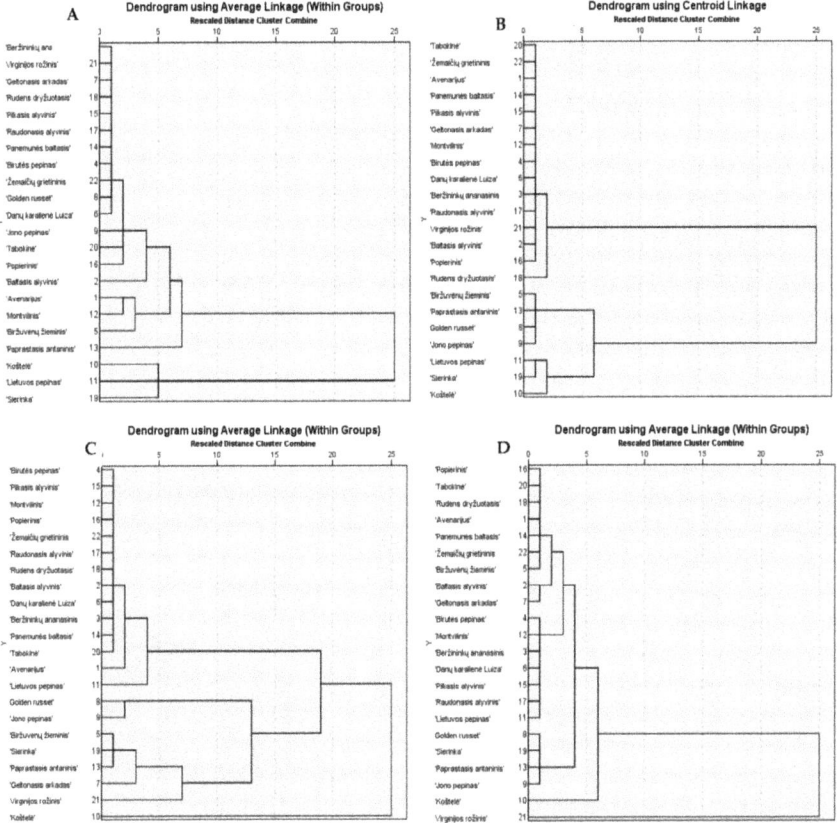

Figure 6. Dendrogram of the similarity of apple samples in terms of the amounts of phenolic compounds. Flavonols were distributed into three clusters (**A**), chlorogenic acid was distributed into four clusters (**B**), (−)-epicatechin, (+)-catechin, and phloridzin were distributed into four clusters (**C**), and compounds of the procyanidin group were distributed into four clusters (**D**).

Fruit samples of heirloom apple cultivars assigned to cluster I (3, 4, 6, 7, 8, 14, 15, 17, 18, 21 and 22) were found to contain lower than average amounts of flavonols. Fruit samples of heirloom apple cultivars assigned to cluster II (1, 2, 5, 9, 12, 16 and 20) were found to contain average amounts of flavonols. Meanwhile, fruit samples of heirloom apple cultivars assigned to cluster III (10, 11, 13 and 19) were found to contain higher than average amounts of flavonols (Figure 6A). Fruit samples of heirloom apple cultivars assigned to cluster I (1, 2, 3, 4, 6, 7, 12, 14, 15, 16, 17, 20, 21 and 22) were found to contain lower than average amounts of chlorogenic acid. Fruit samples of the heirloom apple cultivar assigned to cluster II (18) had average amounts of chlorogenic acid. Meanwhile, fruit samples of heirloom apple cultivars assigned to cluster III (5, 8, 9 and 13) had higher than average amounts of chlorogenic acid. The highest amounts of chlorogenic acid were found in fruit samples of heirloom apple cultivars assigned to cluster IV (10, 11 and 19) (Figure 6B).

Fruit samples of heirloom apple cultivars assigned to cluster I (1, 2, 3, 4, 6, 11, 12, 14, 15, 16, 17, 18, 20 and 22) were found to contain lower than average amounts of (−)-epicatechin, (+)-catechin and phloridzin. Fruit samples of heirloom apple cultivars assigned to cluster II (8 and 9) were found to contain average amounts of (−)-epicatechin, (+)-catechin and phloridzin. Higher than average levels of (−−)-epicatechin, (+)-catechin and phloridzin were found in fruit samples of heirloom apple cultivars assigned to cluster III (5, 7, 13, 19 and 21). The highest levels of (−)-epicatechin, (+)-catechin and phloridzin were found in fruit samples of the heirloom apple cultivar assigned to cluster IV (10) (Figure 6C). Fruit samples of heirloom apple cultivars assigned to cluster I (1, 2, 5, 7, 14, 16, 18, 20 and 22) were found to contain average amounts of procyanidin B1, procyanidin B2 and procyanidin C2. Fruit samples of heirloom apple cultivars assigned to cluster II (3, 4, 6, 11, 12, 15 and 17) contained lower than average amounts of procyanidins. Higher than average amounts of procyanidins were found in fruit samples of heirloom apple cultivars assigned to cluster III (8, 9, 10, 13 and 19). The highest amounts of procyanidin B1, procyanidin B2, and procyanidin C2 were found in fruit samples of heirloom apple cultivars assigned to cluster IV (21) (Figure 6D).

2.3. Principal Component Analysis of Phenolic Compounds of Apple of Heirloom Cultivars

In this study, we analyzed the main components of phenolic compounds in fruit samples of heirloom apple cultivars. Two main components were used for the analysis, as they explain 80.19% of the total variability in the study data (Figure 7).

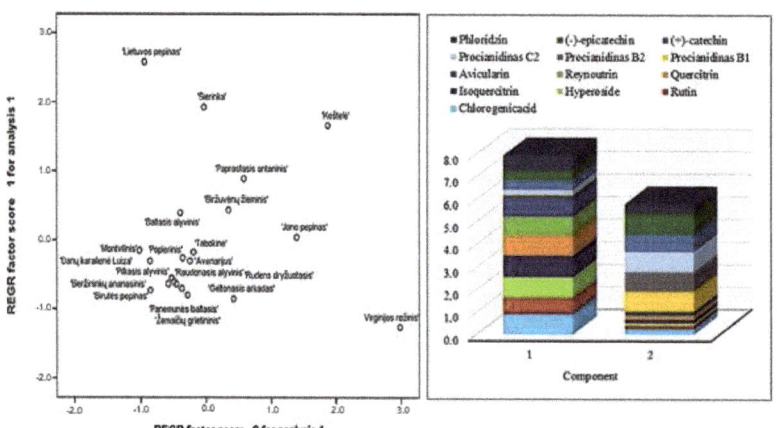

Figure 7. Analysis of the main components of phenolic compounds in apple samples.

The amounts of isoquercitrin (0.939), hyperoside (0.930), avicularin (0.930), quercitrin (0.922), chlorogenic acid (0.902) and reynoutrin (0.815) strongly positively correlated with the first component, which describes 48.53% of the total data variability, while the correlation of the amounts of rutin (0.707) and phloridzin (0.691) with this component was strongly positive (Figure 7). The amounts of procyanidin C2 (0.889), procyanidin B1 (0.887), (−)-epicatechin (0.882), procyanidin B2 (0.878) and (+)-catechin (0.805) very strongly positively correlated with the second component, which describes 31.66% of the dispersion (Figure 7).

Recently, there has been a growing interest in the genetic resources of heirloom cultivars, they are more widely grown, and there is an increasing number of studies on the qualitative and quantitative variability of the composition of their fruit. Fruit samples of some heirloom apple cultivars were found to have a richer quantitative and qualitative composition of phenolic compounds. Heirloom apple cultivars can be used for the selection of new apple cultivars. Apple trees of heirloom cultivars are becoming more popular, and higher levels of biologically active compounds are detected in their fruit [9]. Fruit samples of heirloom apple cultivars grown in Lithuania were found to contain 2.6 times higher amounts of flavonols, 7 times higher amounts of dihydrochalcones, 1.2 times lower amounts of phenolic acids and 1.5 times lower amounts of flavan-3-ols compared to those detected in fruit samples of heirloom apple cultivars grown in Polish orchards [34]. Quantitative differences can be explained by the competitive interaction between the enzymes anthocyanidin reductase and anthocyanidin synthase during flavonoid synthesis, which results in a slower synthesis of flavan-3-ols and their lower accumulation in apples [2].

The results of our study provided new knowledge about apple cultivars from the collection of the Lithuanian heritage of genetic resources and the variability of the qualitative and quantitative composition of the phenolic compounds found in their fruit. The highest sum of the identified phenolic compounds (3.82 ± 0.53 mg/g) was found in apple fruit samples of the 'Koštelė' cultivar. The sum of the identified phenolic compounds was higher than that (0.86 mg/g) found in fruit samples of heirloom apple cultivars grown in Germany [36]. Fruit samples of heirloom apple cultivars included in the collection of the Lithuanian heritage of genetic resources contained higher amounts of phenolic compounds compared to those detected in fruit samples of the 'Jonagold' cultivar grown in the orchards of Lhasa (Italy), Rokietnica (Poland), and Randwijk (the Netherlands) regions (respectively, 2.21 mg/g, 2.69 mg/g, and 3.81 mg/g). However, this amount was lower than that (4.76 mg/g) found in the samples of apples grown in the orchards of the Wieluń region of Poland [37]. In fruit samples of heirloom apple cultivars grown in Lithuania, chlorogenic acid comprised the greatest part of the phenolic compounds. The highest content of chlorogenic acid (2.35 ± 0.03 mg/g) was found in apple fruit samples of the 'Lietuvos pepinas' cultivar. Polish researchers indicated that chlorogenic acid might account for 64–94% of all the identified and quantified phenolic acids in apple fruit samples [34]. Chlorogenic acid in fruit and vegetables determines their sensory properties and has anti-mutagenic and antioxidant effects [34]. The compound phloridzin belonging to the dihydrochalcone group was found in fruit samples of heirloom apple cultivars. Its highest amounts (0.30 ± 0.005 mg/g) were found in apple fruit samples of the 'Golden russet' cultivar. Phloridzin is a biologically active compound with a wide range of biological effects. It regulates blood glucose levels [38,39], antioxidant and anti-aging effects [11,40]. Qualitative and quantitative analysis of dihydrochalcone group compounds is important, as they can be used as chemotaxonomic markers in the taxonomy of apple species as well as for the identification and quality assessment of apple products [6].

3. Materials and Methods

3.1. Plant Materials

The study included 22 heirloom apple cultivars, of which 21 (except for 'Golden russet') are included in the List of the National Plant Genetic Resources (Table 1).

The apple trees were grown in the Collection of the Apple Tree Genetic Resources at the Institute of Horticulture (in Babtai town), a division of the Lithuanian Research Centre for Agriculture and Forestry (henceforth, LAMMC). Coordinates: 55°60′ N, 23°48′ E. The study was conducted during 2019–2020.

Table 1. Origin and properties of the heirloom apple cultivars of Lithuania [4,41].

No.	Apple Cultivar	Year of Release, Finding, or Description, and Country	Other Exclusive Characteristics
1.	'Avenarijus'	1886, Russia, SC	Skin greenish-yellow, flesh pink, sweet; susceptible to canker
2.	'Baltasis alyvinis'	1848, Russia, SC	Skin yellow, flesh white, aromatic; susceptible to scab
3.	'Beržininkų ananasinis'	1886, Lithuania, AC	Skin yellow, flesh crispy, aromatic; scab-resistant
4.	'Birutės pepinas'	1941, Lithuania, AC	Skin reddish-white, flesh white, with suspicion of wine; susceptible to scab
5.	'Biržuvėnų žieminis'	Lithuania, WC	Skin yellow, sweet; scab-resistant
6.	'Danų karalienė Luiza'	1878, Denmark, WC	Skin covered with rust grid, flesh creamy yellow; scab-resistant
7.	'Geltonasis arkadas'	XIX, Russia, SC	Skin yellow, sweet, sometimes astringent; susceptible to scab.
8.	'Golden russet'	1800–1849, USA, WC	Skin strong russet, flesh creamy yellow; resistant to scab
9.	'Jono pepinas'	XIX, Lithuania, WC	Flesh firm, yellow; scab-resistant
10.	'Koštelė'	XIX, Poland, WC	Skin yellow, sweet, flesh firm, creamy; scab-resistant
11.	'Lietuvos pepinas'	XVIII, Lithuania, WC	Skin yellow, vinous taste, flesh white; susceptible to scab
12.	'Montvilinis'	1879, Lithuania, WC	Skin yellow, aromatic; scab-resistant
13.	'Paprastasis antaninis'	XVIII, Russia, AC	Skin greenish-yellow, acidic, very aromatic; moderately scab-resistant
14.	'Panemunės baltasis'	1939, Lithuania, AC	Skin greenish-yellow, flesh white, waxed; scab-resistant
15.	'Pilkasis alyvinis'	1653, Russia, SC	Skin white-yellow, flesh white; susceptible to scab
16.	'Popierinis'	1852, Lithuania or Latvia, SC	Skin white-yellow, flesh white; susceptible to scab
17.	'Raudonasis alyvinis'	XVIII, Russia, SC	Skin reddish-white, aromatic, susceptible to scab
18.	'Rudens dryžuotasis'	1870, Baltic countries, AC	Skin reddish-white, vinous taste, flesh pinkish; moderately scab-resistant
19.	'Sierinka'	1860, Baltic countries, AC	Skin greenish-yellow, fragrant with characteristic aroma, susceptible to canker; moderately scab-resistant
20.	'Tabokinė'	XIX, Baltic countries, WC	Skin reddish-yellow, bitter-sweet, bitterness weakens by spring; scab-resistant
21.	'Virginijos rožinis'	1816, Europe, SC	Skin reddish-white, vinous taste; susceptible to scab
22.	'Žemaičių grietininis'	XIX, Lithuania, SC	Skin white-yellow, flesh white; moderately scab-resistant

SC–summer cultivar, AC–autumn cultivar, WC–winter cultivar.

3.2. Chemicals and Solvents

All solvents, reagents, and standards used were of analytical grade. Acetonitrile and acetic acid were obtained from Sigma-Aldrich GmbH (Buchs, Switzerland), ethanol was obtained from AB Stumbras (Kaunas, Lithuania), hyperoside, rutin, quercitrin, phloridzin, procyanidin B1, procyanidin B2 and chlorogenic acid standards were purchased from Extrasynthese (Genay, France), reynoutrin, (+)-catechin and (−)-epicatechin–from Sigma-Aldrich GmbH (Steinheim, Germany), and avicularin, procyanidin C1 and isoquercitrin–from Chromadex (Santa Ana, CA, USA). Purified deionized water used in the tests was prepared with the Milli-Q® (Millipore, Bedford, MA, USA) water purification system.

3.3. Preparation of Samples

For the analysis, twenty apples at the optimal maturity stage were picked from different parts of the tree crown. Whole apples were immediately frozen in a freezer (at −35 °C) with air circulation. Subsequently, these frozen samples were lyophilized with a ZIRBUS sublimator 3 × 4 × 5/20 (ZIRBUS technology, Bad Grund, Germany) at a pressure of 0.01 mbar (condenser temperature: −85 °C). The lyophilized samples were ground to fine powder using a Retsch 200 mill electric grinder (Haan, Germany). Loss on drying before the analysis was determined by drying the apple lyophilisate in a laboratory drying oven to complete the evaporation of water and volatile compounds (temperature: 105 °C; the difference in weight between measurements: up to 0.01 g) and by calculating the difference in raw material weight before and after the drying. The data were recalculated for the absolute dry lyophilisate weight. The prepared apple samples were stored in dark, tightly closed glass vessels.

3.4. Preparation of the Phenolic Compounds

During the analysis of phenolic compounds, 2.5 g of lyophilizate powder (exact weight) was weighed, added to 30 mL of 70% (v/v) ethanol, and extracted in a Sonorex Digital 10 P ultrasonic bath (Bandelin Electronic GmbH & Co. KG, Berlin, Germany) at room temperature for 20 min. The obtained extract was filtered through a paper filter, and the residue on the filter was washed with 70% (v/v) ethanol in a 50-mL flask until the exact volume was reached. The conditions of the extraction were chosen based on the results of the tests for setting the extraction conditions.

3.5. Qualitative and Quantitative Analysis by HPLC–PDA Method

The qualitative and quantitative HPLC analysis of phenolic compounds was performed with a Waters 2998 PDA detector (Waters, Milford, CT, USA). Chromatographic separations were carried out by using a YMC-Pack ODS-A (5 µm, C18, 250 × 4.6 mm i.d.) column. The column was operated at a constant temperature of 25 °C. The volume of the analyzed extract was 10 µL. The flow rate was 1 mL/min. The mobile phase consisted of 2% (v/v) acetic acid (solvent A) and acetonitrile (solvent B). Gradient variation: 0–30 min 3–15% B, 30–45 min 15–25% B, 45–50 min 25–50% B, and 50–55 min 50–95% B. For the quantitative analysis, the calibration curves were obtained by injecting the known concentrations of different standard compounds. All the identified phenolic compounds were quantified at λ = 200–400 nm wavelength [5].

3.6. Statistical Analysis

The statistical analysis of the study data was performed by using Microsoft Office Excel 2013 (Microsoft, Redmond, WA, USA) and SPSS 25.0 (SPSS Inc., Chicago, IL, USA) computer software. All the results obtained during the ESC analysis were presented as means of three consecutive test results and standard deviations. To evaluate the variance in the quantitative composition, we calculated the coefficient of variation. Univariate analysis of variance (ANOVA) was applied in order to determine whether the differences between the compared data were statistically significant. The hypothesis about the equality of variances was verified by applying Levine's test. If the variances of independent variables were found to be equal, Tukey's multiple comparison test was used. The differences were regarded as statistically significant at $p < 0.05$. The comparison of the chemical composition between the apple fruit samples of the studied heirloom cultivars was carried out by applying the hierarchical cluster analysis, using the squared Euclidean distance. Principal component analysis was performed as well.

4. Conclusions

Apple trees of heirloom cultivars are valuable from the genetic aspect in the selection of new fruit tree cultivars. Their fruit are a source of biologically active compounds and can be used in the development and production of new innovative dietary supplements and medicinal cosmetic products. Apple trees of the heirloom cultivars 'Koštelė', 'Lietuvos pepinas', 'Paprastasis antaninis', 'Virginijos rožinis' and 'Sierinka' grown in the Collection of the Apple Tree Genetic Resources at the Institute of Horticulture of the Lithuanian Research Center for Agriculture and Forestry are not suitable for growing in industrial gardens due to their low fruit yield, poor external quality, small size, and susceptibility to disease. In amateur gardens, growing apples of heirloom cultivars is promising due to their higher content of bioactive substances. Our phytochemical studies of heirloom apple cultivars provide valuable scientific knowledge on the variability of the qualitative and quantitative composition of phenolic compounds. The results of our study will enable a wider cultivation of heirloom apple cultivars in gardens and collections and will help consumers to obtain and use apples with a known chemical composition of phenolic compounds, which determine the use of apples in the healthy food chain and the development of innovative food products.

Author Contributions: Conceptualization, V.J.; methodology, M.L.; formal analysis, A.B.; investigation, A.B.; resources, D.G., D.K.; data curation, A.B.; writing-original draft preparation, A.B.; writing-review and editing, V.J., M.L., D.K., D.G.; visualization, A.B.; supervision, V.J., M.L.; project administration, V.J., M.L. All authors have read and agreed to the published version of the manuscript.

Funding: This research received no external funding.

Conflicts of Interest: The authors declare no conflict of interest.

References

1. De Paepe, D.; Valkenborg, D.; Noten, B.; Servaes, K.; Diels, L.; De Loose, M.; Van Droogenbroeck, B.; Voorspoels, S. Variability of the phenolic profiles in the fruits from old, recent and new apple cultivars cultivated in Belgium. *Metabolomics* **2014**, *11*, 739–752. [CrossRef]
2. Duan, N.; Bai, Y.; Sun, H.; Wang, N.; Thomas, C.; Linyong, M.; Wang, X.; Jiao, C.; LeGall, N.; Mao, L.; et al. Genome re-sequencing reveals the history of apple and supports a two-stage model for fruit enlargement. *Nat. Commun.* **2017**, *8*, 1–11. [CrossRef] [PubMed]
3. Blažytė, A. *National Genetic Resources of Lithuanian Plants: Old Lithuanian Fruit Tree Cultivars, Plant Gene Bank*; Ministry of Environment of the Republic of Lithuania: Lithuanian, Vilnius, 2008; pp. 1–27.
4. Kviklys, D.; Gelvonauskienė, D.; Karklelienė, R.; Juškevičienė, D.; Dambrauskienė, E.; Uselis, N.; Lanauskas, J. Orchards of Heritage: A Catalogue of Cultivars. 2019, pp. 31–83. Available online: https://latlit.eu/wp-content/uploads/2017/06/HG_cultivar-catalog.pdf (accessed on 9 November 2020).
5. Liaudanskas, M.; Viskelis, P.; Kviklys, D.; Raudonis, R.; Janulis, V. A Comparative Study of Phenolic Content in Apple Fruits. *Int. J. Food Prop.* **2015**, *18*, 945–953. [CrossRef]
6. Barreira, J.C.; Arraibi, A.A.; Ferreira, I.C. Bioactive and functional compounds in apple pomace from juice and cider manufacturing: Potential use in dermal formulations. *Trends Food Sci. Technol.* **2019**, *90*, 76–87. [CrossRef]
7. Dobrowolska-Iwanek, J.; Gąstoł, M.; Adamska, A.; Krośniak, M.; Zagrodzki, P. Heirloom Versus Modern Apple Cultivars—A Comparison of Juice Composition. *Folia Hortic.* **2015**, *27*, 33–41. [CrossRef]
8. Belviso, S.; Scursatone, B.; Re, G.; Zeppa, G. Novel Data on the Polyphenol Composition of Italian Ancient Apple Cultivars. *Int. J. Food Prop.* **2013**, *16*, 1507–1515. [CrossRef]

9. Iacopini, P.; Camangi, F.; Stefani, A.; Sebastiani, L. Antiradical potential of ancient Italian apple varieties of Malus×domestica Borkh. in a peroxynitrite-induced oxidative process. *J. Food Compos. Anal.* **2010**, *23*, 518–524. [CrossRef]
10. Pandey, K.B.; Rizvi, S.I. Plant Polyphenols as Dietary Antioxidants in Human Health and Disease. *Oxidative Med. Cell. Longev.* **2009**, *2*, 270–278. [CrossRef]
11. Liddle, D.M.; Kavanagh, M.E.; Wright, A.J.; Robinson, L.E. Apple Flavonols Mitigate Adipocyte Inflammation and Promote Angiogenic Factors in LPS- and Cobalt Chloride-Stimulated Adipocytes, in Part by a Peroxisome Proliferator-Activated Receptor-γ-Dependent Mechanism. *Nutrients* **2020**, *12*, 1386. [CrossRef]
12. Wu, H.; Luo, T.; Li, Y.M.; Gao, Z.P.; Zhang, K.Q.; Song, J.Y.; Xiao, J.S.; Cao, Y.P. Granny Smith apple procyanidin extract upregulates tight junction protein expression and modulates oxidative stress and inflammation in lipopolysaccharide-induced Caco-2 cells. *Food Funct.* **2018**, *9*, 3321–3329. [CrossRef]
13. Zardo, D.M.; Alberti, A.; Zielinski, A.A.F.; Prestes, A.A.; Esmerino, L.A.; Nogueira, A. Influence of solvents in the extraction of phenolic compounds with antibacterial activity from apple pomace. *Sep. Sci. Technol.* **2020**, 1–9. [CrossRef]
14. Han, M.; Li, A.; Shen, T.; Meng, J.; Lei, Y.; Zhang, X.; Liu, P.; Gan, L.; Ao, L.; Li, H. Phenolic compounds present in fruit extracts of Malus spp. show antioxidative and pro-apoptotic effects on human gastric cancer cell lines. *J. Food Biochem.* **2019**, *43*, e13028. [CrossRef] [PubMed]
15. Hecht, F.; Pessoa, C.F.; Gentile, L.B.; Rosenthal, D.; Carvalho, D.P.; Fortunato, R.S. The role of oxidative stress on breast cancer development and therapy. *Tumor Biol.* **2016**, *37*, 4281–4291. [CrossRef] [PubMed]
16. Khurana, S.; Venkataraman, K.; Hollingsworth, A.; Piche, M.; Tai, T.C. Polyphenols: Benefits to the Cardiovascular System in Health and in Aging. *Nutrients* **2013**, *5*, 3779–3827. [CrossRef]
17. Palermo, V.; Mattivi, F.; Silvestri, R.; La Regina, G.; Falcone, C.; Mazzoni, C. Apple Can Act as Anti-Aging on Yeast Cells. *Oxidative Med. Cell. Longev.* **2012**, *2012*, 491759. [CrossRef]
18. Peng, C.; Chan, H.Y.E.; Huang, Y.; Yu, H.; Chen, Z.-Y. Apple Polyphenols Extend the Mean Lifespan of Drosophila melanogaster. *J. Agric. Food Chem.* **2011**, *59*, 2097–2106. [CrossRef]
19. Oszmiański, J.; Lachowicz, S.; Gamsjäger, H. Phytochemical analysis by liquid chromatography of ten old apple varieties grown in Austria and their antioxidative activity. *Eur. Food Res. Technol.* **2019**, *246*, 437–448. [CrossRef]
20. Musacchi, S.; Serra, S. Apple fruit quality: Overview on pre-harvest factors. *Sci. Hortic.* **2018**, *234*, 409–430. [CrossRef]
21. Contessa, C.; Botta, R. Comparison of physicochemical traits of red-fleshed, commercial and ancient apple cultivars. *Hortic. Sci.* **2016**, *43*, 159–166. [CrossRef]
22. Convention on Biological Diversity. Available online: https://www.cbd.int/doc/legal/cbd-en.pdf (accessed on 10 September 2020).
23. Cooper, H.D. The International Treaty on Plant Genetic Resources for Food and Agriculture. *Rev. Eur. Community Int. Environ. Law* **2002**, *11*, 1–16. [CrossRef]
24. Buck, M.; Hamilton, C. The Nagoya Protocol on Access to Genetic Resources and the Fair and Equitable Sharing of Benefits Arising from their Utilization to the Convention on Biological Diversity. *Rev. Eur. Community Int. Environ. Law* **2011**, *20*, 47–61. [CrossRef]
25. Lončarić, A.; Matanović, K.; Ferrer, P.; Kovač, T.; Šarkanj, B.; Babojelić, M.S.; Lores, M. Peel of Heirloom Apple Varieties as a Great Source of Bioactive Compounds: Extraction by Micro-Matrix Solid-Phase Dispersion. *Foods* **2020**, *9*, 80. [CrossRef] [PubMed]
26. Jakobek, L.; Barron, A.R. Ancient apple varieties from Croatia as a source of bioactive polyphenolic compounds. *J. Food Compos. Anal.* **2016**, *45*, 9–15. [CrossRef]
27. Kviklys, D.; Liaudanskas, M.; Viškelis, J.; Buskienė, L.; Lanauskas, J.; Uselis, N.; Janulis, V. Composition and Concentration of Phenolic Compounds of 'Auksis' Apple Grown on Various Rootstocks. *Proc. Latv. Acad. Sci. Sect. B Nat. Exact Appl. Sci.* **2017**, *71*, 144–149. [CrossRef]
28. Liaudanskas, M.; Viškelis, P.; Jakštas, V.; Raudonis, R.; Kviklys, D.; Milašius, A.; Janulis, V. Application of an Optimized HPLC Method for the Detection of Various Phenolic Compounds in Apples from Lithuanian Cultivars. *J. Chem.* **2014**, *2014*, 542121. [CrossRef]
29. Cerutti, A.K.; Bruun, S.; Donno, D.; Beccaro, G.L.; Bounous, G. Environmental Sustainability of Heirloom Foods: The Case of Ancient Apple Cultivars in Northern Italy Assessed by Multifunctional LCA. *J. Clean. Prod.* **2013**, *52*, 245–252. [CrossRef]

30. Morresi, C.; Cianfruglia, L.; Armeni, T.; Mancini, F.; Tenore, G.; D'Urso, E.; Micheletti, A.; Ferretti, G.; Bacchetti, T. Polyphenolic compounds and nutraceutical properties of old and new apple cultivars. *J. Food Biochem.* **2018**, *42*, e12641. [CrossRef]
31. Zardo, D.M.; Zielinski, A.A.F.; Alberti, A.; Nogueira, A. Phenolic Compounds and Antioxidant Capacity of Brazilian Apples. *Food Nutr. Sci.* **2015**, *6*, 727–735. [CrossRef]
32. Piccolo, E.L.; Landi, M.; Massai, R.; Remorini, D.; Conte, G.; Guidi, L. Ancient apple cultivars from Garfagnana (Tuscany, Italy): A potential source for 'nutrafruit' production. *Food Chem.* **2019**, *294*, 518–525. [CrossRef]
33. Bars-Cortina, D.; Macià, A.; Iglesias, I.; Romero, M.P.; Motilva, M.J. Phytochemical Profiles of New Red-Fleshed Apple Varieties Compared with Old and New White-Fleshed Varieties. *J. Agric. Food Chem.* **2017**, *65*, 1684–1696. [CrossRef]
34. Oszmiański, J.; Lachowicz, S.; Gławdel, E.; Cebulak, T.; Ochmian, I. Determination of phytochemical composition and antioxidant capacity of 22 old apple cultivars grown in Poland. *Eur. Food Res. Technol.* **2017**, *244*, 647–662. [CrossRef]
35. Wojdyło, A.; Oszmiański, J.; Laskowski, P. Polyphenolic Compounds and Antioxidant Activity of New and Old Apple Varieties. *J. Agric. Food Chem.* **2008**, *56*, 6520–6530. [CrossRef] [PubMed]
36. Kschonsek, J.; Wiegand, C.; Hipler, U.-C.; Böhm, V. Influence of polyphenolic content on the in vitro allergenicity of old and new apple cultivars: A pilot study. *Nutrients* **2019**, *58*, 30–35. [CrossRef] [PubMed]
37. Łysiak, G.P.; Michalska, A.; Wojdyło, A. Postharvest changes in phenolic compounds and antioxidant capacity of apples cv. Jonagold growing in different locations in Europe. *Food Chem.* **2020**, *310*, 125912. [CrossRef] [PubMed]
38. Raphaelli, C.D.O.; Pereira, E.D.S.; Camargo, T.M.; Vinholes, J.; Rombaldi, C.V.; Vizzotto, M.; Nora, L. Apple Phenolic Extracts Strongly Inhibit α-Glucosidase Activity. *Plant Foods Hum. Nutr.* **2019**, *74*, 430–435. [CrossRef] [PubMed]
39. Kumar, S.; Sinha, K.; Sharma, R.; Purohit, R.; Padwad, Y.S. Phloretin and phloridzin improve insulin sensitivity and enhance glucose uptake by subverting PPARγ/Cdk5 interaction in differentiated adipocytes. *Exp. Cell Res.* **2019**, *383*, 111480. [CrossRef]
40. Xiang, L.; Sun, K.; Lu, J.; Weng, Y.; Taoka, A.; Sakagami, Y.; Qi, J. Anti-Aging Effects of Phloridzin, an Apple Polyphenol, on Yeastviathe SOD and Sir2 Genes. *Biosci. Biotechnol. Biochem.* **2011**, *75*, 854–858. [CrossRef] [PubMed]
41. Tuinyla, V.; Lukoševičius, A.; Bandaravičius, A. *Lithuanian Pomology*. T.1; Apples and Pears Science: Lithuanian, Vilnius, 1990; pp. 1–333.

Publisher's Note: MDPI stays neutral with regard to jurisdictional claims in published maps and institutional affiliations.

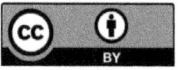

© 2020 by the authors. Licensee MDPI, Basel, Switzerland. This article is an open access article distributed under the terms and conditions of the Creative Commons Attribution (CC BY) license (http://creativecommons.org/licenses/by/4.0/).

Article
Biopharmaceutical Evaluation of Capsules with Lyophilized Apple Powder

Aurita Butkevičiūtė [1,*], Mindaugas Liaudanskas [1], Kristina Ramanauskienė [2] and Valdimaras Janulis [1]

[1] Department of Pharmacognosy, Lithuanian University of Health Sciences, Sukileliu av. 13, LT-50162 Kaunas, Lithuania; Mindaugas.Liaudanskas@lsmu.lt (M.L.); Valdimaras.Janulis@lsmuni.lt (V.J.)
[2] Department of Clinical Pharmacy, Lithuanian University of Health Sciences, Sukileliu av. 13, LT-50162 Kaunas, Lithuania; Kristina.Ramanauskiene@lsmuni.lt
* Correspondence: Aurita.Butkeviciute@lsmu.lt; Tel.: +37-037-621-56190

Abstract: Apples are an important source of biologically active compounds. Consequently, we decided to model hard gelatin capsules with lyophilized apple powder by using different excipients and to evaluate the release kinetics of phenolic compounds. The apple slices of "Ligol" cultivar were immediately frozen in a freezer (at −35°C) with air circulation and were lyophilized with a sublimator at the pressure of 0.01 mbar (condenser temperature, −85°C). Lyophilized apple powder was used as an active substance filled into hard gelatin capsules. We conducted capsule disintegration and dissolution tests to evaluate the quality of apple lyophilizate-containing capsules of different encapsulating content. Individual phenolic compounds can be arranged in the following descending order according to the amount released from the capsules of different compositions: chlorogenic acid > rutin > avicularin > hyperoside > phloridzin > quercitrin > (−)-epicatechin > isoquercitrin. Chlorogenic acid was the compound that was released in the highest amounts from capsules of different encapsulating content: its released amounts ranged from 68.4 to 640.3 µg/mL. According to the obtained data, when hypromellose content ranged from 29% to 41% of the capsule mass, the capsules disintegrated within less than 30 min, and such amounts of hypromellose did not prolong the release of phenolic compounds. Based on the results of the dissolution test, the capsules can be classified as fast-dissolving preparations, as more than 85% of the active substances were released within 30 min.

Keywords: apple; phenolic compounds; dissolution test; HPLC-DAD

1. Introduction

Apples are among the most consumed fruits in Lithuania and worldwide. According to the data of 2020, 84.63 million tons of apples were grown in the world [1]. The greatest amounts of apples are grown in China (around 40.92 million tons). In the US, around 5.19 million tons are grown per year, and in Poland, the amount of apples grown per year is around 3.20 million tons [1]. Apples are widely used in the food industry in the production of various products and beverages (juices, wines, and ciders), and are also used unprocessed [2,3].

In the healthy food chain, apples are an important source of biologically active compounds [4]. They have been found to contain a complex of phenolic (8.2–360.75 mg/g^{-1}) [5], and triterpenic (0.47–3.75 mg/g^{-1}) [6] compounds, glucose (1.96–75.91 mg/g^{-1}), fructose (15.52–342.14 mg/g^{-1}), sucrose (11.81–43.79 mg/g^{-1}), xylitol (1.01–13.79 mg/g^{-1}), pectins (4.05–19.72 mg/g^{-1}), organic acids (malic acid (38.96–107.28 mg/g^{-1}), citric acid (1.84–4.12 mg/g^{-1}), maleic acid (0.17–0.23 mg/g^{-1}), pyruvic acid (0.14–0.34 mg/g^{-1}), shikimic acid (0.04–0.17 mg/g^{-1})) [7,8], vitamins (21.08 mg/g^{-1}) [9], macroelements (K (1.07–1.12 mg/g^{-1}), P (0.074–0.11 mg/g^{-1}), Mg (0.05–0.08 mg/g^{-1}), Ca (0.04–0.06 mg/g^{-1}), Na (0.007–0.04 mg/g^{-1})), microelements (Fe (0.001–0.003 mg/g^{-1}), Zn (0.0004–0.019 mg/g^{-1}),

Mn (0.0003–0.0004 mg/g^{-1}), Cu (0.0003–0.0005 mg/g^{-1}) [10], and fiber (3700–4500 mg/g^{-1}) [5].

Biologically active substances in apples affect the biological systems of the human body. They have an antioxidant effect, neutralizing harmful reactive oxygen and nitrogen species that cause structural damage to the body's molecules, which, in turn, is directly linked to the development and progression of numerous diseases (cardiovascular and neurodegenerative diseases, cancer, diabetes, etc.) [11,12]. The biologically active compounds accumulated in apples are potentially valuable for the prevention of various diseases [13,14]. During the recent period, in order to preserve the chemical composition of high-quality fruit, lyophilization is increasingly used in the food industry. Lyophilized apples with a chemical composition identical to that of fresh apples can be used in the functionalization of food supplements and various pharmaceutical dosage forms.

One important step in modeling a solid pharmaceutical dosage form is the selection of the category of the pharmaceutical form. Hard capsules are a convenient and widely used dosage form in which drugs and excipients content are placed in the capsules. One of the most widely used capsules may not be resistant to and dissolved in gastric juice, so we decided to use this capsules type in the study. In addition, the capsules may be resistant to gastric juice and dissolved in a selected part of the gastrointestinal tract if appropriate excipients are selected. Therefore, one of the most important advantages of capsules is that their use allows for the localization of the gastrointestinal tract site of the release of biologically active compounds from the capsule, thus helping to protect the acid-sensitive biologically active substances from the destructive effects of gastric juice [15].

Another equally important property of hard capsules is that the dissolution kinetics of the active substances can be modified by using different excipients in the modeling of hard capsules. In our study, the active substance in capsules is a lyophilized apple powder rich in phenolic compounds. Excipients are used in the manufacturing process of encapsulated mixtures in order to increase the bulk of the encapsulated substances, to reduce their adhesion, to improve flowability, and/or to promote disintegration or penetrability to water, thus differentially modifying the release of the active ingredients from the capsule. The use of excipients can slow down the release of the capsule contents, thus ensuring a longer and more sustained effect of the biologically active substances in the capsule [15,16]. It is important to select suitable excipients that would ensure adequate dissolution kinetics of the medicinal substance. Microcrystalline cellulose, starch, and D(+)-glucose were used as fillers in the encapsulating mixture. Hypromellose was selected as a drug release modifier that would prolong the release of the active ingredient. Silicon dioxide was selected as the tackifier of the encapsulated mixture.

About 50% of the currently biopharmaceuticals are lyophilized, representing the most common formulation strategy [17]. Lyophilization or freeze drying is a process in which water is frozen, followed by its removal from the sample, initially by sublimation (primary drying) and then by desorption (secondary drying). Freeze-drying is a process of drying in which water is sublimed from the product after it is frozen [17,18]. Although on the pharmacy there are quite a number of medicines, and in particular food supplements, which use various plant extracts as the active ingredients in hard capsules, the use of lyophilized fruits and botanical raw materials in the production of hard capsules is still a rare phenomenon. Lyophilized fruits (apples, pears, plums, peaches), berries (blueberries, cranberries, strawberries), and vegetables (carrots, beets) are used in the food industry and can be added to various types of cocktails, cereals, drinks, meals, juices, yogurts, ice cream; freeze-dried fruit powder can also be added to food supplements thus increasing the content of biologically active compounds [19–22]. Dehydrated, freeze-dried fruit, berries, and vegetables promote long-term storage of freeze-dried food or food supplements. Lyophilization preserves most of the biologically active compounds stored in the fruit, while other methods often destroy thermolabile compounds. Lyophilization does not involve the use of chemical substances, which is crucial for providing the consumers with safe, effective, and environmentally friendly products or food supplements with the highest content of biologically active compounds.

The aim of our study was to model hard gelatin capsules with lyophilized apple powder by using different excipients and to evaluate the release kinetics of phenolic compounds.

2. Results and Discussion

2.1. Qualitative and Quantitative Analysis of Phenolic Compounds of Apple Lyophilisate

During the first stage of the study, the quantitative composition of the lyophilized apple powder was analyzed. Ethanol extracts of the lyophilized apple powder were analyzed by applying high performance liquid chromatography (HPLC). The obtained results allowed for an accurate assessment of the qualitative and quantitative composition of individual phenolic compounds in the studied apple lyophilisate powder. Different groups of phenolic compounds were identified and quantified in the analyzed apple lyophilisate: quercetin glycosides (rutin, hyperoside, isoquercitrin, reynoutrin, avicularin, and quercitrin), flavan-3-ols (procyanidin B1, procyanidin B2, procyanidin C1, (+)-catechin, and (−)-epicatechin), dihydrochalcones (phloridzin), and phenolic acids (chlorogenic acid). The data obtained by Jakobek et al. corroborate to the results of our research [23]. The chromatogram of the tested apple lyophilisate ethanol extract is shown in Figure 1.

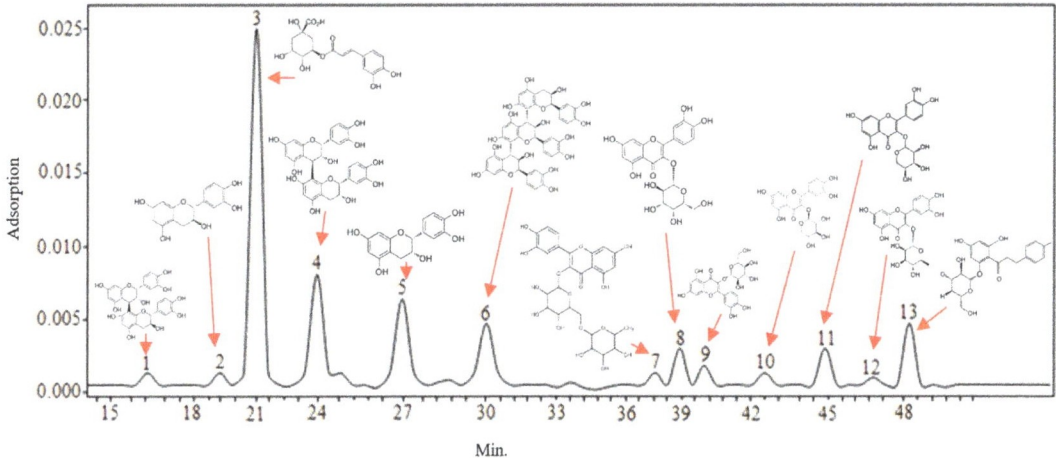

Figure 1. Chromatogram of the ethanol extract of the apple lyophilisate. Analytes determined at $\lambda = 280$ nm wavelength: 1—procyanidin B1; 2—(+)-catechin; 3—chlorogenic acid; 4—procyanidin B2; 5—(−)-epicatechin; 6—procyanidin C1; at $\lambda = 360$ nm wavelength: 7—rutin; 8—hyperoside; 9—isoquercitrin; 10—reynoutrin; 11—avicularin; 12—quercitrin; at $\lambda = 280$ nm wavelength: 13—phloridzin.

The sum of the identified and quantified individual phenolic compounds found in the apple lyophilisate of the "Ligol" cultivar was 1.94 ± 0.05 mg/g. Studies of the fruit samples of apple cultivars grown in the orchards of the Marche region of Italy showed that the total amount of phenolic compounds ranged from 0.82 to 3.60 mg/g and confirm the results of our research [5]. Chlorogenic acid predominated among all the identified phenolic compounds. Its content was 0.67 ± 0.10 mg/g, which accounted for 34.5% of the total content of all the detected phenolic compounds (Figure 2).

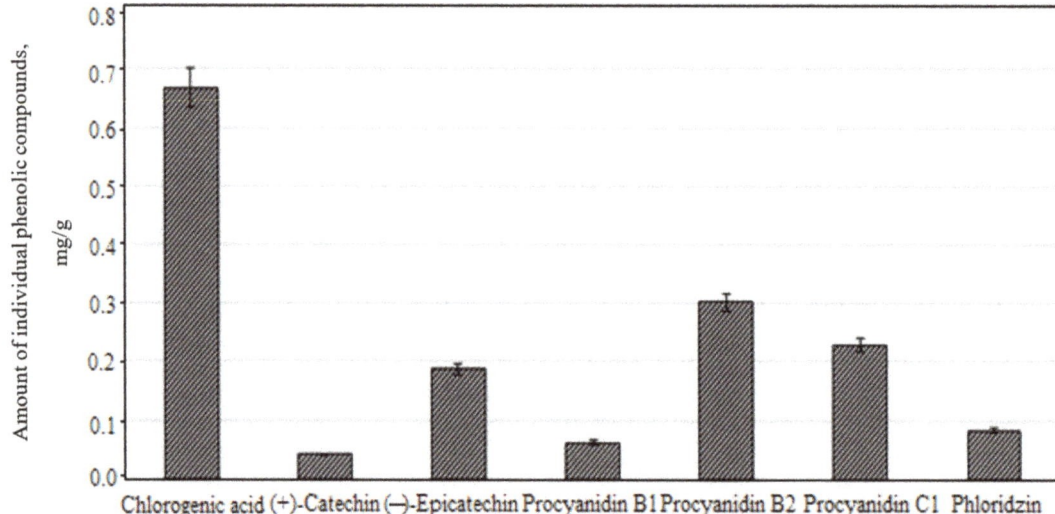

Figure 2. The amount of individual flavan-3-ols, phloridzin, and chlorogenic acid in ethanol extracts obtained from the apple fruit of the "Ligol" cultivar grown in Lithuania.

The results of this study confirmed those of the previous studies reporting that chlorogenic acid is one of the most predominant components in apples [24,25]. The amount of chlorogenic acid in apple samples grown in Italy was found to vary from 0.12 to 0.63 mg/g [26]. In our study, a higher amount of chlorogenic acid compared with the amount described by Italian scientists was determined. Chlorogenic acid has properties important for human health, such as antioxidant activity [27,28], anti-inflammatory activity [29,30], the reduction in the risk of type 2 diabetes [31], the improvement of cardiovascular function [32,33], and the inhibition of the processes of carcinogenesis [34–36].

Another group of flavan-3-ol compounds with diverse biological activity identified in the apple lyophilisate consisted of monomeric compounds ((+)-catechin and (−)-epicatechin) and oligomeric compounds (procyanidin B1, procyanidin B2, and procyanidin C1). The total amount of compounds in flavan-3-ol group was 0.82 ± 0.03 mg/g, which accounted for 42.3% of the total amount of the identified phenolic compounds (Figure 2). The flavan-3-ol content in fruit samples of apple cultivars grown in Croatian orchards was found to vary from 0.02 to 0.69 mg/g [23]. We established the higher amount of total flavan-3-ols compared with the amount determined by Croatian scientists. The variability in the quantitative composition of the individual compounds of the flavan-3-ol group in the apple lyophilisate is shown in Figure 2. The predominant compounds of the flavan-3-ol group in the apple lyophilisate was procyanidins. The highest amount of procyanidin B2 and procyanidin C1 were determined as 0.30 ± 0.08 mg/g and 0.23 ± 0.06 mg/g, respectively (Figure 2). The amount of procyanidin B2 and procyanidin C1 in fruit samples of apple cultivars grown in Polish orchards ranged from 0.07 to 2.00 mg/g and 0.0006 to 0.97 mg/g, accordingly [37]. Our study results confirmed Polish research results. Procyanidins are important for the human body as they exhibit antioxidant, anticancer, anti-inflammatory, platelet aggregation-reducing, and cholesterol-reducing effects [38–40]. Monomeric flavan-3-ols, which together with procyanidins may be responsible for the cholesterol-lowering [41] and vasodilating [42] effect of the apples, also inhibit sulfotransferases, and thus can regulate the biological activity of hydroxysteroids and can act as natural chemopreventive agents [43].

Phloridzin, a compound of the dihydrochalcone group, was detected in the apple lyophilisate as well. Its quantitative content in the sample was 0.08 ± 0.005 mg/g, which accounted for 4.1% of the total amount of phenolic compounds detected in the apple lyophilisate (Figure 2). The amount of phloridzin in fruit samples of apple cultivars grown in orchards in the Garfagnana region of Italy ranged from 0.01 to 0.05 mg/g [44]. The results obtained in these studies confirm the results obtained in our research. Phloridzin exhibits important antidiabetic activity [45,46], and therefore apples, as botanical raw materials accumulating this compound, can be potentially useful for the prevention of diabetes mellitus [14].

The qualitative and quantitative composition of quercetin glycosides is shown in Figure 3. The total amount of quercetin glycosides was 0.37 ± 0.12 mg/g, which accounted for 19.1% of the total amount of phenolic compounds detected in the apple lyophilisate.

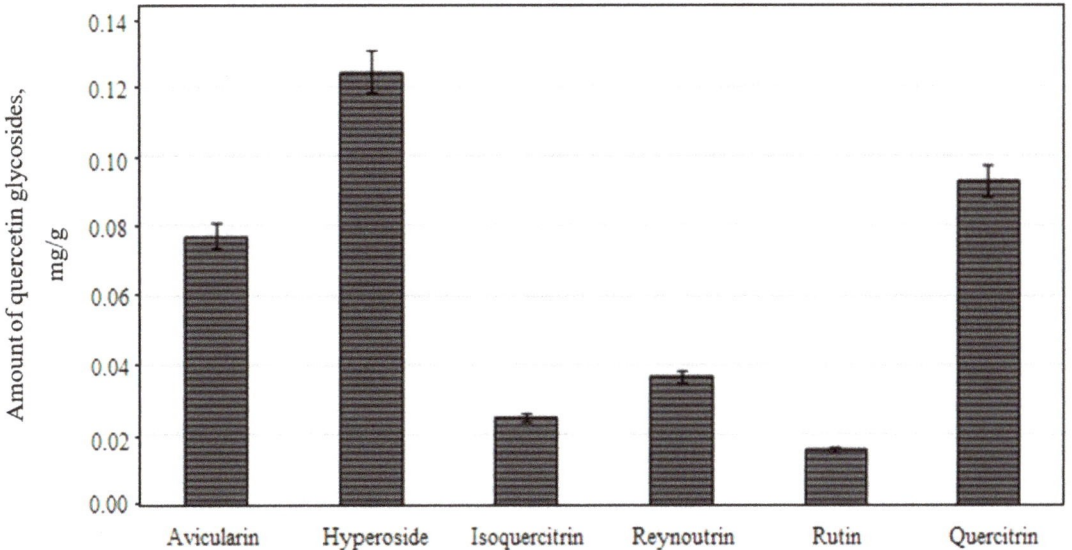

Figure 3. Concentration of individual quercetin glycosides in ethanol extracts obtained from the fruit of the "Ligol" apple cultivar grown in Lithuania.

Studies of fruit samples of apple cultivars grown in Croatian orchards showed that quercetin glycosides levels ranged from 0.20 to 1.22 mg/g [23]. The results of our study are corroborated by research data obtained by Croatian researchers. Hyperoside predominated among all the identified quercetin glycosides. Its content was 0.12 ± 0.06 mg/g, which accounted for 6.2% of the total content of all the detected phenolic compounds (Figure 3). The amount of hyperoside in fruit samples of apple cultivars grown in Italian orchards ranged from 0.0003 to 0.002 mg/g [47]. The apple lyophilisate contained higher amounts of hyperoside compared to these found in fruit samples of apple cultivars grown in Italian orchards. The amount of quercitrin was 0.09 ± 0.04 mg/g and these results confirmed Italian study results that report that the amount of quercitrin found in apple samples ranged from 0.005 to 0.043 mg/g [47].

All the quercetin glycosides identified and quantified in the ethanol extract of the apple lyophilisate can be ranked in the following ascending order by their content: rutin < isoquercitrin < reynoutrin < avicularin < quercitrin < hyperoside. Hyperoside was a predominant component among quercetin glycosides in the ethanol extracts of the fruit samples of apple cultivars selected for this study. Rutin was the minor component among all the quercetin derivatives. These results are consistent with those of the previously published studies, which reported hyperoside to be one of the predominant compounds [3,48].

2.2. Biopharmaceutical Evaluation of Hard Gelatin Capsules

Following the analysis of the composition of biologically active compounds in the apple lyophilisate, the selected amount of the active substance was 0.100 g of lyophilized apple powder per capsule. During the next stage of the research, the selection of excipients was performed. Microcrystalline cellulose, starch, and glucose were chosen as fillers to increase the mass of the encapsulated content when modeling apple lyophilisate-containing capsules (Table 1).

Table 1. Compositions of the apple lyophilisate-containing capsules.

CC	AL, g	SDX, g	MCC, g	HPMC, g	HEC, g	GL, g	ST, g	TCM, g	FQ	MM, g
N1	0.100	0.001	0.019	0.050	-	-	-	0.170		0.171
N2	0.100	0.001	-	0.069	-	-	-	0.170		0.171
N3	0.100	0.001	-	-	-	0.069	-	0.170	The mass	0.069
N4	0.100	0.001	0.069	-	-	-	-	0.170	is	0.171
N5	0.100	0.001	-	-	-	-	0.069	0.170	powdery,	0.171
N6	0.100	-	-	0.070	-	-	-	0.170	the	0.172
N7	0.100	-	-	-	0.070	-	-	0.170	capsule is	0.171
N8	0.100	-	-	0.100	-	-	-	0.200	filled com-	0.202
N9	0.100	-	-	0.150	-	-	-	0.250	pletely	0.251
N10	0.100	-	-	0.250	-	-	-	0.350		0.349
N11	0.100	-	-	0.500	-	-	-	0.600		0.658

CC = capsule compositions; AL = apple lyophilisate; SDX = silicon dioxide; MCC = microcrystalline cellulose; HPMC = hydroxypropyl methylcellulose; HEC = hydroxyethyl cellulose; GL = glucose; ST = starch; TCM = theoretical capsule mass; FQ = filling quality; MM = mean mass.

Microcrystalline cellulose, one of the most commonly used excipients in the manufacture of solid dosage forms, has excellent compressibility and disintegration-enhancing properties [49]. Glucose is well soluble in water and has good sensory properties, but is hygroscopic [50]. Hypromellose was included in the composition of the capsules to prolong their disintegration time and to extend their therapeutic efficacy [51]. All the compositions of the apple lyophilisate-containing capsules are presented in Table 1.

The quality of the manufactured capsules was evaluated according to the following parameters: uniformity of the capsule mass, capsule disintegration time, and the amount of the active substances released from the capsule (the dissolution test). Data presented in Table 1 shows that the indices of the uniformity of the capsule mass were similar. Thus, it can be stated that the selected excipients and their amounts ensured accurate dosage of the encapsulated mixture into the capsules. During the next stage of the study, capsule disintegration and dissolution tests were performed. Based on the results of these tests, the bioavailability of the modeled capsules can be predicted. The results of these tests are presented in Figure 4 and Table 2.

Disintegration time is an important indicator in assessing the quality of capsules. The release of the drug is known to begin only after the disintegration of the capsule. The excipients in the encapsulated mixture must not interfere with the solubility and disintegration of the capsule. According to the test results presented in Figure 4, the capsules of the compositions N1–N9 disintegrated within less than 15 min, the capsules of the composition N10 disintegrated within 20 min, while the capsules of the composition N11 did not disintegrate after more than 60 min (Figure 4). The European Pharmacopoeia states that non-modified capsules must disintegrate within 30 min, and thus it can be stated that capsules N1–N10 meet the requirements of the European Pharmacopoeia [52]. The results of our study were confirmed by the results described by other scientists. Vyas et al. showed that lyophilized *Vasa Swaras* capsules undergo disintegration in more than 4.23 min [53]. Esmaeili et al. confirmed our study results, that hard gelatin capsules from *Pinus eldarica* bark extract disintegrate between 9.4 and 20.0 min [54]. There was no statistically significant difference ($p > 0.05$) between the disintegration time of the N1–N9 capsules compared to the disintegration time of the other tested capsules. The results of the testing showed that capsules disintegrated more slowly when hypromellose was used as a filler (Figure 4). A statistically significant difference ($p < 0.05$) was found between the disintegration time of the N10 capsules and the disintegration time of the other tested capsules. In capsules of this composition, hypromellose made up about 71.4% of the capsule mass. This confirms the literature data indicating that hypromellose has disintegration-prolonging properties [51].

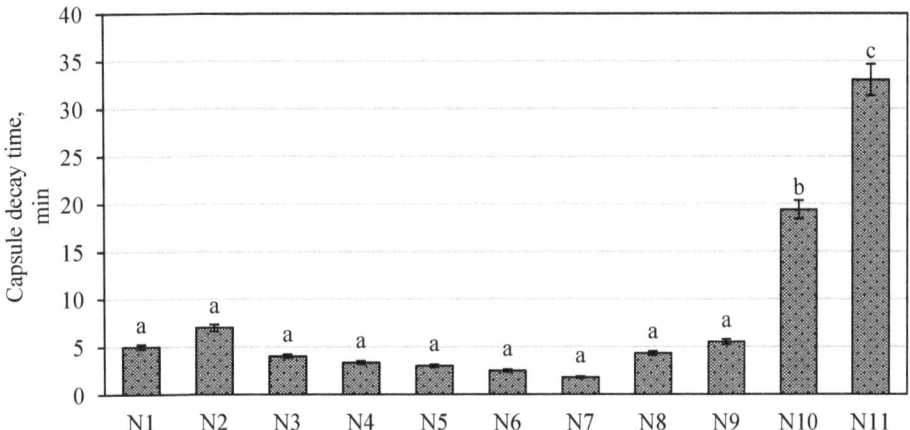

Figure 4. Results of the capsule disintegration test. The means followed by different letters are significantly different at $p < 0.05$.

Table 2. Results of the in vitro dissolution test after 30 min. The means followed by different letters in the columns are significantly different at $p < 0.05$.

CC	Chlorogenic Acid	Rutin	Hyperoside	Isoquercitrin	Quercitrin	Avicularin	(−)-Epicatechin	Phloridzin
				µg/mL				
N1	372.5 [B]	160.0 [B]	144.5 [B]	7.0 [A]	97.5 [B]	149.0 [B]	17.5 [A]	122.5 [B]
N2	367.5 [B]	157.5 [B]	140.0 [B]	6.0 [A]	89.5 [B]	142.5 [B]	9.5 [B]	117.5 [B]
N3	372.5 [B]	149.5 [B]	139.0 [B]	7.5 [A]	91.5 [B]	148.5 [B]	10.0 [B]	121.5 [B]
N4	367.5 [B]	152.5 [B]	140.5 [B]	5.5 [A]	92.5 [B]	142.0 [B]	14.5 [A]	125.0 [B]
N5	385.0 [B]	155.0 [B]	132.5 [B]	4.9 [A]	87.5 [B]	141.5 [B]	8.5 [B]	110.0 [B]
N6	589.5 [A]	265.6 [A]	240.4 [A]	5.0 [A]	170.7 [A]	253.7 [A]	6.3 [B,C]	140.5 [A]
N7	640.3 [A]	268.3 [A]	241.8 [A]	4.9 [A]	166.5 [A]	254.3 [A]	10.2 [B]	119.9 [B]
N8	167.9 [C]	62.1 [C]	60.9 [C]	2.3 [B]	40.3 [C]	61.8 [C]	1.2 [D]	50.6 [C]
N9	128.3 [C]	60.8 [C]	59.6 [C]	2.3 [B]	39.4 [C]	59.6 [C]	1.1 [D]	49.5 [C]
N10	126.4 [C]	39.9 [C]	49.4 [C]	2.9 [B]	33.3 [C]	50.4 [C]	3.8 [C]	40.9 [C]
N11	68.4 [D]	32.4 [D]	31.7 [D]	1.2 [C]	21.0 [D]	31.8 [D]	0.6 [D]	26.4 [D]

CC = capsule compositions.

Dissolution test is one of the most important tests used for capsule quality assessment. The dissolution test evaluates the time taken for a defined amount or part of a drug to be released from a dosage form into a solution. During the test, it is important to choose the right dissolution medium. For this reason, the next stage of the study focused on the selection of a suitable solvent for the active substances. Table 2 presents test results showing that the maximum amount of the active ingredients was released from the capsule when a 1:1 mixture of ethanol and water was used as the solvent.

According to the amount of the active substance released from the capsules of the compositions N1–N11, individual phenolic compounds can be arranged in the following descending order: chlorogenic acid > rutin > avicularin > hyperoside > phloridzin >

quercitrin > (−)-epicatechin > isoquercitrin (Table 2). Based on the results of the study, chlorogenic acid was the compound that was released in the highest amounts from capsules N1–N11, its released amount ranged from 68.4 to 640.3 µg/mL (Table 2).

The results of the testing showed that the selected excipients did not affect the active ingredients because all the capsule formulations released the compounds that were detected in the apple lyophilisate. The amounts of excipients affected the dissolution kinetics of the modeled capsules. The results showed in Table 3 reveals that unequal amounts of the phenolic compounds were released after 30 min.

Table 3. Results of the dissolution test for phenolic compounds released from the N1–N11 capsules after 30 min. The means followed by different letters in the columns are significantly different at $p < 0.05$.

Release Content, %	Chlorogenic Acid	Rutin	Hyperoside	Isoquercitrin	Quercitrin	Avicularin	(−)-Epicatechin	Phloridzin
N1	96.0 [A]	94.0 [A]	88.0 [A]	85.0 [A]	80.0 [A]	90.0 [A]	83.0 [A]	97.0 [A]
N2	94.0 [A]	92.0 [A]	87.0 [A]	84.0 [A]	82.0 [A]	92.0 [A]	80.0 [A]	95.0 [A]
N3	95.0 [A]	85.0 [A]	89.0 [A]	81.0 [A]	80.0 [A]	90.0 [A]	81.0 [A]	94.0 [A]
N4	97.0 [A]	90.0 [A]	89.0 [A]	83.0 [A]	85.0 [A]	88.0 [A]	83.0 [A]	92.0 [A]
N5	94.0 [A]	88.0 [A]	90.0 [A]	85.0 [A]	80.0 [A]	92.0 [A]	85.0 [A]	96.0 [A]
N6	95.0 [A]	96.0 [A]	90.0 [A]	84.0 [A]	84.5 [A]	92.0 [A]	81.0 [A]	94.0 [A]
N7	90.0 [A]	92.0 [A]	88.0 [A]	80.0 [A]	83.0 [A]	91.0 [A]	82.0 [A]	92.0 [A]
N8	55.0 [B]	52.0 [B]	53.0 [B]	35.0 [B]	38.0 [B]	47.0 [B]	35.0 [B]	50.0 [B]
N9	52.0 [B]	55.0 [B]	56.0 [B]	34.0 [B]	37.0 [B]	40.0 [B]	34.0 [B]	54.0 [B]
N10	50.0 [B]	39.0 [B]	42.0 [B]	29.0 [B]	30.0 [B]	40.0 [B]	29.0 [B]	47.0 [B]
N11	29.0 [C]	26.0 [C]	29.0 [C]	19.0 [C]	18.0 [C]	27.0 [C]	19.0 [C]	28.0 [C]

There was no statistically significant difference ($p > 0.05$) between the amount of phenolic compounds released from the N1–N7 capsules after 30 min (Table 3). Thus, it can be argued that the amount of hypromellose used in capsules N1–N7 did not prolong the release of the active substance [55]. The results of the testing revealed that the amount of hypromellose used in capsule production did not prolong the release of the active substance when its amount in the capsules ranged from 29% to 41%. The selected excipients with different properties such as glucose, microcrystalline cellulose and starch did not affect the release of the active ingredients, and no statistically significant ($p > 0.05$) difference was found between the amount of the active compounds released from capsules N3, N4, and N5.

The results of the investigation exposed that the higher amount of hypromellose ranging from 50% to 83% in capsules did prolong the release of the active substance. The results show that after 30–60 min the lowest amount of the phenolic compounds is released from capsule N11 containing 0.500 g of the hypromellose. Of studied N8–N11 composition capsules was released than 85% of active compounds after 75 min (Table 4).

There was no statistically significant difference determined between the amount of released active compounds of capsules N8–N11 after 75 and 90 min ($p > 0.05$). The testing results confirmed the literature data indicating that the dissolution test is an informative tool for assessing the quality of solid dosage forms, helping to evaluate how the dosage form releases the active ingredients [56]. The results of the study showed that the selected excipients were suitable for the modeling of capsules with lyophilized apple powder. The results of this study proved that hypromellose is an appropriate excipient for prolonging the release of an active substance. Active compounds release and disintegration rate depends on the quantity of hypromellose in a capsule. The corresponding amount of hypromellose in capsule N1–N7 neither prolonged the disintegration of the capsules nor affected the dissolution rate of the active compounds. The results of the study showed that the use of hypromellose as a filler in higher amounts (N8–N11) prolongs the release of the active compounds.

Table 4. Results of the dissolution test. Released content of the individual phenolic compounds after 60, 75, 90 min. The means followed by different letters in the columns are significantly different at $p < 0.05$.

Release Content, %	Chlorogenic Acid	Rutin	Hyperoside	Isoquercitrin	Quercitrin	Avicularin	(−)-Epicatechin	Phloridzin
				After 60 min				
N8	88.0 [A]	85.0 [A]	83.0 [A]	76.0 [A]	80.0 [A]	83.0 [A]	81.0 [A]	86.0 [A]
N9	82.0 [A]	82.0 [A]	86.0 [A]	79.0 [A]	80.0 [A]	81.0 [A]	79.0 [A]	82.0 [A]
N10	79.0 [A]	74.0 [A]	76.0 [A]	70.0 [A]	73.0 [A]	77.0 [A]	69.0 [A]	78.0 [A]
N11	57.0 [B]	55.0 [B]	51.0 [B]	45.0 [B]	40.0 [B]	57.0 [B]	39.0 [B]	55.0 [B]
				After 75 min				
N8	90.0 [A]	86.0 [A]	87.0 [A]	81.0 [A]	82.0 [A]	87.0 [A]	83.0 [A]	88.0 [A]
N9	91.0 [A]	89.0 [A]	88.0 [A]	81.0 [A]	83.0 [A]	88.0 [A]	82.0 [A]	90.0 [A]
N10	88.0 [A]	88.0 [A]	86.0 [A]	83.0 [A]	82.0 [A]	87.0 [A]	81.0 [A]	89.0 [A]
N11	92.0 [A]	86.0 [A]	87.0 [A]	85.0 [A]	83.0 [A]	87.0 [A]	81.0 [A]	88.0 [A]
				After 90 min				
N8	95.0 [A]	92.0 [A]	93.0 [A]	89.0 [A]	88.0 [A]	91.0 [A]	88.0 [A]	96.0 [A]
N9	97.0 [A]	94.0 [A]	96.0 [A]	92.0 [A]	90.0 [A]	93.0 [A]	91.0 [A]	96.0 [A]
N10	96.0 [A]	95.0 [A]	90.0 [A]	89.0 [A]	87.0 [A]	90.0 [A]	89.0 [A]	97.0 [A]
N11	94.0 [A]	93.0 [A]	92.0 [A]	88.0 [A]	89.0 [A]	91.0 [A]	88.0 [A]	93.0 [A]

The literature has demonstrated concerning data related to herbal medicinal product dissolution tests. A study performed with phytomedicines based on *Ginkgo biloba* extract capsules and tablets found marked differences in dissolution behavior were established, with values of 99% and 33% dissolution, on average, after 15 min and 60 min, respectively [57]. The dissolution profile of *Senna* sp. was less than 10% sennoside release from capsules containing dry extract, in a period of 60 min, in contrast to lyophilized *Senna* sp. extract, which attained around 90% dissolution after the same period. Data on the dissolution test of *Passiflora* sp. showed that capsules containing the crude extract presented 50% dissolution while lyophilized extract and other standardized extract reached around 100% for the same period [58].

The modeled capsules are suitable for internal use as a food supplement that contains all the components of the chemical composition of the phenolic compounds found in lyophilized apples, as these components have a wide range of biological effects on the human body. Given the fact that the bioavailability of phenolic compounds is not particularly high, compounds with a lower molecular weight are more readily absorbed in the gastrointestinal tract [59]. According to scientific literature, various groups of phenolic compounds are absorbed at a rate of 0.3–43%, and the metabolite content circulating in the plasma can be low [60]. Chlorogenic acid absorption is approximately 33%, and the majority of chlorogenic acid will reach the large intestine, while (+)-catechin and (−)-epicatechin are both absorbed by small intestinal epithelial cells [11]. The route of administration, the release of a dosage form, and absorption are known to affect bioavailability [61]. The bioavailability of flavonoids depends on their physicochemical properties. Flavonoids with complex structures and larger molecular weights, bioavailability may be even lower [62,63]. The absorption of flavonoids in the small intestine is limited owing to their molecular weight and hydrophilicity of their glycosides. It is therefore important to select suitable excipients that do not limit the therapeutic efficacy of the active compounds [64].

Since the active compounds in the apple lyophilisate were not highly soluble, we tried to model capsules whose excipients would not impair their solubility. When modeling capsules that contain active substances of botanical origin, it is expedient to avoid possible interactions between the lyophilized apple powder and the excipients, since dissolution, base structure, molecular size, and interaction with other components are the major physiochemical properties that lower the effectiveness of phenolic compounds [59]. According to the scientific literature, lyophilisate of *Vasa Swaras* capsules improved the stability and oral bioavailability of vasicine as well as reduced its conversion to vasicinone. The pharmacokinetic profiles of the various formulations inferred that the highest bioavailability of vasicine was obtained from hard gelatin capsules of lyophilized *Vasa Swaras* [53].

Considering the increasing consumption of herbal medicines, food supplements, there is a need for studies to ensure quality from raw material to finished product. Quality control is essential for the safety of functional food or nutrition supplements. Thus, biopharmaceutical studies of capsules with apple lyophilisate are of great importance since they can contribute toward ensuring future research for the planning and manufacture of innovative nutrition supplements.

3. Materials and Methods

3.1. Plant Materials

The study included "Ligol" apple cultivar (a winter cultivar bred in Poland). The apple trees were grown in the experimental orchard (block 2, row 4, trees 21–40) of the Institute of Horticulture, Lithuanian Research Centre for Agriculture and Forestry, Babtai, Lithuania (55°60′ N, 23°48′ E). The altitude of Babtai town is 57 m above sea level. Trees were trained as a slender spindle. Pest and disease management was carried out according to the rules of integrated plant protection. The experimental orchard was not irrigated. Tree fertilization was performed based on the results of soil and leaf analysis. Nitrogen was applied before flowering at the rate of 80 kg ha^{-1}, and potassium was applied after the harvest at the rate of 90 kg ha^{-1}. Soil conditions of the experimental orchard were the following: clay loam, pH—7.3, humus—2.8%, P_2O_5—255 mg kg^{-1}, and K_2O—230 mg kg^{-1}. The apples harvested in September 2019 were immediately lyophilized and used for the study.

3.2. Chemicals and Solvents

All solvents, reagents, and standards used were of analytical grade. Acetonitrile, acetic acid, D(+)-glucose monohydrate, hypromellose, Aerosil^{TM} 200, microcrystalline cellulose, silicon dioxide and starch were obtained from Sigma-Aldrich GmbH (Buchs, Switzerland), and ethanol was obtained from Stumbras AB (Kaunas, Lithuania). Hyperoside, rutin, quercitrin, phloridzin, procyanidin B1, procyanidin B2, and chlorogenic acid standards were purchased from Extrasynthese (Genay, France), reynoutrin, (+)-catechin and (−)-epicatechin were purchased from Sigma-Aldrich GmbH (Buchs, Switzerland), and avicularin, procyanidin C1, and isoquercitrin were purchased from Chromadex (Santa Ana, USA). In this study, we used deionized water produced by the Milli-Q® (Millipore, Bedford, MA, USA) water purification system.

3.3. Preparation of Apple Lyophilisate

The apples were cut into slices of equal size (up to 1 cm in thickness), and the stalks and the seeds were removed. The apple slices were immediately frozen in a freezer (at −35 °C) with air circulation. Apple samples were lyophilized with a ZIRBUS sublimator 3 × 4 × 5/20 (ZIRBUS technology, Bad Grund, Germany) at the pressure of 0.01 mbar (condenser temperature, −85 °C). The lyophilized apple slices were ground to fine powder (particle size about 100 µm) by using a knife mill Grindomix GM 200 (Retsch, Haan, Germany).

3.4. Preparation of Phenolic Extracts

During the analysis of phenolic compounds, 2.5 g of lyophilizate powder (exact weight) was weighed, added to 30 mL of 70% (v/v) ethanol, and extracted in a Sonorex Digital 10 P ultrasonic bath (Bandelin Electronic GmbH & Co. KG, Berlin, Germany) at room temperature for 20 min. The obtained extract was filtered through a paper filter, and the residue on the filter was washed with 70% (v/v) ethanol in a 50 mL flask until the extract volume was reached. The conditions of the extraction were chosen based on the results of the tests for setting the extraction conditions [65].

3.5. Qualitative and Quantitative Analysis by HPLC-PDA Method

The qualitative and quantitative HPLC analysis of phenolic compounds was performed with a Waters 2998 PDA detector (Waters, Milford, USA). Chromatographic separations were carried out by using a YMC-Pack ODS-A (5 µm, C18, 250 × 4.6 mm i.d.) column. The column was operated at a constant temperature of 25 °C. The volume of the analyzed extract was 10 µL. The flow rate was 1 mL/min. The mobile phase consisted of 2% (v/v) acetic acid (solvent A) and acetonitrile (solvent B). Gradient variation: 0–30 min 3–15% B, 30–45 min 15–25% B, 45–50 min 25–50% B, and 50–55 min 50–95% B. For the quantitative analysis, the calibration curves were obtained by injecting the known concentrations of different standard compounds. All the identified phenolic compounds were quantified at λ = 200–400 nm wavelength [66,67].

3.6. Encapsulation Process

Compositions of capsules fillings are given in Table 1. Powder was prepared by simple mixing of the mixture of apple lyophilizate with excipient. Filled capsules were prepared using the manual capsule filling machine (Capsuline, Davie, FL, USA).

3.6.1. Test of the Uniformity of Mass of Single-Dose Preparations

The tested capsules were weighed, and the mean weight of 1 capsule was determined [68]. One capsule was weighed, apple lyophilizate and excipients mixture were poured out, and then the capsule shell was weighed. Subsequently, the mass of the content—i.e., the difference between the weight of the capsule and the weight of the shell—was calculated. This procedure was applied to each modeled capsule. The allowed deviation for capsules weighing not more than 250 mg was 7.5%.

3.6.2. Capsule Disintegration Test

The capsule disintegration time was determined based on the methodology outlined in Ph. Eur. 2.9.1. [69]. The device C-MAG HS7 (IKA®-Werke GmbH & Co, Staufen, Germany) was used to determine the disintegration time. The disintegration medium was 0.1 M hydrochloric acid solution, temperature 37 ± 0.50 °C, observed for 30 min.

3.6.3. Capsule Dissolution Test

The capsule dissolution test was performed using a Sotax AT 7smart dissolution tester (SOTAX AG, Allschwil, Switzerland). The acceptor medium was an ethanol-water mixture at the ratio of 1:1, the temperature being 37.0 ± 0.5 °C. The volume of the medium was 250 mL. The samples were taken after 15, 30, 60, 75 and 90 min. The sample volume was 10 mL. The analysis of the active compounds was performed by applying HPLC.

3.7. Statistical Analysis

The statistical analysis of the study data was performed by using Microsoft Office Excel 2013 (Microsoft, Redmond, WA, USA) and SPSS 25.0 (SPSS Inc., Chicago, IL, USA) computer software. All the results obtained during the HPLC analysis were presented as means of three consecutive test results and standard deviations. To evaluate the variance in the quantitative composition, we calculated the coefficient of variation. Univariate analysis of variance (ANOVA) was applied in order to determine whether the differences between the compared data were statistically significant. The hypothesis about the equality of variances was verified by applying Levine's test. If the variances of independent variables were found to be equal, Tukey's multiple comparison test was used. The differences were regarded as statistically significant at $p < 0.05$.

4. Conclusions

Excipients and their amounts may affect the dissolution kinetics of the phenolic compounds. Hypromellose prolonged the disintegration time of the modeled capsules when its amount reached 50–83% of the capsule weight. The selected fillers did not affect the kinetics of the release of the phenolic compounds from the capsules. Based on the results of the dissolution test, the capsules can be classified as fast-dissolving preparations since more than 85% of the active substance was released within 30 min.

According to the amount released from the capsules of different encapsulating content, individual phenolic compounds can be arranged in the following descending order: chlorogenic acid > rutin > avicularin > hyperoside > phloridzin > quercitrin > (−)-epicatechin > isoquercitrin. Chlorogenic acid was the compound that was released in the highest amounts from capsules of different encapsulating content: its released amounts ranged from 68.4 to 640.3 μg/mL.

The results of the solubility and disintegration tests proved that the capsules of the proposed composition are appropriate for internal use. The proposed product could serve as a basis for the development of food supplements with lyophilized apple powder.

Author Contributions: Conceptualization, V.J. and K.R.; methodology, K.R. and M.L.; formal analysis, A.B. and M.L.; investigation, A.B.; resources, K.R. and M.L.; data curation, A.B.; writing—original draft preparation, A.B., M.L. and K.R. writing—review and editing, V.J.; visualization, A.B.; supervision, V.J. and K.R. All authors have read and agreed to the published version of the manuscript.

Funding: This research received no external funding.

Institutional Review Board Statement: Not applicable.

Informed Consent Statement: Not applicable.

Data Availability Statement: All datasets generated for this study are included in the article.

Acknowledgments: The authors wish to thank the LSMU Science Foundation for the support of this study.

Conflicts of Interest: The authors declare no conflict of interest.

Sample Availability: The samples for this paper's experiment are available from the authors.

References

1. Food and Agriculture Organization. FAOSTAT. Available online: http://www.fao.org/faostat/en/#data/QL (accessed on 23 May 2020).
2. Marks, S.C.; Mullen, W.; Crozier, A. Flavonoid and chlorogenic acid profiles of English cider apples. *J. Sci. Food Agric.* **2007**, *87*, 719–728. [CrossRef]
3. Price, K.; Prosser, T.; Richetin, A.; Rhodes, M. A comparison of the flavonol content and composition in dessert, cooking and cider-making apples; distribution within the fruit and effect of juicing. *Food Chem.* **1999**, *66*, 489–494. [CrossRef]
4. Wu, J.; Gao, H.; Zhao, L.; Liao, X.; Chen, F.; Wang, Z.; Hu, X. Chemical compositional characterization of some apple cultivars. *Food Chem.* **2007**, *103*, 88–93. [CrossRef]
5. Morresi, C.; Cianfruglia, L.; Armeni, T.; Mancini, F.; Tenore, G.C.; D'Urso, E.; Micheletti, A.; Ferretti, G.; Bacchetti, T. Polyphenolic compounds and nutraceutical properties of old and new apple cultivars. *J. Food Biochem.* **2018**, *42*, e12641. [CrossRef]
6. Oszmiański, J.; Lachowicz, S.; Gławdel, E.; Cebulak, T.; Ochmian, I. Determination of phytochemical composition and antioxidant capacity of 22 old apple cultivars grown in Poland. *Eur. Food Res. Technol.* **2017**, *244*, 647–662. [CrossRef]
7. Berni, R.; Cantini, C.; Guarnieri, M.; Nepi, M.; Hausman, J.-F.; Guerriero, G.; Romi, M.; Cai, G. Nutraceutical Characteristics of Ancient Malus x domestica Borkh. Fruits Recovered across Siena in Tuscany. *Medicines* **2019**, *6*, 27. [CrossRef]
8. Oszmiański, J.; Lachowicz, S.; Gamsjäger, H. Phytochemical analysis by liquid chromatography of ten old apple varieties grown in Austria and their antioxidative activity. *Eur. Food Res. Technol.* **2019**, *246*, 437–448. [CrossRef]
9. Ferretti, G.; Turco, I.; Bacchetti, T. Apple as a Source of Dietary Phytonutrients: Bioavailability and Evidence of Protective Effects against Human Cardiovascular Disease. *Food Nutr. Sci.* **2014**, *5*, 1234–1246. [CrossRef]
10. Nour, V.; Trandafir, I.; Ionica, M.E. Compositional characteristics of fruits of several apple (*Malus domestica* Borkh.) cultivars. *Not. Bot. Hort. Agrobot.* **2010**, *38*, 228–233.
11. Boyer, J.; Liu, R.H. Apple phytochemicals and their health benefits. *Nutr. J.* **2004**, *3*, 5. [CrossRef]
12. Pandey, K.B.; Rizvi, S.I. Plant Polyphenols as Dietary Antioxidants in Human Health and Disease. *Oxidative Med. Cell. Longev.* **2009**, *2*, 270–278. [CrossRef]
13. Hyson, D.A. A Comprehensive Review of Apples and Apple Components and Their Relationship to Human Health. *Adv. Nutr.* **2011**, *2*, 408–420. [CrossRef]
14. Francini, A.; Sebastiani, L. Phenolic Compounds in Apple (*Malus x domestica* Borkh.): Compounds Characterization and Stability during Postharvest and after Processing. *Antioxidants* **2013**, *2*, 181–193. [CrossRef] [PubMed]

15. Wagner, B.; Brinz, T.; Otterbach, S.; Khinast, J. Rapid automated process development of a continuous capsule-filling process. *Int. J. Pharm.* **2018**, *546*, 154–165. [CrossRef] [PubMed]
16. Ullmann, P. Excipient selection for compounded pharmaceutical capsules: They're only fillers, right? *Aust. J. Pharm.* **2017**, *1164*, 78–83.
17. Nireesha, G.R.; Divya, L.; Sowmya, C.; Venkateshan, N.; Babu, M.N.; Lavakumar, V. Lyophilization/freeze drying—A review. *IJNTPS* **2013**, *4*, 87–98.
18. Cock, L.S.; Munoz, D.P.V.; Aponte, A.A. Structural, physical, functional and nutraceutical changes of freeze-dried fruit. *Afr. J. Biotechnol.* **2015**, *14*, 442–450.
19. Čakste, I.; Augšpole, I.; Cinkmanis, I.; Kuka, P. Bioactive Compounds in Latvian Wild Berry Juice. *Mater. Sci. Appl. Chem.* **2014**, *30*, 5–9. [CrossRef]
20. Bajića, A.; Pezo, L.L.; Stupara, A.; Filipčeva, B.; Cvetkovića, B.R.; Horeckic, A.T.; Mastilović, J. Application of lyophilized plum pomace as a functional ingredient in a plum spread: Optimizing texture, colour and phenol antioxidants by ANN modelling. *LWT* **2020**, *130*, 109588. [CrossRef]
21. Delpino-Rius, A.; Eras, J.; Vilaró, F.; Cubero, M.Á.; Balcells, M.; Canela-Garayoa, R. Characterisation of phenolic compounds in processed fibres from the juice industry. *Food Chem.* **2015**, *172*, 575–584. [CrossRef] [PubMed]
22. Ruszkowska, M.; Kropisz, P.; Wiśniewska, Z. Evaluation of the stability of the storage of selected fruit and vegetables freeze-dried powder based on the characteristics of the sorption properties. *SJ GMU* **2019**, *19*, 55–63.
23. Jakobek, L.; Barron, A.R. Ancient apple varieties from Croatia as a source of bioactive polyphenolic compounds. *J. Food Compos. Anal.* **2016**, *45*, 9–15. [CrossRef]
24. Tsao, R.; Yang, R.; Young, A.J.C.; Zhu, H. Polyphenolic Profiles in Eight Apple Cultivars Using High-Performance Liquid Chromatography (HPLC). *J. Agric. Food Chem.* **2003**, *51*, 6347–6353. [CrossRef] [PubMed]
25. Duda-Chodak, A.; Tarko, T.; Satora, P.; Sroka, P.; Tuszy'nski, T. The profile of polyphenols and antioxidant properties of selected apple cultivars grown in Poland. *J. Fruit Ornam. Plant Res.* **2010**, *18*, 39–50.
26. Iacopini, P.; Camangi, F.; Stefani, A.; Sebastiani, L. Antiradical potential of ancient Italian apple varieties of *Malus x domestica* Borkh. in a peroxynitrite-induced oxidative process. *J. Food Compos. Anal.* **2010**, *23*, 518–524. [CrossRef]
27. Bandoniene, D.; Murkovic, M. On-Line HPLC-DPPH Screening Method for Evaluation of Radical Scavenging Phenols Extracted from Apples (Malus domesticaL.). *J. Agric. Food Chem.* **2002**, *50*, 2482–2487. [CrossRef] [PubMed]
28. Bai, X.; Zhang, H.; Ren, S. Antioxidant activity and HPLC analysis of polyphenol-enriched extracts from industrial apple pomace. *J. Sci. Food Agric.* **2013**, *93*, 2502–2506. [CrossRef]
29. Hwang, S.J.; Kim, Y.-W.; Park, Y.; Lee, H.-J.; Kim, K.-W. Anti-inflammatory effects of chlorogenic acid in lipopolysaccharide-stimulated RAW 264.7 cells. *Inflamm. Res.* **2014**, *63*, 81–90. [CrossRef] [PubMed]
30. Dos Santos, M.D.; Almeida, M.C.; Lopes, N.P.; De Souza, G.E.P. Evaluation of the Anti-inflammatory, Analgesic and Antipyretic Activities of the Natural Polyphenol Chlorogenic Acid. *Biol. Pharm. Bull.* **2006**, *29*, 2236–2240. [CrossRef]
31. Thomas, T.; Pfeiffer, A.F.H. Foods for the prevention of diabetes: How do they work? *Diabetes Metab. Res. Rev.* **2012**, *28*, 25–49. [CrossRef]
32. Suzuki, A.; Yamamoto, N.; Jokura, H.; Yamamoto, M.; Fujii, A.; Tokimitsu, I.; Saito, I. Chlorogenic acid attenuates hypertension and improves endothelial function in spontaneously hypertensive rats. *J. Hypertens.* **2006**, *24*, 1065–1073. [CrossRef]
33. Kanno, Y.; Watanabe, R.; Zempo, H.; Ogawa, M.; Suzuki, J.-I.; Isobe, M. Chlorogenic acid attenuates ventricular remodeling after myocardial infarction in mice. *Int. Heart. J.* **2013**, *54*, 176–180. [CrossRef]
34. Yang, J.-S.; Liu, C.-W.; Ma, Y.-S.; Weng, S.-W.; Tang, N.-Y.; Wu, S.-H.; Ji, B.-C.; Ma, C.-Y.; Ko, Y.-C.; Funayama, S.; et al. Chlorogenic acid induces apoptotic cell death in U937 leukemia cells through caspase- and mitochondria-dependent pathways. *In Vivo.* **2012**, *26*, 971–978.
35. Cinkilic, N.; Çetintas, S.K.; Zorlu, T.; Vatan, O.; Yilmaz, D.; Çavaş, T.; Tunc, S.; Özkan, L.; Bilaloğlu, R.; Yılmaz, D. Radioprotection by two phenolic compounds: Chlorogenic and quinic acid, on X-ray induced DNA damage in human blood lymphocytes in vitro. *Food Chem. Toxicol.* **2013**, *53*, 359–363. [CrossRef]
36. Yan, Y.; Li, J.; Han, J.; Hou, N.; Song, Y.; Dong, L. Chlorogenic acid enhances the effects of 5-fluorouracil in human hepatocellular carcinoma cells through the inhibition of extracellular signal-regulated kinases. *Anti-Cancer Drugs* **2015**, *26*, 540–546. [CrossRef]
37. Wojdyło, A.; Oszmiański, J.; Laskowski, P. Polyphenolic Compounds and Antioxidant Activity of New and Old Apple Varieties. *J. Agric. Food Chem.* **2008**, *56*, 6520–6530. [CrossRef] [PubMed]
38. Carnésecchi, S.; Schneider, Y.; A Lazarus, S.; Coehlo, D.; Gossé, F.; Raul, F. Flavanols and procyanidins of cocoa and chocolate inhibit growth and polyamine biosynthesis of human colonic cancer cells. *Cancer Lett.* **2002**, *175*, 147–155. [CrossRef]
39. Lotito, S.B.; Actis-Goretta, L.; Renart, M.; Caligiuri, M.; Rein, D.; Schmitz, H.H.; Steinberg, F.M.; Keen, C.L.; Fraga, C.G. Influence of Oligomer Chain Length on the Antioxidant Activity of Procyanidins. *Biochem. Biophys. Res. Commun.* **2000**, *276*, 945–951. [CrossRef] [PubMed]
40. Terra, X.; Valls, J.; Vitrac, X.; Mérrillon, J.M.; Arola, L.; Ardèvol, A.; Blade, C.; Larrea, J.F.; Pujadas, G.; Salvadó, J.; et al. Grape-seed procyanidins act as anti-inflammatory agents in endotoxin stimulated RAW 264.7 macrophages by inhibiting NFkB signaling pathway. *J. Agric. Food Chem.* **2007**, *55*, 4357–4365. [CrossRef] [PubMed]

41. Serra, T.; Rocha, J.; Sepodes, B.; Matias, A.A.; Feliciano, R.P.; Carvalho, A.; Bronze, M.R.; Duarte, C.M.M.; Figueira, M.E. Evaluation of cardiovascular protective effect of different apple varieties correlation of response with composition. *Food Chem.* **2012**, *135*, 2378–2386. [CrossRef] [PubMed]
42. Lina, B.; Reus, A.; Hasselwander, O.; Bui, Q.; Tenning, P. Safety evaluation of EvesseTM EPC, an apple polyphenol extract rich in flavan-3-ols. *Food Chem. Toxicol.* **2012**, *50*, 2845–2853. [CrossRef]
43. Huang, C.; Chen, Y.; Zhou, T.; Chen, G. Sulfation of dietary flavonoids by human sulfotransferases. *Xenobiotica* **2009**, *39*, 312–322. [CrossRef]
44. Piccolo, E.L.; Landi, M.; Massai, R.; Remorini, D.; Conte, G.; Guidi, L. Ancient apple cultivars from Garfagnana (Tuscany, Italy): A potential source for 'nutrafruit' production. *Food Chem.* **2019**, *294*, 518–525. [CrossRef]
45. Kobori, M.; Masumoto, S.; Akimoto, Y.; Oike, H. Phloridzin reduces blood glucose levels and alters hepatic gene expression in normal BALB/c mice. *Food Chem. Toxicol.* **2012**, *50*, 2547–2553. [CrossRef] [PubMed]
46. Najafian, M.; Jahromi, M.Z.; Nowroznejhad, M.J.; Khajeaian, P.; Kargar, M.M.; Sadeghi, M.; Arasteh, A. Phloridzin reduces blood glucose levels and improves lipids metabolism in streptozotocin-induced diabetic rats. *Mol. Biol. Rep.* **2011**, *39*, 5299–5306. [CrossRef]
47. Belviso, S.; Scursatone, B.; Re, G.; Zeppa, G. Novel Data on the Polyphenol Composition of Italian Ancient Apple Cultivars. *Int. J. Food Prop.* **2013**, *16*, 1507–1515. [CrossRef]
48. Schieber, A.; Keller, P.; Carle, R. Determination of phenolic acids and flavonoids of apple and pear by high-performance liquid chromatography. *J. Chromatogr. A* **2001**, *910*, 265–273. [CrossRef]
49. Elsakhawy, M.; Hassan, M. Physical and mechanical properties of microcrystalline cellulose prepared from agricultural residues. *Carbohydr. Polym.* **2007**, *67*, 1–10. [CrossRef]
50. Alves, L.A.; Silva, J.B.A.; Giulietti, M. Solubility of D-glucose in water and ethanol/water mixtures. *J. Chem. Eng. Data.* **2007**, *52*, 2166–2170. [CrossRef]
51. Li, C.; Martini, L.G.; Ford, J.L.; Robe, M. The use of hypromellose in oral drug delivery. *J. Pharm. Pharmacol.* **2005**, *57*, 533–546. [CrossRef]
52. *Supplement 6.1*; European Pharmacopoeia; Council of Europe 2007: Strasbourg, France, 2007.
53. Vyas, T.; Dash, R.P.; Anandjiwala, S.; Nivsarkar, M. Formulation and pharmacokinetic evaluation of hard gelatin capsule encapsulating lyophilized Vasa Swaras for improved stability and oral bioavailability of vasicine. *Fitoterapia* **2011**, *82*, 446–453. [CrossRef]
54. Esmaeili, S.; Dayani, L.; Taheri, A.; Zolfaghari, B. Phytochemical standardization, formulation and evaluation of oral hard gelatin capsules from *Pinus eldarica* bark extract. *Avicenna J. Phytomed.* **2020**, *11*, 168–179.
55. Dressman, J.; Butler, J.; Hempenstall, J.; Reppas, C. The BCS: Where do we go from here? *Pharm. Technol.* **2001**, *5*, 68–76.
56. Brown, C.K.; Friedel, H.D.; Barker, A.R.; Buhse, L.F.; Keitel, S.; Cecil, T.L.; Kraemer, J.; Morris, J.M.; Reppas, C.; Stickelmeyer, M.P.; et al. FIP/AAPS joint workshop report: Dissolution in vitro release testing of novel/special dosage forms. *Pharm. Sci. Tech.* **2011**, *12*, 782–794. [CrossRef]
57. Kressmann, S.; Biber, A.; Wonnemann, M.; Schug, B.; Blume, H.H.; Muller, W.E. Influence of pharmaceutical quality on the bioavailability of active components from *Ginkgo biloba* preparations. *J. Pharm. Pharmacol.* **2002**, *54*, 1507–1514. [CrossRef]
58. Taglioli, V.; Bilia, A.R.; Ghiara, C.; Mazzi, G.; Mercati, V.; Vincieri, F.F. Evaluation of the dissolution behaviour of some commercial herbal drugs and their preparations. *Die Pharm.* **2001**, *56*, 868–870.
59. Carbonell-Capella, J.M.; Buniowska, M.; Barba, F.J.; Esteve, M.J.; Frígola, A. Analytical Methods for Determining Bioavailability and Bioaccessibility of Bioactive Compounds from Fruits and Vegetables: A Review. *Compr. Rev. Food Sci. Food Saf.* **2014**, *13*, 155–171. [CrossRef] [PubMed]
60. Manach, C.; Scalbert, A.; Morand, C.; Rémésy, C.; Jiménez, L. Polyphenols: Food sources and bioavailability. *Am. J. Clin. Nutr.* **2004**, *79*, 727–747. [CrossRef] [PubMed]
61. Porrini, M.; Riso, P. Factors influencing the bioavailability of antioxidants in foods: A critical appraisal. *Nutr. Metab. Cardiovasc. Dis.* **2008**, *18*, 647–650. [CrossRef] [PubMed]
62. Landete, J.M. Updated Knowledge about Polyphenols: Functions, Bioavailability, Metabolism, and Health. *Crit. Rev. Food Sci. Nutr.* **2012**, *52*, 936–948. [CrossRef]
63. Scalbert, A.; Morand, C.; Manach, C.; Rémésy, C. Absorption and metabolism of polyphenols in the gut and impact on health. *Biomed. Pharmacother.* **2002**, *56*, 276–282. [CrossRef]
64. Appleton, J. Evaluating the bioavailability of isoquercetin. *Nat. Med. J.* **2010**, *2*, 1–6.
65. Liaudanskas, M.; Viškelis, P.; Jakštas, V.; Raudonis, R.; Kviklys, D.; Milašius, A.; Janulis, V. Application of an Optimized HPLC Method for the Detection of Various Phenolic Compounds in Apples from Lithuanian Cultivars. *J. Chem.* **2014**, *2014*, 1–10. [CrossRef]
66. Liaudanskas, M.; Viškelis, P.; Kviklys, D.; Raudonis, R.; Janulis, V. A Comparative Study of Phenolic Content in Apple Fruits. *Int. J. Food Prop.* **2015**, *18*, 945–953. [CrossRef]
67. Kviklys, D.; Liaudanskas, M.; Janulis, V.; Viskelis, P.; Rubinskienė, M.; Lanauskas, J.; Uselis, N. Rootstock genotype determines phenol content in apple fruits. *Plant, Soil Environ.* **2014**, *60*, 234–240. [CrossRef]
68. *Monograph: 2.9.5. Uniformity of Mass of Single-Dose Preparations*; European Pharmacopoeia 6.0; Council of Europe 2007: Strasbourg, France, 2007.
69. *Monograph: 2.9.1. Disintegration of Tablets and Capsules*; European Pharmacopoeia 6.0; Council of Europe 2007: Strasbourg, France, 2007.

Article

Hydrogel Emulsion with Encapsulated Safflower Oil Enriched with Açai Extract as a Novel Fat Substitute in Beef Burgers Subjected to Storage in Cold Conditions

Monika Hanula [1,*], Arkadiusz Szpicer [1], Elżbieta Górska-Horczyczak [1], Gohar Khachatryan [2], Grzegorz Pogorzelski [1], Ewelina Pogorzelska-Nowicka [1] and Andrzej Poltorak [1]

1. Department of Technique and Food Development, Institute of Human Nutrition Sciences, Warsaw University of Life Sciences, Nowoursynowska 159c Street 32, 02-776 Warsaw, Poland; arkadiusz_szpicer@sggw.edu.pl (A.S.); elzbieta_gorska_horczyczak@sggw.edu.pl (E.G.-H.); grzegorz.t.pogorzelski@gmail.com (G.P.); ewelina_pogorzelska@sggw.edu.pl (E.P.-N.); andrzej_poltorak@sggw.edu.pl (A.P.)
2. Department of Food Analysis and Evaluation of Food Quality, Faculty of Food Technology, University of Agriculture in Krakow, Mickiewicz Ave. 21, 31-120 Krakow, Poland; gohar.khachatryan@urk.edu.pl
* Correspondence: monika_hanula@sggw.edu.pl

Abstract: This study evaluates the effects of using a fat substitute in beef burgers composed of a hydrogel emulsion enriched with encapsulated safflower oil and açai extract. The influences of the fat substitute on the chemical (TBARS, fatty acids, and volatile compounds profile) and physical (weight loss, cooking loss, water-holding capacity, color, and texture analyses) characteristics of the burgers were analyzed after 0, 4 and 8 days of storage at 4 ± 1 °C. The obtained results were compared with control groups (20 g of tallow or 8 g of safflower oil). The fat substitute used improved burger parameters such as chewiness, hardness and the a* color parameter remained unchanged over storage time. The addition of açai extract slowed the oxidation rate of polyunsaturated fatty acids and reduced the changes in the volatile compounds profile during the storage of burgers. The utilization of a fat substitute enriched the burgers with polyunsaturated fatty acids and lowered the atherogenic index (0.49 raw, 0.58 grilled burger) and the thrombogenicity index (0.8 raw, 1.09 grilled burger), while it increased the hypocholesterolemic/hypercholesterolemic ratio (2.59 raw, 2.09 grilled burger) of consumed meat. Thus, the application of the presented fat substitute in the form of a hydrogel enriched with açai berry extract extended the shelf life of the final product and contributed to the creation of a healthier meat product that met the nutritional recommendations.

Keywords: konjac; linseed flour; fat substitute; volatile compounds; lipid oxidation; encapsulation

1. Introduction

The current literature suggests that the development of many human diseases stems from a variety of factors, in which diet type is prominent [1]. Over the last 40 years, the prevalence of obesity has doubled, resulting in ischemic heart disease, strokes, and numerous other diseases. Consumers and international health organizations (the World Health Organization and the European Food Safety Authority) have demanded changes in food quality and content in order to improve the level of human health. Meat products belong to a category of food that is a rich source of saturated and trans fatty acids that can increase the risk of cardiovascular diseases. Due to the evolution of human lifestyles, greater demands for easily accessible and fast-food preparation are observed, for example, beef burgers. Recent studies have focused on meeting these demands through the preparation of burgers with potential health benefits that consider consumers' needs and the nutritional recommendations of global organizations. This has been achieved through a combination of functional ingredients or by using fat substitutes [1–3].

The main challenge of fat substitutes is finding an oil that improves the nutritional profile without affecting consumer acceptability of the final product. To overcome such drawbacks of fat substitutes, many strategies have been proposed such as oil encapsulation and immobilization in oleogels or hydrogels [1]. The conversion of liquid vegetable oils into a solid gel has been the subject of many scientific studies. However, this technique, due to high production cost and the destructive effect of organogelators at high temperatures on the fatty acid profile of the oils, is problematic in the food industry. Unlike oleogels, emulsion hydrogel creation is cheap, simple and requires lower temperatures. Hence, this approach is suitable for heat-sensitive or bioactive compounds that undergo oxidative degradation. Moreover, emulsion hydrogels contain $\leq 50\%$ oil. Thus, they improve the fatty acid profile and also effectively reduce the total fat and caloric content in modified meat products. Furthermore, this method allows for the incorporation of both hydrophilic and hydrophobic functional components into the hydrogel matrix [1]. Researchers have used various emulsifiers, biocomposites, and polysaccharides to create emulsion hydrogels that may be used as fat substitutes. Konjac flour, which is a low-calorie ingredient, has been proposed as a promising biocomposite, as it has been successfully used in dry sausages as a fat substitute in pork [4], salchichón enriched with n-3 [5], and pork liver pates [6].

Current trends in the production of functional foods include the designs of products with lower fat content or with additional health benefits using bioactive compounds and dietary fiber. Açai berries are a popular bioactive additive, due to their antioxidant, antilipidemic, anti-inflammatory, and antiproliferative activities; açai berries have been classified as a "superfood" [7,8]. In contrast, dietary fibre is one of the most common functional ingredients in foods. The incorporation of fiber into meat can increase the daily intake of dietary fiber with food, which is recommended to be >25 g/day. Clinical and epidemiological studies have shown that dietary fiber can increase the feeling of satiety. Moreover, fiber has been shown to reduce hyperlipidaemia, total cholesterol, and the risk of cancer occurrence, as well as to improve glucose tolerance and gastrointestinal health [9]. Flaxseed flour is another ingredient that possesses health-promoting properties, which contains numerous functional compounds. Flaxseed has a favorable profile of fatty acids (polyunsaturated fatty acids) and is a rich source of dietary fiber, protein, and antioxidants (lignans). Moreover, flaxseed is gluten free and can be used to enrich the diet of people suffering from celiac disease [10].

Therefore, the aim of this study was to develop a healthier burger recipe by using a hydrogel emulsion and to study its effect on chemical and physical parameters of raw and grilled meat during storage. To the best of our knowledge, according to the literature, this type of low-fat burger formulation has not yet been tested.

2. Results and Discussion

2.1. Effect of Encapsulated Safflower Oil Concentration on the Physical Characteristics of Emulsion Hydrogel

2.1.1. Texture and Rheological Analysis

The values of the hydrogel texture parameters with safflower oil concentrations of 29–48% and a control without oil (0%) are shown in Table 1. The values for the firmness parameter ranged from 5.65 (N) to 11.91 (N). The encapsulated oil content (29%, 33%, and 38%) in the hydrogel emulsion resulted in a statistically significant increase in firmness; a similar trend was observed for the lubricity parameter, where the highest value was 11.22 (N × n). The viscosity and adhesion parameters decreased with increasing oil concentration up to 38%. In contrast, the addition of 42%, 45%, and 48% oil increased these parameters ($p < 0.05$). Hence, the obtained analysis showed that oil concentration influenced the hydrogel texture parameters [11,12].

Table 1. Effect of oil concentration on the hydrogel texture parameters.

Oil (%)	Firmness (N)	Lubricity (N × s)	Viscosity (N)	Adhesiveness (N × s)
0	5.65 ± 0.34 [A]	4.81 ± 0.39 [A]	−3.38 ± 0.21 [D]	−1.02 ± 0.04 [E]
29	10.15 ± 0.44 [C]	9.41 ± 0.55 [C,D]	−6.01 ± 0.59 [C]	−2.10 ± 0.25 [B,C]
33	11.17 ± 0.69 [D]	10.37 ± 1.02 [D,E]	−7.03 ± 0.56 [B]	−2.42 ± 0.29 [B]
38	11.91 ± 0.43 [D]	11.22 ± 0.61 [E]	−8.03 ± 0.30 [A]	−2.45 ± 0.32 [A]
42	10.20 ± 1.03 [C]	9.17 ± 1.04 [C]	−7.10 ± 0.69 [B]	−1.90 ± 0.35 [C,D]
45	9.31 ± 0.61 [B,C]	8.66 ± 0.90 [B,C]	−6.61 ± 0.24 [B,C]	−1.87 ± 0.41 [C,D]
48	8.89 ± 1.16 [B]	8.07 ± 1.10 [B]	−6.37 ± 0.82 [C]	−1.47 ± 0.66 [D]

[A–E]—Mean values between variants in the same column indicated by different letters indicate a statistically significant difference.

The analysis of the rheological parameters of the hydrogel with encapsulated safflower oil are shown in Table 2. The analyzed samples all behaved as non-Newtonian, pseudoplastic liquids. Based on the Ostwald–de Waele model fitted to the upper flow curves and n values obtained, it was determined that the addition of oil to the hydrogel emulsion promoted a statistically significant increase in pseudoplasticity. The addition of oil increased the shear stress, which was characterized by a higher shear resistance. This was confirmed by a statistically significant increase in the consistency coefficient (K) value. The highest K value was recorded for the sample with 38% oil (139.42 (Pa×s^n)). A further increase in oil concentration of the hydrogel decreased the K value. A similar trend was observed for the thixotropy parameter. The report by Cano et al. [13] showed that an increase in the lipid phase content in the studied emulsion increased the K parameter.

Table 2. Parameters of the Ostwald–de Waele rheological model and area of the hysteresis loop of the hydrogel with encapsulated safflower oil.

Oil (%)	Ostwald–de Waele Model			Area of Hysteresis Loop (Pa × s)	
	K (Pa × s^n)	n (−)	R^2	Thixotropy	Area
0	53.51 ± 2.18 [A]	0.34 ± 0.02 [D]	0.98 ± 0.01	1157.33 ± 52.45 [A]	26,801.67 ± 1615.65 [A]
29	117.05 ± 2.33 [B,C]	0.25 ± 0.02 [A,B]	0.97 ± 0.02	3566.67 ± 76.48 [B]	41,850.00 ± 1800.13 [BC]
33	125.92 ± 1.79 [E]	0.24 ± 0.04 [A,B]	0.97 ± 0.01	4516.00 ± 124.61 [E]	44,446.67 ± 2536.03 [B,C]
38	139.42 ± 0.67 [F]	0.24 ± 0.02 [A,B]	0.98 ± 0.01	4562.83 ± 167.84 [E]	53,178.33 ± 3242.89 [D]
42	122.05 ± 2.19 [C]	0.21 ± 0.03 [A]	0.98 ± 0.01	4223.83 ± 109.58 [D]	45,855.00 ± 1596.82 [C]
45	120.57 ± 2.11 [C,D]	0.23 ± 0.02 [A,B]	0.97 ± 0.01	3980.50 ± 89.72 [C]	42,505.00 ± 2921.69 [B,C]
48	114.95 ± 2.83 [B]	0.26 ± 0.01 [C]	0.98 ± 0.01	3413.67 ± 93.66 [B]	40,705.00 ± 2564.98 [B]

[A–F]—Mean values between variants in the same column indicated by different letters indicate a statistically significant difference.

2.1.2. SEM and FT-IR Analysis

Figure 1 shows the FT-IR spectra of the analyzed hydrogels with encapsulated safflower oil. The absorbance band characteristics of the oil were recorded for 45% and 0% oil content samples. The spectra showed peaks corresponding to the −CH_3 groups in the range of 1350–1150 cm^{-1}. The C−O bond stretching vibrations belonging to ester groups consisted of two coupled asymmetric vibrations, i.e., C−C(=O)-O and O−C−C, which were observed between 1300 and 1000 cm^{-1}. The bands corresponding to C−C(=O) −O vibrations of saturated esters were found between 1240 and 1163 cm^{-1}, whereas unsaturated esters were observed at lower wave numbers. The vibrational bands of the O−C−C bonds from esters of primary alcohols were found at 1064−1031 cm^{-1} and from secondary alcohols at 1100 cm^{-1}, both types of esters were present in triacylglycerol molecules [14]. The low-intensity band at 1390 cm^{-1} was related to C−H combination vibrations. The bands at 1726 cm^{-1} and 1760 cm^{-1} corresponded to C−H stretching vibrations of the methyl, methylene and ethylene groups. The band at 1725 cm^{-1} corresponded to oleic acid, while saturated and trans-unsaturated triacylglycerols exhibited absorption bands at 1725 cm^{-1} and 1760 cm^{-1}. The band at 2145 cm^{-1} was related to C−C and C−H stretching vibrations, and the following vibrations at 2952, 2921, and 2855 cm^{-1} corresponded to the valence $-C-H$ vibrations from $-CH_3$ and $-CH_2$ groups of triglycerides, respectively [15]. The results indicated that the encapsulation process had no effect on the oil's structure.

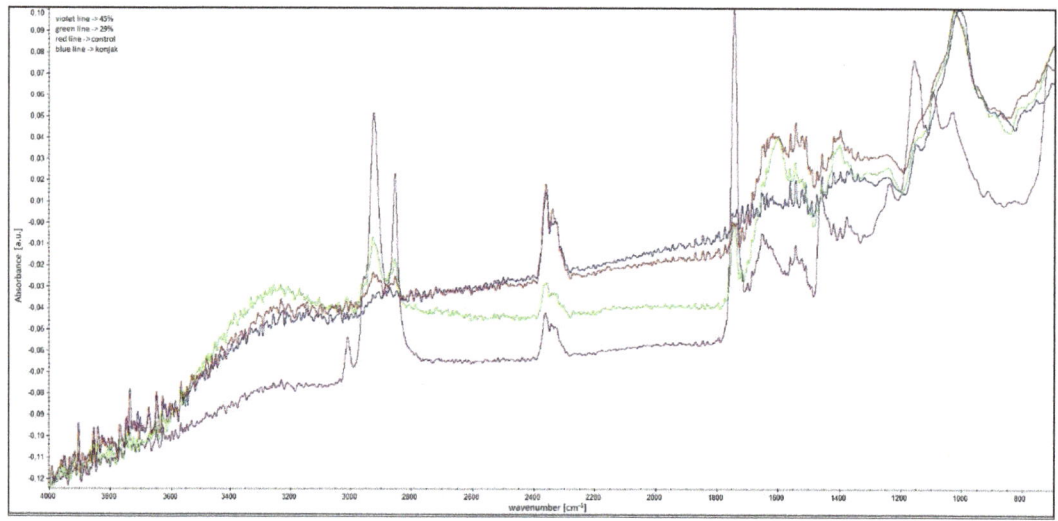

Figure 1. FT-IR analysis of hydrogels with encapsulated safflower oil.

The images of scanning electron microscope SEM are shown in Figure 2 and show that nanocapsules were successfully obtained in a polysaccharide matrix. The size and shape of the capsules varied depending on the oil concentration. The results indicated that, in the case of 29% and 33% oil content samples, the capsule envelope was multi-layered (Figure 2A,B). The size of the capsules decreased with increasing oil concentration (Figure 2C,D). The capsules in the hydrogel emulsion were present throughout the matrix and their distribution was uniform.

Despite slight statistical differences in the tested variants, the hydrogels with concentrations ranging from 29% to 45% were characterized with similar texture parameters. A 48% oil content was too high and differed significantly from other concentrations. Furthermore, the success of hydrogel applications in food depends largely on the ability of the oleogelator to form a network that traps liquid oil [16]. Therefore, the hydrogel with 45% concentration encapsulated oil was selected for further study as a fat substitute.

2.1.3. Biochemical Analysis of Oil and Açai Extract

The results of the TPC analysis and antioxidant activity of oil and açai extract are shown in Table 3. The concentration of the extract used in the main study was determined based on the study conducted by Mokhtar et al. [17]. Safflower oil containing polyphenols accounted for 0.27 mg gallic acid/g of oil, whereas the antioxidant activity was 0.09 mg ascorbic acid/g of oil according to the ABTS analysis and 0.32 mg ascorbic acid/g of oil according to the FRAP analysis. Nimrouzi et al. [18] reported similar results.

The fatty acid profile analysis showed that safflower oil was characterized by a high PUFA content, especially n-6. This result was also confirmed by a study conducted by Rutkowska et al. [19].

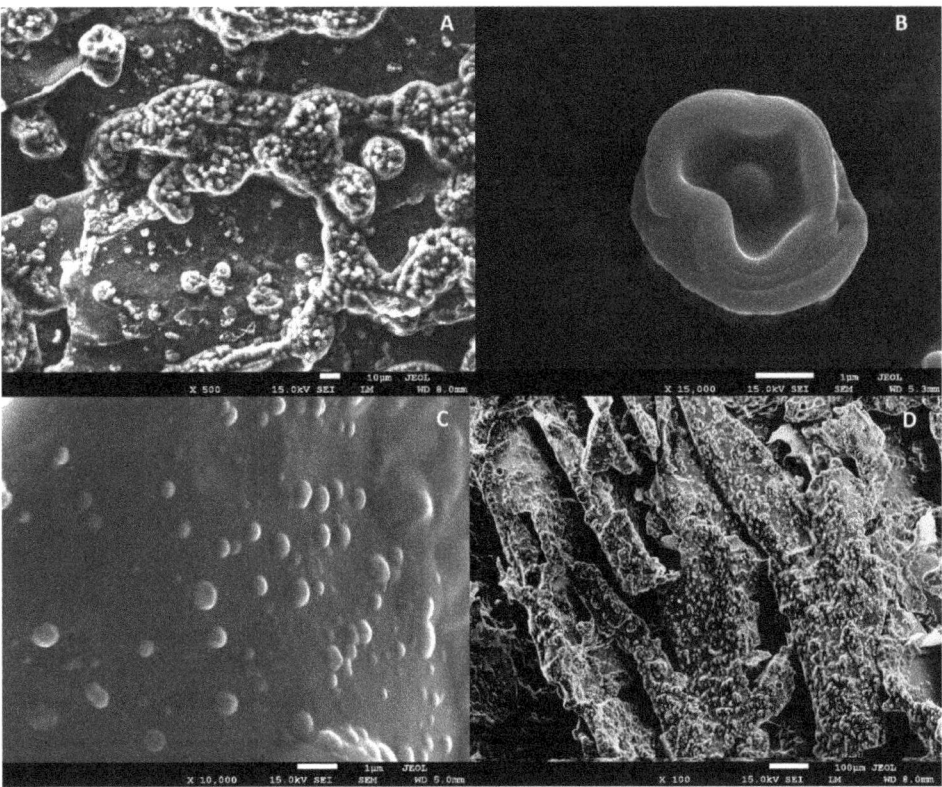

Figure 2. SEM analysis of hydrogels with encapsulated oil: (**A**,**B**) Concentration of 29%; (**C**,**D**) concentration in the range of 45%.

Table 3. Characteristics of açai extract and safflower oil.

	Safflower Oil	Açai Extract
TPC (mg gallic acid/g of sample)	0.27 ± 0.011	31.36 ± 1.220
ABTS (mg ascorbic acid/g of sample0	0.09 ± 0.003	50.54 ± 0.296
FRAP (mg ascorbic acid/g of sample)	0.32 ± 0.004	38.05 ± 1.268
Fatty acid profile (%)		
SFA		10.88 ± 1.36
MUFA		9.74 ± 1.13
PUFA		79.19 ± 0.95
$\sum$n-6		78.91 ± 0.98
$\sum$n-3		0.15 ± 0.02

TPC—total phenolic compounds; ABTS—2,2′-azino-bis-3-ethylbenzthiazoline-6-sulphonic acid; FRAP—ferric reducing antioxidant power; SFA—saturated fatty acid; MUFA—monounsaturated fatty acid; PUFA—polyunsaturated fatty acid.

2.2. Main Study

2.2.1. TBARS Analysis

A TBARS analysis is a commonly used indicator of oxidative lipid rancidity in meat, which quantifies the amount of secondary oxidation products. The analysis of the lipid peroxidation content in the studied burgers after 0, 4, and 8 days of storage is shown in Figure 3. The results indicated that, depending on the day of storage and variant, the lipid peroxidation content ranged from 1.14 to 6.92 mg MA/100 g sample. At Day 0, depending on the variant used, the lipid oxidation values ranged from 1.14 (CO) to 5.2 mg MA/100 g sample (GE), hence, the application of a fat substitute in the form of a hydrogel with encapsulated oil and flaxseed flour increased the TBARS values as compared with the control variants (CT and CO). This result was probably due to the presence of flaxseed flour which contained high PUFA levels [20]. The defatted flaxseed flour used in the experiment contained 10 g of fat per 100 g of flour. The manufacturing process of the flaxseed flour could have influenced the generation of free radicals, aldehydes, and ketones upon exposure of PUFAs to light, heat, and oxygen. A study performed by Hautrive et al. [9] revealed that the addition of defatted flaxseed flour elevated TBARS values as compared with a control variant. Furthermore, our results showed that between 0 and 4 days of storage, the highest increase in lipid oxidation (1.85–2.08) was observed in CT and CO. Therefore, using a fat substitute in the form of gel (konjac flour and sodium alginate) with encapsulated oil and flaxseed flour (G, GT, GE, and GET) exerted a positive effect on the reduction in the peroxidation rate. Thus, structuring the added fat significantly reduced the TBARS value ($p < 0.05$, Figure 3) as compared with the product containing animal or vegetable fat [21]. Additionally, our research showed that the MA value increased with storage time, regardless of variant type. As a result, lipid oxidation contributed to the development of rancidity while reducing the quality of meat products during storage [22]. The threshold value that dictates the loss of sensory quality of food is >1.0 mg malondialdehyde/kg burger [23]. In our case, despite the observed increase in fat oxidation, all values obtained were below the threshold value.

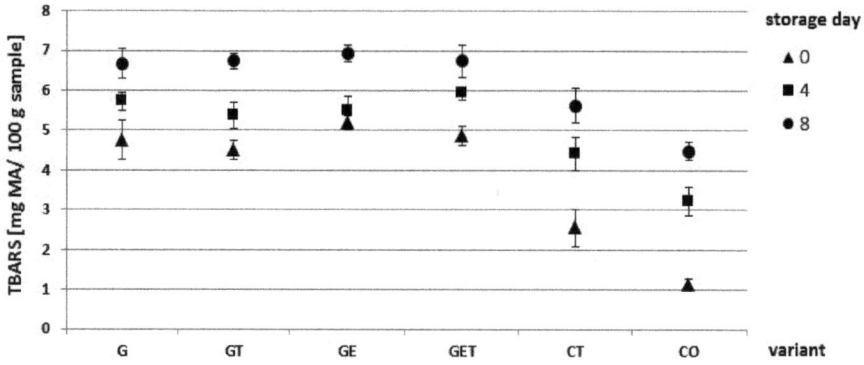

Figure 3. Analysis of lipid oxidation (TBARS) in burgers with a fat substitute after 0, 4, and 8 days of storage. G—encapsulated oil; GT—encapsulated oil + tallow; GE—encapsulated oil with açai extract; GET—encapsulated oil with açai extract + tallow; CT—control with tallow; CO—control with oil.

2.2.2. Color and pH Analysis

The pH parameter of meat can affect certain characteristics such as color, flavor, aroma, tenderness, and nutritional value. An analysis of the meat pH parameter was carried out on raw burgers after each storage time. Table 4 lists the obtained pH values, which, depending on the variant and storage time, range from 5.56 to 5.81. The addition of a hydrogel and flaxseed flour contributed to the observed increase in pH on Day 0 as compared with the controls (CT and CO). This effect was possibly due to the addition of fiber in the form of flaxseed flour. Hautrive et al. [9] and Sánchez-Zapata et al. [24] also reported higher pH values in modified fiber burgers as compared with control variants. Our study demonstrated that the addition of tallow to the studied meat increased the pH values of the burgers more than the addition of safflower oil (5.64, respectively, 5.56 $p < 0.05$). The observed increase on Day 4 of storage, especially in the G, GT, GE, and GET variants, may have been due to the accumulation of volatile bases such as trimethylamine and ammonia, which formed during protein hydrolysis and amino acid degradation by endogenous enzymes or microorganisms [25].

Table 4. Effect of fat substitute in the form of a hydrogel with encapsulated safflower oil, açai extract, and linseed flour on color parameters, browning index (BI), and pH in raw and grilled burgers at 0, 4, and 8 days of storage.

Variant	Day	Raw				
		L*	a*	b*	BI	pH
G	0	44.5 ± 2.85 B,C,b	22.6 ± 2.36 B	14.7 ± 1.52 A,B,b	75.32 ± 6.83 A	5.70 ± 0.04 C
GT	0	46.2 ± 3.06 A,b	22.7 ± 2.80 B	15.2 ± 1.52 A,b	74.20 ± 7.75 A,B	5.71 ± 0.04 C
GE	0	45.0 ± 3.25 A,B,a,b	21.9 ± 1.93 B	14.7 ± 2.01 A,B,b	73.38 ± 5.89 A,B	5.72 ± 0.03 C
GET	0	43.2 ± 3.02 C,D,c	22.8 ± 2.20 B,b	14.0 ± 1.50 B,a	75.57 ± 7.24 A	5.71 ± 0.05 C
CT	0	42.0 ± 2.66 D,E,b	24.1 ± 1.81 A,a	11.5 ± 0.97 C	71.30 ± 7.18 B,a	5.64 ± 0.04 A
CO	0	40.4 ± 2.40 E,b	22.0 ± 1.61 B,a	10.4 ± 0.86 D	67.10 ± 5.54 C,a	5.56 ± 0.04 B
G	4	44.2 ± 3.13 A,b	22.3 ± 1.87 A	14.7 ± 1.31 A,b	75.57 ± 5.06 A	5.81 ± 0.06 C
GT	4	45.3 ± 4.24 A,b	22.3 ± 2.45 A	14.6 ± 1.9 A,b	73.42 ± 7.15 A	5.77 ± 0.03 C
GE	4	43.7 ± 3.85 A,b	21.6 ± 2.09 A,B	14.0 ± 1.5 A,b	73.09 ± 7.35 A	5.76 ± 0.05 C
GET	4	44.9 ± 3.78 A,b	21.8 ± 2.32 A,B,a	14.4 ± 1.52 A,a,b	72.87 ± 8.00 A	5.76 ± 0.05 C
CT	4	41.4 ± 3.64 B,b	22.8 ± 2.29 A,b	11.0 ± 1.42 B	68.89 ± 7.57 B,a	5.63 ± 0.09 A
CO	4	41.0 ± 3.06 B,b	20.8 ± 1.68 B,b	10.2 ± 1.11 C	63.50 ± 6.32 C,b	5.57 ± 0.07 B
G	8	46.9 ± 3.16 a	22.7 ± 2.18 A	16.3 ± 1.51 A,a	76.35 ± 6.28 A	5.73 ± 0.04 B
GT	8	48.6 ± 3.55 a	21.1 ± 2.47 A	16.6 ± 1.45 A,a	72.36 ± 6.68 A	5.73 ± 0.03 B
GE	8	46.9 ± 3.02 a	21.1 ± 1.15 A	16.0 ± 1.51 A,a	73.44 ± 5.66 A	5.75 ± 0.01 B
GET	8	47.5 ± 4.00 a	20.9 ± 2.54 A,a,c	15.4 ± 1.69 A,b	70.18 ± 8.77 A	5.75 ± 0.03 B
CT	8	46.9 ± 6.54 a	18.5 ± 2.94 B,b	10.9 ± 1.76 B	55.01 ± 11.42 B,b	5.58 ± 0.03 A
CO	8	44.9 ± 5.44 a	18.6 ± 2.03 B,c	10.8 ± 1.51 B	56.83 ± 7.73 B,c	5.58 ± 0.03 A

Variant	Day	Grilled			
		L*	a*	b*	BI
G	0	52.2 ± 1.68 A	7.4 ± 0.75 A,B,a,b	13.5 ± 0395 A	39.87 ± 2.66 A,b
GT	0	52.7 ± 1.71 A	7.0 ± 0.40 A,a	13.7 ± 1.25 A	39.27 ± 2.38 A
GE	0	51.4 ± 1.92 A,a	7.3 ± 0.81 A,B,a	12.6 ± 1.47 A,a	38.09 ± 2.95 A,b
GET	0	52.7 ± 1.38 A,a	7.3 ± 0.56 A,B,a	13.5 ± 1.32 A	39.27 ± 2.80 A,b
CT	0	51.6 ± 2.25 A	7.7 ± 1.00 B,a	10.0 ± 0.88 B,a	32.18 ± 1.75 B,a
CO	0	49.1 ± 2.37 B,a	7.9 ± 0.66 B	9.8 ± 0.62 B,a	33.72 ± 2.53 B,a
G	4	52.5 ± 1.61	7.0 ± 0.41 A,C,b	13.0 ± 0.84 A	37.83 ± 1.69 B,b
GT	4	52.3 ± 2.378	7.3 ± 0.45 A,b	13.7 ± 1.30 A	40.03 ± 2.32 A
GE	4	53.9 ± 1.81 b	6.7 ± 0.35 C,D,b,c	13.7 ± 1.16 A,b	37.96 ± 2.87 B,b
GET	4	53.3 ± 1.85 a	6.2 ± 0.50 D,b	13.9 ± 0.62 B	38.43 ± 2.16 A,B,b
CT	4	53.1 ± 2.04	7.1 ± 0.45 A,C,b	9.6 ± 1.04 B,a	29.23 ± 1.94 D,b
CO	4	51.0 ± 1.44 b	7.8 ± 0.23 B	9.4 ± 0.55 B,b,c	31.21 ± 1.80 C,b
G	8	51.4 ± 4.93 A	10.7 ± 5.29 A,a	12.7 ± 1.73 A	43.74 ± 9.60 A,a
GT	8	52.7 ± 2.38 A	7.7 ± 0.72 A,b	13.6 ± 1.10 A	40.02 ± 2.54 B
GE	8	48.6 ± 4.44 B,C,a	6.8 ± 0.59 B,a,c	13.5 ± 1.14 A,b	42.62 ± 4.18 A,B,a
GET	8	51.0 ± 2.12 A,C,b	7.0 ± 0.56 B,a	13.7 ± 0.85 A	41.03 ± 2.60 A,B,a
CT	8	52.2 ± 1.40 A	8.1 ± 0.63 A,a	9.0 ± 0.80 B,b	29.84 ± 2.10 D,b
CO	8	47.6 ± 1.64 B,c	8.0 ± 0.37 A	9.6 ± 0.70 B,a,c	34.54 ± 1.97 C,a

A-E Mean values between variants on the same storage day with different letters indicate a significant difference. a-c Mean values of the same variants between storage day with different letters indicate a significant difference. G—encapsulated oil; GT—encapsulated oil + tallow; GE—encapsulated oil with açai extract; GET—encapsulated oil with açai extract + tallow; CT—control with tallow; CO—control with oil. L*—lightness; a*—redness; b*—yellowness; BI—browning index.

The effects of hydrogel with encapsulated safflower oil and flaxseed flour on the color parameters of grilled and raw burgers after 0, 4, and 8 days of storage are shown in Table 4. The color parameter of meat influences the willingness of consumers to buy a product due to a growing appreciation for bright red products. The color parameter was significantly affected by storage time and formulation ingredients. The values of the L* parameter in raw burgers increased with increasing storage time regardless of the variant type. A similar trend was observed by Carvalho et al. [26]. However, as compared with the L* color parameter on Day 4, the control variants (CT and CO) had lower values ($p < 0.05$) than the experimental variants (G, GT, GE, and GET). This trend was also observed for a* and b* parameters on Days 4 and 8. Furthermore, the addition of açai extract (GE and GET) had no significant effect on the color parameter regardless of storage time. The fat substitute with microencapsulated oil and flaxseed flour contributed to an improved color parameter of raw burgers after Days 4 and 8 of storage. The analysis of the browning index showed that for both raw and grilled meat, the BI was higher in the G, GT, GE, and GET groups. Probably this effect was caused by the addition of flaxseed flour, which was characterized by a brown color. The color analysis performed on the grilled burgers after each storage day showed no differences among the variants. This was also confirmed by Summo et al. [27] and Gök et al. [28]. However, in the case of the study reported by Lucas-González et al. [29], an increase in the a* color parameter and a decrease in the L* color parameter in grilled burgers with a fat substitute (chestnut flour, emulsion gel, and chia oil) were noted. Grilling changed the color of the meat due to heat-induced denaturation of myoglobin. Currently, the role of fat type used for grilled burger formulation is not fully understood, but it should have less of an effect on the color than other parameters such as storage conditions or pH [27].

2.2.3. TPA Analysis

Texture changes (chewiness, springiness, and hardness) that occur in meat products as a result of replacing animal fat with vegetable fats are becoming an interesting area of research, especially because texture is importance in sensory attributes. The TPA analysis of the grilled burgers is shown in Table 5. The texture parameter values, regardless of variant used and storage time, were significantly ($p < 0.05$) lower (5.3–15.0 (N)) than those of the control samples (24.8–90.9 (N0). This was also observed by Afshari et al. [30], where a fat substitute was applied as an emulsion of soy protein, inulin, β-glucan, canola oil, and olive oil. Similarly, Lucas-González et al. [29] showed that as the degree of fat substitute (chestnut flour emulsion gel and chia oil in pork burgers) increased, texture parameters decreased as compared with control samples. However, Moghtadaei et al. [31] applied a hydrogel (sesame oil and ethyl cellulose) as a fat substitute in a burger and observed the opposite effect as compared with our results. According to the literature, there are many conflicting reports regarding the effect of hydrogel type on the texture parameters of grilled burgers. These differences may occur due to the method of vegetable oil incorporation into the product, its concentration, and the type of hydrogel used [32]. The grilled burgers (G, GT, GE, and GET) had lower hardness values than that of the CT and CO samples. As expected, the grilling process increased hardness of the control samples due to protein denaturation, water loss, and fat loss [33]. In general, the hardness of meat products is related to the size of the fat molecules therein, allowing the formation of an interfacial protein film around the fat globules by salt-soluble proteins (actin, myosin). Thus, an exponential relationship exists between the size of fat globules and the amount of interfacial protein layer [34,35]. In the case of the studied hydrogel, the fat was encapsulated in a polymer blend, whereas in the control samples, an interfacial protein film likely formed and denaturation occurred because of grilling. The variation in hardness between the control samples was probably due to the amount of interfacial protein layer formed, the type of fat used (beef tallow in tissue form, liquid vegetable oil), and its thermal stability. The higher thermal stability of the hydrogel contributed to a greater decrease in hardness of the product after grilling as compared with beef fat or safflower oil. In addition, the values of grilled burger parameters such as springiness and cohesiveness decreased with increasing storage time, whereas the values of chewiness and firmness parameters increased. This effect was related to natural leakage in burgers, which consequently influenced texture parameters [36]. From the consumer's point of view, reductions in hardness or chewiness parameters are considered to be a favorable characteristics due to their association with enhanced meat quality of the burger [29].

Table 5. Effect of a hydrogel emulsion with capsulated safflower oil, açai extract, and linseed flour as a fat substitute, on texture parameters (TPA) of grilled burgers at 0, 4, and 8 days of storage.

Variant	Springiness (−)	Chewiness (N)	Cohesiveness (−)	Hardness (N)
G	0.4 ± 0.20	0.6 ± 0.26 [B,a,b]	0.1 ± 0.04 [C,a]	6.4 ± 1.59 [B]
GT	0.4 ± 0.11 [a]	0.3 ± 0.17 [B]	0.0 ± 0.05 [B,C]	5.3 ± 1.23 [B]
GE	0.8 ± 0.30 [a]	0.4 ± 0.26 [B]	0.1 ± 0.04 [B,C]	5.5 ± 0.98 [B]
GET	0.5 ± 0.2	0.5 ± 0.24 [B]	0.1 ± 0.10 [B,C]	5.6 ± 1.53 [B]
CT	0.9 ± 0.22	10.6 ± 2.30 [A,b]	0.4 ± 0.03 [A]	27.5 ± 5.25 [A,b]
CO	0.5 ± 0.12 [a]	8.8 ± 1.50 [A,c]	0.4 ± 0.04 [A]	24.8 ± 1.95 [A,c]
G	0.2 ± 0.05 [C]	1.0 ± 0.49 [B,a]	0.1 ± 0.03 [C,a]	9.5 ± 2.16 [B]
GT	0.2 ± 0.03 [C,b]	0.4 ± 0.59 [B]	0.0 ± 0.07 [B,C]	7.8 ± 2.68 [B]
GE	0.1 ± 0.03 [C,b]	0.5 ± 0.62 [B]	0.0 ± 0.07 [B,C]	7.9 ± 2.46 [B]
GET	0.1 ± 0.04 [C]	0.0 ± 0.36 [B]	0.0 ± 0.09 [B,C]	5.8 ± 1.20 [B]
CT	0.4 ± 0.06 [A]	17.1 ± 4.73 [A,a,b]	0.4 ± 0.03 [A]	47.3 ± 12.23 [A,a,b]
CO	0.3 ± 0.04 [B,b]	21.4 ± 4.25 [A,b]	0.4 ± 0.02 [A]	58.6 ± 12.04 [A,b]
G	0.1 ± 0.03 [C]	−0.3 ± 0.90 [C,b]	−0.1 ± 0.14 [B,b]	10.4 ± 3.34 [C]
GT	0.1 ± 0.03 [C,b]	−0.5 ± 0.70 [C]	−0.1 ± 0.08 [B]	10.2 ± 2.51 [C]
GE	0.2 ± 0.04 [C,b]	−0.1 ± 0.99 [C]	0.0 ± 0.10 [B]	11.6 ± 3.93 [C]
GET	0.1 ± 0.03 [C]	0.5 ± 1.43 [C]	0.0 ± 0.12 [B]	15.0 ± 7.16 [C]
CT	0.5 ± 0.04 [A]	19.6 ± 6.80 [B,a]	0.3 ± 0.04 [A]	58.6 ± 17.54 [B,a]
CO	0.3 ± 0.01 [B,b]	29.1 ± 6.22 [A,a]	0.3 ± 0.03 [A]	90.9 ± 18.76 [A,a]

[A–C] Mean values between variants on the same storage day with different letters indicate a significant difference.
[a–c] Mean values of the same variants between storage day with different letters indicate a significant difference.
G—encapsulated oil; GT—encapsulated oil + tallow; GE—encapsulated oil with açai extract; GET—encapsulated oil with açai extract + tallow; CT—control with tallow; CO—control with oil.

2.2.4. WHC Analysis, Weight Loss, and Cooking Loss Analysis

The food industry demands the appropriate technological properties of a burger related to mass retention after storage and grilling, and therefore, retention of intrinsic water is of key importance. Adequate water retention in meat products not only reduces mass loss, but also causes accumulation of liquid in the package and consequently changes the texture, color, and ultimately, consumer acceptance of the meat product [37]. Figure 4 shows the analysis of water retention in raw and grilled burgers after 0, 4, and 8 days of storage. The values for the variants G, GT, GE, and GET, regardless of storage time, were in the range of 93.5–98.8%. In contrast, the values of the control samples were 31.8–43.2% depending on the period of storage. Our study showed that a fat substitute with flaxseed flour (G, GT, GE, and GET) improved the WHC about 54–60% as compared with those of the control samples, depending on the storage period and variant. A similar trend was observed by Zinina et al. [38], who observed an increased WHC parameter when flaxseed flour was used. In contrast, a study by Sharefiabadi et al. [39] revealed that the addition of flaxseed flour and coconut flour did not improve the WHC parameter in chicken pasties. The difference in the aforementioned studies may have been the type of fat substitute added to the meat products.

The analysis of mass loss conducted in this study showed that mass loss increased with storage time ($p < 0.05$) in the burgers with a fat substitute as well as the control variants. Nevertheless, the G, GT, GE, and GET variants had much lower mass loss (0.5–0.6%) than that of the CT and CO variants (1.3–2.6%). The replacement of fat with a hydrogel (konjac flour and sodium alginate) enriched with encapsulated oil with flaxseed flour helped to reduce mass changes during storage. The significant difference ($p < 0.05$) observed between the tallow and liquid oil controls was possibly due to the form of added fat [40]. Similar trends were observed for grilled samples after 0, 4, and 8 days of storage, where the fat substitute based on konjac flour and sodium alginate enriched with encapsulated safflower oil showed statistically significant ($p < 0.05$) reduction in the percentage mass loss of the burger. A study by Salcedo-Sandaval et al. [41] showed that konjac gel with added oils (olive oil, flaxseed oil, and fish oil) showed lower mass loss after grilling and baking as compared with control variants. The limiting role in mass changes during grilling was also supported by Moghtadaei et al. [35]. The analysis showed that the addition of tallow (GT and GET) increased the percentage mass loss of the grilled burgers, which could be due to changes in the consistency of the tallow under the influence of the grilling process.

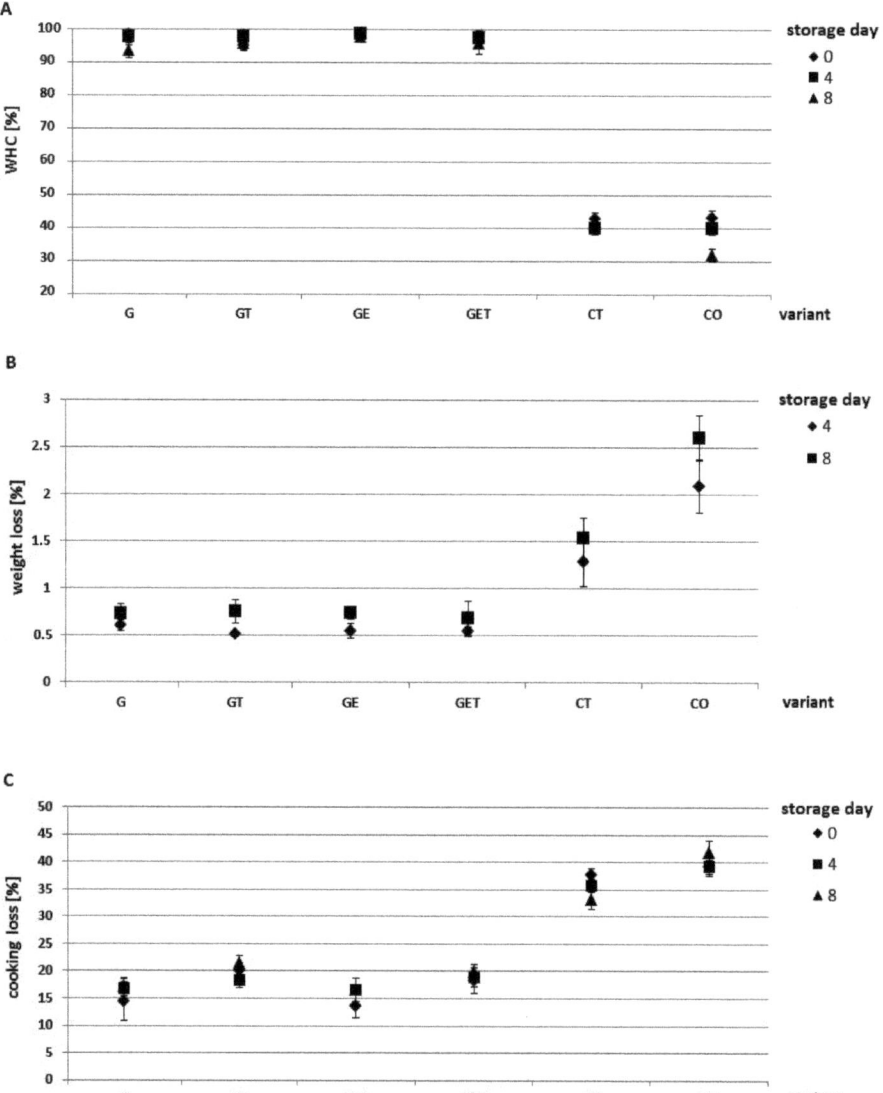

Figure 4. Effect of a fat substitute on water retention (WHC) (**A**); weight loss (**B**); and cooking loss (**C**), after 0, 4, and 8 days of storage. G—encapsulated oil; GT—encapsulated oil + tallow; GE—encapsulated oil with açai extract; GET—encapsulated oil with açai extract + tallow; CT—control with tallow; CO—control with oil.

2.2.5. Analysis of the Volatile Compounds Profile

Fat is a precursor to many aromatic compounds, and it also acts as a solvent for these compounds. Changes in the amount and composition of fat can affect the rate and type of processes that occur during burger storage [1]. The analysis of changes to the profile of volatile compounds in raw and grilled burgers after 0, 4, and 8 days of storage is shown in Figure 5. The obtained results displayed differences in the volatile compounds profile between G and GT, between G and GE, between GET and CT, and between GET and CO variants on Day 0. The data revealed that the presence of the extract affected the aroma profile of the raw burger by reducing the changes in compound growth (Figure 5A), thus, slowing down changes that naturally occur in the burger during storage. The alterations in the volatile compounds profile of burgers with a fat substitute after 4 and 8 days of storage were comparable. The opposite was observed for burgers with tallow and oil, where changes increased with storage time, and the process of changes progressed fastest between 4 and 8 days of storage. In contrast, for grilled burgers (Figure 5B), the variants used showed no difference in the volatile compounds profile regardless of storage time, with only a slight variation at Day 0 in GET. However, this may stem from the presence of both extract and tallow. Fluctuations in volatile compounds profile for the CT variant changed dramatically at Day 8, which was possibly due to the progressive oxidative processes of high tallow content (20%), especially after 4 days of storage. In contrast, the CT variant with safflower oil displayed linear changes, which indicated gradual changes that progressed with storage time.

Table 6 shows the component analysis of the volatile compounds profile of raw burgers with a fat substitute (G, GT, GE, and GET) and control variants (CT and CO) after 0, 4, and 8 days of storage. The analysis revealed that the number of compounds, especially corresponding to aldehydes, alcohols, esters, and ketones, increased with storage time. The addition of oils with increased amounts of unsaturated fatty acids promotes oxidative processes in meat and consequently increases the content of volatile compounds formed by lipid oxidation [26]. Volatile compounds such as alcohols, aldehydes, and ketones are mainly responsible for reducing the sensory quality of meat products [42]. Wantanabe et al. [43] confirmed our findings, where the number of volatile compounds related to alcohols increased with storage time. In contrast, alcohols such as 1−hexanol, 1−pentanol, and 1−octen−3−ol have been considered to be key indicators of lipid oxidation in meat [26]. The component analysis of the volatile compounds profile in grilled burgers was dominated by aldehyde and alcohol group bearing compounds. Emerging compounds such as benzaldehyde, 3−methylbutanal, 2−methylpropanal, pyrazine, and dimethyl sulphide are typical compounds that arise from the Maillard reaction, which is induced by a thermal process [44,45]. The obtained results showed that, apart from lipid degradation and the Maillard reaction, the applied product components were the main factors that influenced the formation of volatile substance characteristics for a particular variant, for example, compounds such as benzaneacetaldehyde, 1−propanol−2 methyl, and pyrazine for variants G, GT, GE, and GET; pentan−2−ol for GE and GET; 2−furanmethanol for CO; and dimethyl sulphide for CT.

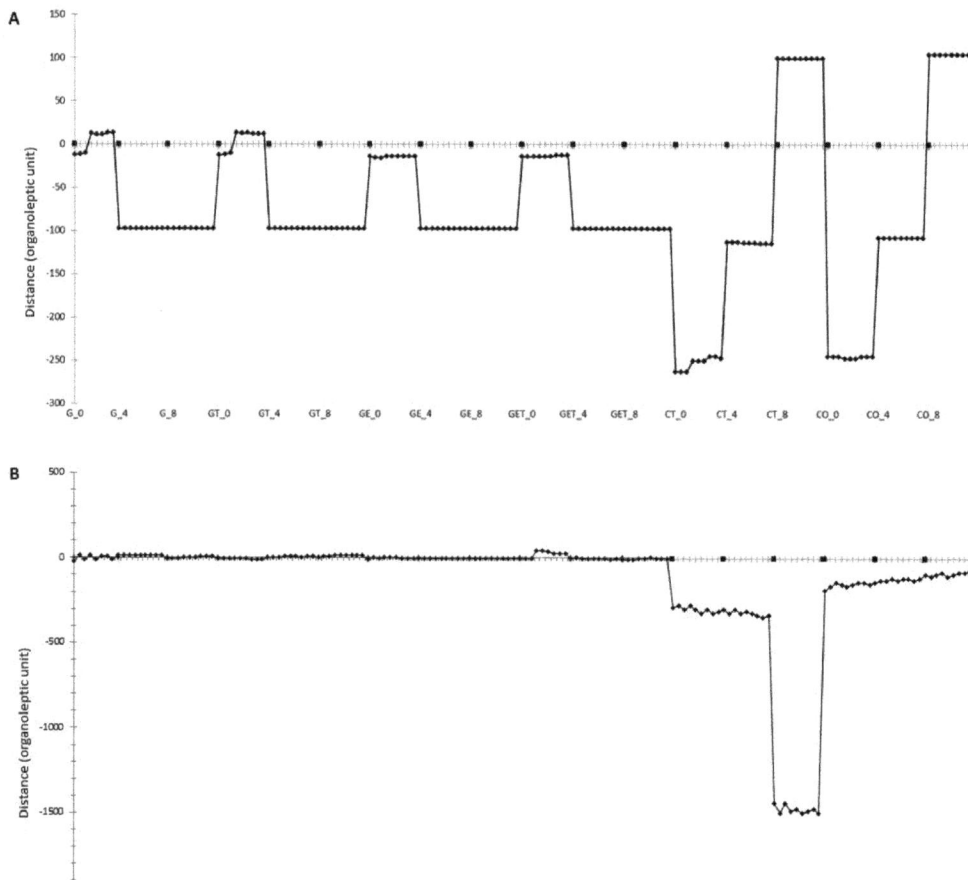

Figure 5. Changes in the volatile compounds profile of raw burgers (**A**); grilled burgers (**B**), after 0, 4, and 8 days of storage (4 ± 1 °C). G—encapsulated oil; GT—encapsulated oil + tallow; GE—encapsulated oil with açai extract; GET—encapsulated oil with açai extract + tallow; CT—control with tallow; CO—control with oil.

Table 6. Effects of a fat substitute on the volatile compounds profile in raw and grilled burger after 0, 4, and 8 days of storage in cold conditions.

Volatile Compounds	Raw Burger 0						Raw Burger 4						Raw Burger 8					
	G	GT	GE	GET	CT	CO	G	GT	GE	GET	CT	CO	G	GT	GE	GET	CT	CO
aldehyde																		
(E,E)–2,4–hexadienal	+																	
2--Methylpropanal		+	+	+	+	+	+	+	+	+	+		+	+	+	+	+	+
3–Methylbutanal						+						+						
Benzaldehyde																		+
Benzeneacetaldehyde							+	+	+	+		+	+	+	+	+	+	+
Propanal	+	+	+	+	+	+	+	+	+	+	+	+						
alcohol																		
1–Hexanol							+	+	+	+	+	+	+	+	+	+	+	+
1–Hexen–3–ol			+	+					+						+	+		
1–Penten–3–ol										+						+		
1–Propanol	+	+	+	+	+	+	+	+	+	+	+	+	+	+	+	+	+	+
1–Propanol, 2–methyl	+	+	+				+	+	+	+		+		+	+	+	+	+
2–Nonen–1–ol									+								+	+
Pentan–2–ol								+		+								+
ester																		
Ethyl 2–methylbutyrate										+						+		
Ethyl isobutyrate	+	+	+	+	+	+				+								
Hexyl propionate												+						
Methyl isobutyrate	+	+	+	+	+	+												
Propyl propanoate							+	+	+	+		+		+		+	+	+
ketone																		
1–Hexen–3–one										+						+		
2,3–Butanediol																	+	+
Sotolon							+	+	+						+			
acid																		
Acetic acid	+	+		+	+	+	+	+	+	+	+	+	+	+	+	+	+	+
Pentanoic acid							+	+	+	+		+				+		
Propanoic acid		+	+				+	+	+	+				+	+			

Table 6. Cont.

Volatile Compounds	Raw Burger																	
	G	GT	GE⁰	GET⁰	CT	CO	G	GT	GE⁴	GET⁴	CT	CO	G	GT	GE⁸	GET⁸	CT	CO
acetate																		
Bezyl acetate	+						+					+						
Isoamyl acetate		+	+	+	+												+	+
Isopropyl acetate			+	+	+	+												
terpene																		
Alpha–phellandrene												+						
Alphapinene			+	+		+			+	+		+			+			
Limonene				+					+	+								
sulphur compounds																		
Dimethyl sulfide							+		+	+	+		+		+		+	+
2–Methyl–2–propanethiol									+	+								

Volatile compounds	Grilled Burger																	
	G	GT	GE⁰	GET⁰	CT	CO	G	GT	GE⁴	GET⁴	CT	CO	G	GT	GE⁸	GET⁸	CT	CO
aldehyde																		
(E)–3–hexenal	+	+					+	+			+							
(E,E)–2,4–hexadienal	+	+					+	+	+						+			
2–Methylpropanal			+	+	+									+				
3–Methylbutanal		+		+	+		+											
Benzaldehyde		+						+										
Benzeneacetaldehyde	+	+	+	+		+	+	+	+	+		+			+	+		+
Methional						+				+		+						+
Propanal						+		+				+			+			+
alcohol																		
1–Hexanol										+	+					+		
1–Hexen–3–ol	+		+	+		+		+	+	+		+			+	+		+
1–Propanol			+	+		+		+	+	+		+			+	+	+	+
1–Propanol, 2-methyl	+	+	+					+	+			+						
2–Furanmethanol						+			+	+								+
n–Butanol																	+	
Pentan–2–ol			+	+				+		+					+			

Table 6. Cont.

Volatile compounds	Grilled Burger																	
	0						4						8					
	G	GT	GE	GET	CT	CO	G	GT	GE	GET	CT	CO	G	GT	GE	GET	CT	CO
ethyl 2–methylbutyrate propyl propanoate				+						+							+	
ketone																		
1–Hexen–3–one																+		
2,3-Butanediol					+												+	+
2–Acetyl–1–pyrroline					+						+						+	
Acetophenone						+						+						+
acid																		
3–Methylbutanoic acid	+							+										
Acetic acid		+	+	+	+			+		+							+	
Benzoic acid																	+	+
acetate																		
Ethyl acetate	+	+	+	+		+			+	+		+		+	+	+		
terpene																		
Alpha–phellandrene										+							+	
Alphapinene			+	+		+			+	+	+				+	+		+
nitrogenous compounds																		
Pyrazine	+	+	+	+				+	+	+	+			+	+	+	+	
Pyrrole	+	+	+	+	+			+	+	+	+			+		+	+	
sulphur compounds																		
2–Methyl–2–propanethiol										+								
Dimethyl sulfide					+												+	

G—encapsulated oil; GT—encapsulated oil + tallow; GE—encapsulated oil with açai extract; GET—encapsulated oil with açai extract + tallow; CT—control with tallow; CO—control with oil.

2.2.6. Analysis of Fatty Acid Profile and Nutritional Indexes AI, TI, and h/H

The analysis of the fatty acid profile and nutritional indexes of raw and grilled burgers after 0, 4, and 8 days of storage are shown in Table 7. The fatty acid profile was influenced by the type of formulation used. The analysis of saturated fatty acids (SFA) and unsaturated fatty acids (MUFA and PUFA) in raw burgers showed that SFA increased and MUFA and PUFA decreased with storage time, regardless of the variant used. Our results were consistent with the theory that as the number of double bonds in a fatty acid increased, the susceptibility to oxidation increased [26]. As predicted, the addition of safflower oil significantly increased the PUFA content of the raw burgers from 1% (CT) to 24% (GET). The analysis of PUFAs and MUFAs in reformulated raw burgers showed that the addition of açai extract (GE) contributed to lower oxidation levels. Carvalho et al. [26] and Rutkowska et al. [46] confirmed a positive effect of extracts (pitanga leaves, guarana seeds, and chokeberry fruit) on reducing the rate of oxidative changes in fat. Safflower oil used in the experiment was characterized by high PUFA content (79%), with an $n-6/n-3$ ratio of 526. In contrast, the applied reformulation of the burger with cassava oil with the addition of flaxseed flour reduced the $n-6/n-3$ ratio by as much as 10-fold (50 for CO and 5 for GE), while maintaining high PUFA values. According to dietary recommendations, this ratio should be 5-4:1 [19]. For other nutritional indexes, it is recommended that meat products should have the lowest possible AI and TI values, while the h/H ratio should be as high as possible [47]. In our study, independent of storage time, the burger variants with the fat substitute used had the lowest AI and TI values as compared with CT. Furthermore, hydrogel emulsion with flaxseed flour significantly increased the h/H ratio from 1.3 (CT) to 2.5 (GE). Considering the indexes of healthiness that were analyzed, the best results were obtained for raw burgers with the addition of açai extract (GE) in relation to hydrogel without extract (G). The correlation analysis among SFA, MUFA, PUFA, and CLA and storage day, showed that SFA had a very high positive correlation (0.736, $p < 0.05$). In contrast, the correlation analysis of MUFA and CLA showed moderately high negative correlations (-0.359 and -0.488, $p < 0.05$, respectively). In contrast, the PUFA analysis showed no correlation with storage time. The correlations obtained indicated that changes occurred during storage related to the fat oxidation process as a result of which, polyunsaturated acids were converted to a saturated form [26]. The analysis of the fatty acid profile of grilled burgers showed that the use of reformulated burgers contributed to an increase in PUFA content as compared with CT and CO. In addition, usage of hydrogels contributed to lowering $n-6/n-3$ acid ratios, from 24 (CO) to 5 (GE), which was extremely important to maintain proper nutritional standards. Furthermore, the use of reformulation resulted in improved health values of the grilled burger by lowering the AI and TI values and increasing the h/H ratio.

Table 7. Effects of a fat substitute (hydrogel emulsion with encapsulated oil and acai extract) on the fatty acid profile of raw and grilled burgers at 0, 4, and 8 days of storage in cold conditions.

		Raw Burger					
		G	GT	GE	GET	CT	CO
SFA							
	0	38.2 ± 0.46 [A]	36.3 ± 2.62 [A,B]	35.0 ± 0.51 [B]	38.9 ± 1.00 [A]	39.4 ± 0.37 [A]	32.7 ± 0.18 [C]
	4	41.5 ± 0.16 [B]	40.7 ± 0.52 [B]	41.6 ± 1.61 [B]	42.7 ± 0.62 [B]	50.1 ± 0.03 [A]	37.7 ± 0.29 [C]
	8	43.8 ± 0.60 [B]	45.3 ± 1.08 [B]	40.3 ± 0.48 [C]	44.1 ± 1.65 [B]	50.5 ± 0.64 [A]	51.6 ± 2.13 [A]
MUFA							
	0	35.9 ± 0.26 [D]	43.4 ± 2.47 [B]	39.7 ± 0.32 [B]	41.2 ± 0.92 [B]	58.8 ± 0.45 [A]	37.5 ± 0.42 [C]
	4	36.7 ± 1.26 [C]	39.9 ± 0.26 [B]	32.5 ± 0.52 [E]	38.2 ± 0.27 [C]	48.5 ± 0.01 [A]	34.2 ± 0.79 [D]
	8	33.6 ± 1.09 [C]	36.5 ± 0.51 [B]	36.7 ± 0.55 [B]	37.1 ± 1.32 [B]	48.0 ± 0.68 [A]	28.9 ± 1.70 [D]

Table 7. Cont.

		Raw Burger					
		G	GT	GE	GET	CT	CO
PUFA	0	25.4 ± 0.78 [B]	19.7 ± 0.12 [C]	24.8 ± 0.14 [B]	19.5 ± 0.07 [C]	1.0 ± 0.02 [D]	28.8 ± 0.10 [A]
	4	21.4 ± 1.39 [C]	18.9 ± 0.75 [D]	24.0 ± 1.09 [B]	18.7 ± 0.67 [D]	0.9 ± 0.01 [E]	27.6 ± 0.51 [A]
	8	20.2 ± 1.69 [B]	17.7 ± 0.58 [C]	22.6 ± 0.10 [A]	18.3 ± 0.21 [C]	1.0 ± 0.02 [D]	19.1 ± 0.44 [B]
CLA	0	0.46 ± 0.06 [C]	0.57 ± 0.04 [B]	0.50 ± 0.05 [C]	0.49 ± 0.01 [C]	0.72 ± 0.06 [A]	0.49 ± 0.00 [C]
	4	0.50 ± 0.02 [A]	0.48 ± 0.04 [B]	0.38 ± 0.00 [C]	0.45 ± 0.00 [B]	0.54 ± 0.01 [A]	0.40 ± 0.02 [C]
	8	0.45 ± 0.00 [B]	0.41 ± 0.01 [B]	0.41 ± 0.03 [B]	0.47 ± 0.06 [A,B]	0.54 ± 0.02 [A]	0.40 ± 0.01 [B]
∑n3	0	3.24 ± 0.46 [B]	3.16 ± 0.06 [B]	3.95 ± 0.16 [A]	3.25 ± 0.01 [B]	0.52 ± 0.01 [C]	0.58 ± 0.04 [C]
	4	3.15 ± 0.69 [A,B]	2.69 ± 0.46 [B]	3.91 ± 0.16 [A]	3.12 ± 0.05 [B]	0.46 ± 0.01 [D]	0.53 ± 0.01 [C]
	8	3.33 ± 0.72 [A]	2.18 ± 0.07 [B]	3.53 ± 0.05 [A]	3.15 ± 0.27 [A]	0.60 ± 0.07 [C]	0.46 ± 0.05 [D]
∑n6	0	21.98 ± 0.31 [B]	16.35 ± 0.11 [C]	20.65 ± 0.02 [B]	16.00 ± 0.06 [C]	0.31 ± 0.02 [D]	28.01 ± 0.06 [A]
	4	18.01 ± 0.69 [C]	16.04 ± 0.28 [D]	19.88 ± 0.92 [B]	15.40 ± 0.62 [D]	0.30 ± 0.00 [E]	26.88 ± 0.50 [A]
	8	18.73 ± 0.96 [A]	15.39 ± 0.51 [B]	18.86 ± 0.06 [A]	16.48 ± 1.44 [A,B]	0.25 ± 0.05 [C]	18.45 ± 0.51 [A]
∑n6/∑n3	0	6.92 ± 0.89 [B]	5.18 ± 0.03 [C]	5.24 ± 0.22 [C]	4.92 ± 0.01 [C]	0.60 ± 0.04 [D]	48.29 ± 3.04 [A]
	4	5.95 ± 1.08 [B]	6.12 ± 0.93 [B]	5.09 ± 0.03 [C]	4.94 ± 0.12 [C]	0.66 ± 0.02 [D]	50.57 ± 0.35 [A]
	8	5.84 ± 0.98 [C]	7.06 ± 0.01 [B]	5.35 ± 0.05 [C]	5.23 ± 0.00 [C]	0.44 ± 0.13 [D]	41.22 ± 5.84 [A]
TI	0	0.95 ± 0.05 [B]	0.88 ± 0.09 [B,C]	0.80 ± 0.02 [C]	0.97 ± 0.04 [B]	1.16 ± 0.02 [A]	0.91 ± 0.00 [B]
	4	1.08 ± 0.06 [B]	1.09 ± 0.06 [B]	1.10 ± 0.08 [B]	1.13 ± 0.02 [B]	1.78 ± 0.01 [A]	1.13 ± 0.01 [B]
	8	1.17 ± 0.09 [D]	1.34 ± 0.06 [C]	1.01 ± 0.02 [D]	1.17 ± 0.01 [D]	1.72 ± 0.02 [B]	1.99 ± 0.15 [A]
AI	0	0.49 ± 0.01 [B]	0.54 ± 0.04 [B]	0.49 ± 0.01 [B]	0.55 ± 0.01 [B]	0.69 ± 0.04 [A]	0.44 ± 0.03 [C]
	4	0.58 ± 0.01 [B]	0.57 ± 0.01 [B]	0.52 ± 0.02 [B]	0.60 ± 0.00 [B]	0.85 ± 0.00 [A]	0.49 ± 0.00 [B]
	8	0.59 ± 0.02 [CD]	0.65 ± 0.03 [C]	0.54 ± 0.00 [D]	0.61 ± 0.02 [C]	0.90 ± 0.02 [A]	0.72 ± 0.09 [B]
h/H	0	2.53 ± 0.01 [B]	2.37 ± 0.21 [B,C]	2.59 ± 0.02 [B]	2.21 ± 0.06 [C]	1.77 ± 0.08 [C]	2.93 ± 0.03 [A]
	4	2.14 ± 0.02 [B]	2.11 ± 0.02 [B]	2.29 ± 0.10 [B]	1.99 ± 0.01 [C]	1.33 ± 0.01 [D]	2.50 ± 0.01 [A]
	8	2.06 ± 0.10 [B]	1.89 ± 0.08 [C]	2.24 ± 0.03 [A]	1.91 ± 0.02 [C]	1.25 ± 0.02 [D]	1.63 ± 0.19 [C]
		Grilled Burger					
		G	GT	GE	GET	CT	CO
SFA	0	42.93 ± 0.69 [A]	40.86 ± 2.47 [A]	50.20 ± 1.25 [A]	48.88 ± 4.36 [A]	50.21 ± 1.06 [A]	47.47 ± 10.32 [A]
	4	43.81 ± 1.28 [A,B,C]	41.06 ± 1.86 [B,C]	38.56 ± 1.89 [C]	45.35 ± 0.83 [A,B]	50.21 ± 1.67 [A]	42.85 ± 1.84 [B,C]
	8	43.92 ± 0.71 [A]	40.86 ± 2.47 [A]	51.66 ± 0.81 [A]	47.48 ± 2.38 [A]	50.04 ± 0.84 [A]	51.41 ± 15.90 [A]
MUFA	0	34.06 ± 3.32 [B,C]	38.54 ± 0.57 [A,B]	31.52 ± 2.71 [B,C]	32.32 ± 0.27 [B,C]	46.85 ± 1.32 [A]	28.64 ± 2.58 [C]
	4	34.94 ± 0.11 [B]	39.55 ± 0.90 [B]	37.00 ± 1.74 [B]	35.81 ± 1.53 [B]	47.95 ± 0.74 [A]	40.66 ± 2.50 [B]
	8	35.33 ± 1.50 [B,C]	38.34 ± 0.85 [B]	32.73 ± 0.99 [C,D]	32.32 ± 0.27 [C,D]	47.36 ± 0.60 [A]	28.64 ± 2.58 [D]
PUFA	0	20.55 ± 0.53 [A]	19.40 ± 0.36 [A]	19.86 ± 1.49 [A]	18.73 ± 4.20 [A]	2.76 ± 0.00 [B]	12.65 ± 3.00 [A]
	4	21.25 ± 1.39 [B]	18.46 ± 0.36 [B,C]	27.01 ± 0.00 [A]	17.89 ± 1.01 [C]	3.91 ± 0,03 [D]	18.27 ± 0.22 [C]
	8	20.75 ± 0.79 [A]	19.40 ± 0.36 [A]	20.11 ± 1.14 [A]	20.20 ± 2.11 [A]	2.77 ± 0.00 [C]	12.65 ± 3.00 [B]
CLA	0	0.21 ± 0.04 [B]	0.26 ± 0.02 [A,B]	0.26 ± 0.02 [A,B]	0.20 ± 0.01 [B]	0.33 ± 0.03 [A]	0.23 ± 0.04 [A,B]
	4	0.25 ± 0.01 [A]	0.27 ± 0.03 [A]	0.30 ± 0.03 [A]	0.24 ± 0.01 [A]	0.32 ± 0.02 [A]	0.25 ± 0.04 [A]
	8	0.21 ± 0.04 [B]	0.26 ± 0.02 [A,B]	0.25 ± 0.02 [A,B]	0.20 ± 0.01 [B]	0.33 ± 0.03 [A]	0.23 ± 0.04 [A,B]
∑n3	0	3.56 ± 0.13 [A]	2.80 ± 0.61 [A]	3.28 ± 0.21 [A]	3.45 ± 0.37 [A]	0.46 ± 0.03 [B]	0.61 ± 0.27 [B]
	4	3.40 ± 0.41 [A,B]	2.51 ± 0.01 [B]	4.26 ± 0.00 [A]	3.95 ± 0.53 [A]	0.52 ± 0.08 [C]	0.74 ± 0.03 [C]
	8	3.03 ± 0.63 [A]	3.01 ± 0.32 [A]	3.28 ± 0.21 [A]	3.45 ± 0.37 [A]	0.46 ± 0.03 [B]	0.48 ± 0.09 [B]

195

Table 7. Cont.

		Grilled Burger					
		G	GT	GE	GET	CT	CO
$\sum$n6							
	0	16.34 ± 0.49 [A]	15.96 ± 0.28 [A]	15.31 ± 0.38 [A]	14.89 ± 3.55 [A]	1.76 ± 0.24 [B]	11.59 ± 2.83 [A]
	4	19.28 ± 4.15 [A,B]	15.29 ± 0.35 [A,B]	22.05 ± 0.00 [A]	13.32 ± 0.52 [B]	2.49 ± 0.38 [C]	16.78 ± 0.10 [A,B]
	8	17.07 ± 1.51 [A]	17.53 ± 2.51 [A]	16.02 ± 1.27 [A]	16.19 ± 1.71 [A]	1.59 ± 0.01 [C]	11.59 ± 2.83 [B]
$\sum$n6/$\sum$n3							
	0	4.59 ± 0.03 [C]	6.86 ± 0.09 [B]	4.96 ± 0.03 [B,C]	4.61 ± 0.12 [C]	3.77 ± 0.27 [C]	24.08 ± 1.33 [A]
	4	5.48 ± 0.76 [B,C]	6.10 ± 0.11 [B]	5.18 ± 0.00 [B,C,D]	3.39 ± 0.32 [D]	3.70 ± 0.20 [C,D]	22.55 ± 0.88 [A]
	8	5.82 ± 1.71 [B]	5.90 ± 1.45 [B]	4.96 ± 0.02 [B]	4.64 ± 0.07 [B]	3.60 ± 0.02 [B]	24.08 ± 1.33 [A]
TI							
	0	1.19 ± 0.08 [A]	1.09 ± 0.11 [A]	1.38 ± 0.21 [A]	1.42 ± 0.29 [A]	1.90 ± 0.03 [A]	2.16 ± 0.33 [A]
	4	1.02 ± 0.26 [B]	1.15 ± 0.02 [B]	0.85 ± 0.00 [B]	1.18 ± 0.08 [B]	1.87 ± 0.14 [A]	1.37 ± 0.11 [A,B]
	8	1.19 ± 0.09 [A]	1.14 ± 0.03 [A]	1.60 ± 0.52 [A]	1.32 ± 0.15 [A]	1.87 ± 0.07 [A]	2.16 ± 0.33 [A]
AI							
	0	0.63 ± 0.01 [A]	0.58 ± 0.03 [A]	0.63 ± 0.02 [A]	0.70 ± 0.17 [A]	0.85 ± 0.01 [A]	0.94 ± 0.14 [A]
	4	0.54 ± 0.11 [A,B]	0.57 ± 0.04 [A,B]	0.50 ± 0.00 [B]	0.65 ± 0.09 [A,B]	0.76 ± 0.03 [A]	0.57 ± 0.00 [A,B]
	8	0.62 ± 0.02 [A]	0.56 ± 0.05 [A]	0.69 ± 0.10 [A]	0.58 ± 0.05 [A]	0.84 ± 0.02 [A]	0.79 ± 0.35 [A]
h/H							
	0	1.93 ± 0.04 [A]	2.09 ± 0.12 [A]	1.91 ± 0.06 [A]	1.98 ± 0.11 [A]	1.32 ± 0.00 [B]	1.21 ± 0.20 [B]
	4	2.38 ± 0.35 [A]	2.17 ± 0.15 [A,B]	2.50 ± 0.00 [A]	1.82 ± 0.30 [A,B]	1.42 ± 0.20 [B]	2.11 ± 0.01 [A,B]
	8	2.00 ± 0.05 [A]	2.17 ± 0.23 [A]	1.85 ± 0.15 [A,B]	1.98 ± 0.11 [A]	1.34 ± 0.02 [B,C]	1.21 ± 0.20 [C]

[A–E] Mean values between variants on the same storage day with different letters indicate a significant difference. SFA—saturated fatty acid; MUFA—monounsaturated fatty acid; PUFA—polyunsaturated fatty acid; CLA—conjugated linoleic acid; AI—atherogenic index; TI—thrombogenicity index; h/H—hypocholesterolemic/hypercholesterolemic ratio; G—encapsulated oil; GT—encapsulated oil + tallow; GE—encapsulated oil with açai extract; GET—encapsulated oil with açai extract + tallow; CT—control with tallow, CO—control with oil.

2.2.7. Analysis Correlation Coefficients among Color Parameters (L*, a*, b*, BI), Textural (Springiness, Chewiness, Cohesiveness, and Hardness), Cooking Loss, Weight Loss, Fatty Acid Profile (SFA, MUFA, and PUFA), WHC, pH, and TBARS in Raw and Grilled Burgers

The correlation analysis among fatty acid profiles (SFA, MUFA, and PUFA), color parameters (L*, a*, b*, and BI), WHC, pH, weight loss, and TBARS in raw burgers is presented in Table 8. The analysis showed a high negative correlation between PUFA and SFA and between PUFA and MUFA (-0.580 and -0.790, $p < 0.05$, respectively). These correlation are probably related to the change in the number of bonds in fatty acids associated with oxidation processes. In addition, the amount of SFA in the raw burger is negatively correlated with the color parameter a* and BI; this may indicate an oxidative process during which the color of the fat changes. The analysis of the burger brightness parameter (L*) showed positive correlations with b*, WHC, pH, TBARS (0.727, 0.539, 0.497, and 0.848, $p < 0.05$, respectively). Moreover, the correlation analysis showed high positive correlations of the parameter b* with BI, WHC, pH, and the TBARS analyses (0.751, 0.928, 0.880, and 0.765, $p < 0.05$, respectively). The correlation analysis among fatty acid profiles (SFA, MUFA, and PUFA), color parameters (L*, a*, b*, and BI), WHC, pH, weight loss, and TBARS in raw burgers is presented in Table 8. The analysis showed a high negative correlation between PUFA and SFA and between PUFA and MUFA (-0.580 and -0.790, $p < 0.05$, respectively). This correlation is probably related to the change in the number of bonds in fatty acids associated with oxidation processes. In addition, the amount of SFA in the raw burger was negatively correlated with the color parameter a* and BI; this may indicate an oxidative process during which the color of the fat changes. The analysis of the burger brightness parameter (L*) showed positive correlations with b*, WHC, pH, and TBARS (0.727, 0.539, 0.497, and 0.848, $p < 0.05$, respectively). Moreover, the correlation analysis showed high positive correlations of the parameter b* with BI, WHC, pH, and the TBARS analyses (0.751, 0.928, 0.880, and 0.765, $p < 0.05$, respectively).

Table 8. Analysis of correlations among fatty acid profile (SFA, MUFA, and PUFA), color parameters (L*, a*, b*, and BI) and WHC, pH, weight and cooking loss, TBARS, and TPA parameters (springiness, chewiness, cohesiveness, and hardness) with raw and/or grilled burgers.

Raw Burger

	SFA	MUFA	PUFA	L*	a*	b*	BI	WHC	pH	Weight Loss	TBARS
SFA	1										
MUFA	−0.040	1									
PUFA	−0.580 *	−0.790 *	1								
L*	0.345	−0.230	−0.020	1							
a*	−0.523 *	0.396	−0.001	−0.343	1						
b*	−0.116	−0.282	0.307	0.727 *	0.277	1					
BI	−0.474 *	−0.027	0.318	0.112	0.809 *	0.751 *	1				
WHC	−0.292	−0.309	0.438	0.539 *	0.345	0.928 *	0.810 *	1			
pH	−0.108	−0.201	0.236	0.497 *	0.381	0.880 *	0.797 *	0.925 *	1		
Weight loss	0.677 *	−0.311	−0.162	0.008	−0.750 *	−0.473 *	−0.764 *	−0.588 *	−0.487 *	1	
TBARS	0.445	−0.319	−0.006	0.848 *	−0.226	0.765 *	0.281	0.654 *	0.698 *	0.072	1

Grilled burger

	SFA	MUFA	PUFA	Springiness	Chewiness	Cohesiveness	Hardness	Cooking loss	L*	a*	b*	BI
SFA	1											
MUFA	−0.040	1										
PUFA	−0.611 *	−0.612 *	1									
Springiness	0.401	0.129	−0.408	1								
Chewiness	0.435	0.285	−0.657 *	0.139	1							
Cohesiveness	0.416	0.391	−0.765 *	0.437	0.850 *	1						
Hardness	0.440	0.210	−0.594 *	0.031	0.985 *	0.759 *	1					
Cooking loss	0.395	0.306	−0.739 *	0.176	0.891 *	0.901 *	0.845 *	1				
L*	−0.546 *	0.506 *	0.133	−0.026	−0.428	−0.268	−0.492 *	−0.433	1			
a*	0.035	−0.004	−0.125	−0.007	0.185	0.060	0.220	0.181	−0.267	1		
b*	−0.492 *	−0.384	0.790 *	−0.329	−0.905 *	−0.936 *	−0.848 *	−0.920 *	0.382	−0.302	1	
BI	−0.345	−0.565 *	0.782 *	−0.367	−0.811 *	−0.937 *	−0.716 *	−0.830 *	0.024	0.076	0.887 *	1

*—$p < 0.05$.

3. Materials and Methods

3.1. Preliminary Studies

Preliminary studies were conducted to verify the maximum amount of oil absorbed by the base hydrogel without affecting the gel structure. The base for gel formulation consisted of konjac flour (green essence) and sodium alginate (Agnex 1999). Preparation of the gel with encapsulated safflower oil (gold press) was conducted in a multistep process. Gelation involved dissolving 2% sodium alginate and konjac flour in H_2O at 60 °C with constant stirring until a clear emulsion was obtained. An emulsion was obtained of the mixture of safflower oil and water at a ratio of 2:1. Next, homogenization of the emulsion in base gel was performed using an immersion homogenizer (IKA T18 digital, Ultra Turrax, Germany). The concentrations of encapsulated oil in the emulsion hydrogels were 0% (control), 29%, 33%, 38%, 42%, 45%, and 48%. The biocomposites obtained through this approach were used for further studies: SEM image analysis, FT-IR spectroscopy analysis, texture, and rheology analysis, from which the optimal hydrogel was selected for further analysis and application (see Results and Discussion section).

3.2. Beef Burgers Formation and Packaging

The beef (neck muscles, Zakłady Mięsne Wierzejki, Poland) without excess fat and connective tissue was minced. Then, the beef and beef fat (tallow) were ground separately using a meat grinder with an 8 mm hole diameter plate (PI-22-TU-T, Edesa, Greece). Table 9 shows the composition of the prepared burgers with encapsulated oil without/with addition of açai extract (superfoods, PL-EKO-07) in hydrogel and defatted flaxseed flour (LenVitol, Oleofarm, Wrocław, Poland) (variants G, GT, GE, and GET). An emulsion hydrogel containing 45% encapsulated oil was prepared according to the recipe presented in the preliminary studies. The control variant was a burger with tallow (CT) as the conventional source of fat in meat products and oil (CO) as an alternative source of fat. All ingredients, according to the specified proportions, were mixed and burgers (120 g ± 1) of 10 cm diameter were formed. Then, the burgers were placed on 137 × 187 × 50 mm trays made from polyethylene terephthalate (PET) with an absorbent pad (absorbency 1700 mL/m^2). The trays were then sealed with 35 μm thick PSF films (PSF35ZAC, PolTechPack, Olstzn, Poland). Burgers were packed in modified atmosphere (80% O_2 and 20% CO_2) and stored for 0, 4, and 8 days at a temperature of 4 ± 1 °C. Color, pH, fatty acid profile, thiobarbituric acid reactive substances (TBARS), weight loss, water-holding capacity (WHC), and volatile compounds profile analyses were performed on the raw burgers. After the specified storage time (0, 4, and 8 days), the burgers were grilled on an electric grill (silex), heated to 190 °C (bottom plate) and 210 °C (top plate) until 75 °C at the geometric center of each burger (measured with a thermocouple), and then cooled to 25 °C. The prepared burgers were used for the following analyses: color, fatty acid profile, cooking loss, volatile compounds and texture profile analysis (TPA) test. The experimental set-up covered 3 biological replicates (162 samples).

Table 9. Beef burger composition.

Variant	Component			
	Type of Fat Added	Linseed Flour (g)	Meat (g)	Salt (g)
G	9.5 g Hydrogel with encapsulated oil	10.5	100	1.7
GT	9.5 g Hydrogel with encapsulated oil + 5 g beef tallow	10.5	95	1.7
GE	9.5 g Hydrogel with encapsulated oil with açai extract	10.5	100	1.7
GET	9.5 g Hydrogel with encapsulated oil with açai extract + 5 g beef tallow	10.5	95	1.7
CT	20 g Beef tallow	-	100	1.7
CO	8 g Oil	-	112	1.7

G—encapsulated oil; GT—encapsulated oil + tallow; GE—encapsulated oil with açai extract; GET—encapsulated oil with açai extract + tallow; CT—control with tallow; CO—control with oil.

3.3. Rheology Analysis

Melt flow curves were measured using a MARS III rheometer (MTMC—MARS Temperature Module) in CR mode with a coaxial cylinder measuring system (CC25 DIN Ti) with a 5.3 mm gap, wherein the measurements were determined at 5 °C. The shear rate was increased from 0 to 80 s^{-1}, for 5 min, and then decreased from 80 to 0 s^{-1}, for 5 min. The Ostwald–de Waele rheological analysis (Steffe 1996) was used to describe the melt flow curves. Thixotropy and hysteresis loop areas were calculated according to the method described by Sikora et al. [48].

3.4. Analysis of the Textural Parameters of Hydrogel Emulsion

Analysis of the hydrogel emulsion and burger texture textural parameters of the hydrogel were analyzed using a texture analyzer (TA.XTplusC Texture Analyzer) by penetration using Perspex 45° TTC Spreadability Rig Cone Sensors (Stable Micro System, Ltd., Goldaming, UK), according to method described by Öğütcü and Yilmaz [12] with some modifications. Initially, the temperature of the sample was maintained at 5 °C for 24 h, then, penetration was carried out to a depth of 23 mm, at a speed of 3 mm/s. From the data obtained, the following parameters were determined using exponent connect software: firmness (N), lubricity (N × s), viscosity (Pa s) and stickiness (N × s).

The texture profile analysis (TPA) of the grilled beef burgers after 0, 4, and 8 days of storage at 4 ± 1 °C was conducted in a double compression cycle using an Instron 5965 universal testing machine (Instron, USA) with a 500 (N) load cell connected to the Bluehill®2 software, following the methodology described by Afshari et al. [13]. Samples of 2.45 cm in diameter and 2.50 cm height, cut out from the center of the burger, were subjected to double compression with 3 s relaxation time until their initial height was reduced by 50%. The analysis was performed at a constant head travel speed of 200 mm·min^{-1}, at a temperature of 4 ± 1 °C. Six measurements were made for each group. Texture parameters, such as cohesiveness (−) (the ratio of the area under the curve from the second compression to the area under the curve from the first compression), hardness (N0 the maximum force of the first compression), elasticity (−), and chewiness (N) (hardness × cohesiveness × elasticity) were calculated using methodology described by Półtorak et al. [49].

3.5. Scanning Electron Microscope (SEM) Analysis

The morphology of the prepared oil-encapsulated gels was examined using a JEOL JSM-7500F high-resolution scanning electron microscope.

3.6. Fourier Transform Infrared Spectroscopy (FT-IR) Analysis

The FT-IR spectra of the biocomposites were recorded in the range of 4000–700 cm^{-1} using a MATTSON 3000 FT-IR spectrophotometer (Madison, Wisconsin, USA). The instrument was equipped with a 30SPEC 30 Degree Reflectance adapter and a MIRacle ATR accessory (PIKE Technologies Inc., Madison, WI, USA). The FT-IR spectra were performed on dried gels (films were obtained).

3.7. Water-Holding Capacity (WHC) Analysis

The WHC of raw burgers after 0, 4 and 8 days of storage was analyzed according to the method reported by Grau and Hamm [50]. Three hundred milligrams of the sample was placed on Whatman No. 1 filter paper between two glass plates under a weight of 2000 g for 5 min. In order to take press stain images, a Kaiser system (Germany) equipped with the OImaging MicroPublisher 5.0 RTV software (Canada) was used. Meat and fluid areas were evaluated using the Image-Pro Plus software (v.7.0). The WHC values were calculated using the following formula:

$$WHC\% = (Am)/Ap \times 100 \qquad (1)$$

Am—meat areas; Ap—fluid areas.

3.8. Color and pH Analysis

The color evaluation was performed on raw and grilled burgers after 0, 4, and 8 days of storage. Measurements were obtained at 5 different locations on the burgers' surfaces. The analysis was performed in a CIE L*a*b* system using a Minolta CR-400 chromameter with a CA-A98 attachment (Konica Minolta Inc., Tokyo, Japan) and D65 illuminant. The browning index (BI) was calculated using L*, a*, and b* values according to the following formula [51]:

$$BI = 100 (x - 0.31)/0.17 \qquad (2)$$

where $x = (a^* + 1.75 L^*)/(5.645 L^* + a^* - 3.012 b^*)$.

The pH was measured using a digital pH meter (FiveEasy F20, Mettler Toledo, Warsaw, Poland).

3.9. Weight Loss and Cooking Loss during Storage Analysis

The technological properties of the tested burgers were determined in 3 biological replicates using 2 samples for each variant. Raw burgers were weighed on Day 0 and after each day of storage to determine mass loss during storage. Samples were also weighed after grilling and cooling the burgers to room temperature (25 °C). Mass loss after both storage (F) and grilling (G) were calculated according to the following equations:

$$\text{weight loss}\% = (BR0 - BRx)/BR0 \times 100 \qquad (3)$$

$$\text{cooking loss}\% = (BRx - BGx)/BRx \times 100 \qquad (4)$$

BR0—raw burger weight on day 0; BRx—raw burger weight after each day of storage; BGx—grilled burger weight after each day of storage

3.10. Analysis of Total Phenolic Content (TPC) and Antioxidant Activity of the 2,2-Azinobis(3-ethylbenzothiazoline-6-suslfonic Acid (ABTS) and Ferric Reducing Antioxidant Power (FRAP)

3.10.1. Extraction Process

Safflower oil extraction for the analysis of TPC and antioxidant activity was prepared according to the procedure described by Ablay et al. [52]. Briefly, 5 g of oil was shaken in 5 mL of n-hexane for 5 min. Then, 5 mL of MeOH/H_2O (80:20, v/v) was added, centrifuged, and the resulting extract was stored at 4 °C. TPC and antioxidant activity of the açai extract (superfoods, PL-EKO-07) was analyzed after extraction according to the study reported by Hanula et al. [8] with minor modifications. First, 1 g of lyophilized extract was shaken in 25 mL of H_2O for 1 h. Then, the extraction process was carried out using ultrasound for 5 min. The obtained extract was centrifuged and stored at 4 °C for further analysis.

3.10.2. TPC Analysis

The TPC analysis of the studied oil and açai extract was carried out using the method described by Singleton and Rossi [53] with some modifications. First, 0.1 mL of extract, 0.5 mL of Folin–Ciocalteu, 2.9 mL of H_2O, and 1.5 mL of 7% Na_2CO_3 were mixed and incubated for 40 min in the dark. The absorbance was measured at 765 nm using a UV-Vis spectrophotometer. The obtained results were expressed as mg gallic acid/g sample.

3.10.3. ABTS and FRAP Analyses

The ABTS and FRAP analyses were performed according to the methods described by Belwal et al. [54] with slight modifications. The ABTS analysis was conducted mixing 0.1 mL of extract with 2.9 mL of ABTS and incubation for 30 min. The FRAP analysis was based on mixing 2.9 mL of FRAP solution (20 mM ferric chloride in H_2O, 10 mM 2,4,6-tri(2-pyridyl)-s-triazine in 40 mM hydrochloric acid, and 300 mM sodium acetate buffer at a 1:1:10 ratio) with 0.1 mL of the extract and further incubation in the dark for 15 min. The ABTS and FRAP concentrations were measured at 520 nm and 593 nm, respectively, using a UV-Vis spectrophotometer. The results were expressed as mg ascorbic acid/g sample.

3.11. Thiobarbituric Acid Reactive Substances (TBARS) Analysis

The analysis of lipid oxidation was evaluated by TBARS changes and was performed according to the procedure described by Brodowska et al. [55]. 1,1,3,3-Tetramethoxypropane was used to prepare the standard curve. The absorbance of the resulting color complex was measured using a UV-Vis spectrophotometer (UV-1800, Shimadzu Corp., 115 VAC, Tokyo, Japan). The TBARS values were calculated in mg of malondialdehyde (MDA) per 100 g sample.

3.12. Fatty Acid Profile Analysis, Thrombogenicity Index (TI), Atherogenic Index (AI), and Hypocholesterolemic/Hypercholesterolemic (h/H) Ratio Analysis

The fatty acid profile analysis was performed for safflower oil in each burger variant (raw and grilled) after 0, 4, and 8 days of storage. Lipids were directly methylated as described by Wojtasik-Kalinowska et al. [56] and Heck et al. [3] with slight modifications. The fatty acid methyl ester composition was analyzed using gas chromatography (Shimadzu GC-2010) with a flame ionization detector (FID) equipped with a Zebron ZB-FAME column (GC Cap. Column, 60 mL × 0.25 mm ID × 0.2 µm df). The initial column temperature was 100 °C held for 3 min, which was increased to 240 °C at a rate of 2.5 °C/min, and held for 10 min. The detector was maintained at 260 °C. In order to identify the FAME composition in burgers or oils, FAME Mix-37 standard (Supelco, TraceCERT®, EC:200-838-9, SKU: CRM47885) was used. The obtained results were presented as a fatty acid profile. In addition, TI and AI were determined according to the method described by Ulbricht and Southgate [57] and the hypocholesterolemic/hypercholesterolemic (h/H) ratio was calculated according to Fernandez et al. [58] as follows:

$$TI = (C14:0 + C16:0 + 18:0)/((0.5 \times \Sigma MUFA) + (0.5 \times \Sigma n - 6) + (3 \times \Sigma n-3) + ((\Sigma n - 3)/(\Sigma n - 6))) \quad (5)$$

$$AI = (C12:0 + (4 \times C14:0) + 16:0)/((\Sigma PUFA\ n - 3) + (\Sigma PUFA\ n - 6) + (\Sigma MUFA)) \quad (6)$$

$$h/H = (C18:1n9 + \Sigma PUFA)/(C14:0 + C16:0) \quad (7)$$

3.13. Analysis of the Volatile Compounds Profile

The analysis of the volatile compounds profile was performed using a Heracles II e-nose (Alpha MOS Co., Toulouse, France) based on ultrafast gas chromatograph with a flame ionization detector and a retention index counting application using the AroChemBase library (AlphaSoft software, Alpha MOS Co., Toulouse, France). The gas chromatograph was equipped with two capillary columns of different polarities, i.e., DB-5 and DB-1701, with 10 m × 0.18 mm ID x 0.4 µm film thickness. The analysis was conducted according to the methodology reported by Górska-Horczyczak et al. [59]. Calibration was performed on a standard mixture of C6-C16 alkanes (Restek, ANCHEM Plus, Warsaw, Poland).

3.14. Statistical Analysis

The results were analyzed using the Statistica software version 13.3 (StatSoft, Tulsa, OK, USA). The normality of data distribution was verified using the Shapiro–Wilk test. Factorial analysis of variance (ANOVA) was performed in the case of the TBARS analysis. The results of hydrogel texture and rheology as well as color of meat were analyzed with one-way ANOVA. Texture parameters of the burgers were subjected to the Kruskal–Wallis ANOVA, followed by multiple comparisons of mean ranks. Moreover, the strengths of the relationships among fatty acid profile (SFA, MUFA, and PUFA), texture parameters (springiness, chewiness, cohesiveness, and hardness), cooking loss, weight loss, WHC, pH, and color parameters (L*, a*, b*, and BI) methods were determined using Pearson's correlation coefficients. For all analyses, 95% confidence intervals were established. The AlfaSoft package with statistical quality control was used in order to perform a comparative analysis and to evaluate the chromatographic fingerprints of the volatile compounds.

4. Conclusions

In conclusion, an emulsion hydrogel formulated based on konjac flour and sodium alginate with encapsulated oil was used as a functional ingredient in beef burgers enriched with flaxseed flour to develop a healthier alternative. Each variant of the fat substitute containing extract contributed to a reduction in the changes of volatile compounds profile rate and preserved a* color parameter. In addition, the fat substitute reduced the hardness and chewiness parameters of the grilled burgers. According to the obtained results, the applied fat substitute promoted a reduction in the nutritional AI and TI indexes, as well as increased the amount of the PUFAs and h/H ratio. Thus, a hydrogel emulsion enriched with encapsulated oil and açai extract along with the addition of flaxseed flour in a burger recipe instead of beef fat results in a healthier alternative that is rich in fiber.

Author Contributions: M.H., conceptualization, formal analysis, investigation, methodology, supervision, writing—original draft, visualization, writing—review and editing; A.S., formal analysis, investigation, methodology; E.G.-H., formal analysis, methodology; G.K., formal analysis, methodology; G.P., formal analysis; E.P.-N., formal analysis, investigation, methodology, supervision, writing—review and editing; A.P.; funding acquisition, supervision, writing—review and editing. All authors have read and agreed to the published version of the manuscript.

Funding: The research reported in this manuscript has been financed by the Polish Ministry of Science and Higher Education within the fund from the Institute of Human Nutrition Sciences, Warsaw, University of Life Sciences (WULS), for scientific research.

Institutional Review Board Statement: Not applicable.

Informed Consent Statement: Not applicable.

Data Availability Statement: Available from the authors.

Conflicts of Interest: The authors declare no conflict of interest. The funders had no role in the design of the study; in the collection, analyses, or interpretation of data; in the writing of the manuscript, or in the decision to publish the results.

Sample Availability: Samples of the compounds are available from the authors.

References

1. Domínguez, R.; Munekata, P.E.; Pateiro, M.; López-Fernández, O.; Lorenzo, J.M. Immobilization of oils using hydrogels as strategy to replace animal fats and improve the healthiness of meat products. *Curr. Opin. Food Sci.* **2021**, *37*, 135–144. [CrossRef]
2. Bahmanyar, F.; Hosseini, S.M.; Mirmoghtadaie, L.; Shojaee-Aliabadi, S. Effects of replacing soy protein and bread crumb with quinoa and buckwheat flour in functional beef burger formulation. *Meat Sci.* **2020**, *172*, 108367. [CrossRef] [PubMed]
3. Heck, R.T.; Vendruscolo, R.G.; Etchepare, M.D.A.; Cichoski, A.J.; de Menezes, C.R.; Barin, J.S.; Lorenzo, J.M.; Wagner, R.; Campagnol, P.C.B. Is it possible to produce a low-fat burger with a healthy n − 6/n − 3 PUFA ratio without affecting the technological and sensory properties? *Meat Sci.* **2017**, *130*, 16–25. [CrossRef] [PubMed]

4. Jiménez-Colmenero, F.; Triki, M.; Herrero, A.M.; Rodríguez-Salas, L.; Ruiz-Capillas, C. Healthy oil combination stabilized in a konjac matrix as pork fat replacement in low-fat, PUFA-enriched, dry fermented sausages. *LWT Food Sci. Technol.* **2013**, *51*, 158–163. [CrossRef]
5. Lorenzo, J.M.; Munekata, P.E.S.; Pateiro, M.; Campagnol, P.C.B.; Domínguez, R. Healthy Spanish salchichón enriched with encapsulated n − 3 long chain fatty acids in konjac glucomannan matrix. *Food Res. Int.* **2016**, *89*, 289–295. [CrossRef] [PubMed]
6. Delgado-Pando, G.; Cofrades, S.; Ruiz-Capillas, C.; Triki, M.; Jiménez-Colmenero, F. Enriched n−3 PUFA/konjac gel low-fat pork liver pâté: Lipid oxidation, microbiological properties and biogenic amine formation during chilling storage. *Meat Sci.* **2012**, *92*, 762–767. [CrossRef]
7. Melo, P.S.; Arrivetti, L.D.O.R.; de Alencar, S.M.; Skibsted, L.H. Antioxidative and prooxidative effects in food lipids and synergism with α-tocopherol of açaí seed extracts and grape rachis extracts. *Food Chem.* **2016**, *213*, 440–449. [CrossRef]
8. Hanula, M.; Wyrwisz, J.; Moczkowska, M.; Horbańczuk, O.K.; Pogorzelska-Nowicka, E.; Wierzbicka, A. Optimization of Microwave and Ultrasound Extraction Methods of Açai Berries in Terms of Highest Content of Phenolic Compounds and Antioxidant Activity. *Appl. Sci.* **2020**, *10*, 8325. [CrossRef]
9. Hautrive, T.P.; Piccolo, J.; Rodrigues, A.S.; Campagnol, P.C.B.; Kubota, E.H. Effect of fat replacement by chitosan and golden flaxseed flour (wholemeal and defatted) on the quality of hamburgers. *LWT Food Sci. Technol.* **2019**, *102*, 403–410. [CrossRef]
10. Karakurt, G.; Özkaya, B.; Saka, I. Chemical composition and quality characteristics of cookies enriched with microfluidized flaxseed flour. *LWT Food Sci. Technol.* **2022**, *154*, 112773. [CrossRef]
11. Zetzl, A.K.; Marangoni, A.G. Structured Emulsions and Edible Oleogels as Solutions to Trans Fat. *Trans Fats Repl. Solut.* **2014**, 215–243. [CrossRef]
12. Frolova, Y.; Sobolev, R.; Kochetkova, A. Influence of oil combinations on the structural properties of oleogels. *E3S Web Conf.* **2021**, *285*, 05009. [CrossRef]
13. Cano, Y.; García-Zapateiro, L.A.; Zárate, Y. Emulsiones alimentarias del tipo aceite en agua preparadas con harina con alto contenido proteico a partir de cabezas de camarón (*Penaeus vannamei*). *Ing. Investig.* **2017**, *37*, 17–22. [CrossRef]
14. Hourant, P.; Baetan, V.; Morales, M.T.; Meurens, M.; Aparicio, R. Oil and Fat Classification by Selected Bands of Near-infrared Spectroscopy. *Appl. Spectrosc.* **2000**, *54*, 1168–1174. [CrossRef]
15. Rohman, A.; Man, Y.B.C.; Yusof, F.M. The Use of FTIR Spectroscopy and Chemometrics for Rapid Authentication of Extra Virgin Olive Oil. *J. Am. Oil Chem. Soc.* **2014**, *91*, 207–213. [CrossRef]
16. Si, H.; Cheong, L.-Z.; Huang, J.; Wang, X.; Zhang, H. Physical Properties of Soybean Oleogels and Oil Migration Evaluation in Model Praline System. *J. Am. Oil Chem. Soc.* **2016**, *93*, 1075–1084. [CrossRef]
17. Mokhtar, S.M.; Eldeep, G.S.S. Impact of Mango Peel Extract on the Physicochemical Properties, Microbiological Stability and Sensory Characteristics of Beef Burgers During Cold Storage. *Egypt. J. Food Sci.* **2020**, *48*, 245–258. [CrossRef]
18. Nimrouzi, M.; Ruyvaran, M.; Zamani, A.; Nasiri, K.; Akbari, A. Oil and extract of safflower seed improve fructose induced metabolic syndrome through modulating the homeostasis of trace elements, TNF-α and fatty acids metabolism. *J. Ethnopharmacol.* **2020**, *254*, 112721. [CrossRef]
19. Rutkowska, J.; Antoniewska, A.; Baranowski, D.; Rasińska, E. Analiza profilu kwasów tłuszczowych wybranych olejów "nietypowych". *Bromat. Chem. Toksykol.* **2016**, *3*, 385–389.
20. Goyal, A.; Sharma, V.; Upadhyay, N.; Gill, S.; Sihag, M. Flax and flaxseed oil: An ancient medicine & modern functional food. *J. Food Sci. Technol.* **2014**, *51*, 1633–1653. [CrossRef]
21. Alejandre, M.; Astiasarán, I.; Ansorena, D.; Barbut, S. Using canola oil hydrogels and organogels to reduce saturated animal fat in meat batters. *Food Res. Int.* **2019**, *122*, 129–136. [CrossRef] [PubMed]
22. Jin, S.; Hwang, J.; Hur, S.J.; Kim, G. Quality changes in fat-reduced sausages by partial replacing sodium chloride with other chloride salts during five weeks of refrigeration. *LWT Food Sci Technol.* **2018**, *97*, 818–824. [CrossRef]
23. Rather, S.A.; Masoodi, F.A.; Akhter, R.; Gani, A.; Wani, S.M.; Malik, A.H. Effects of guar gum as fat replacer on some quality parameters of mutton goshtaba, a traditional Indian meat product. *Small Rumin. Res.* **2016**, *137*, 169–176. [CrossRef]
24. Sánchez-Zapata, E.; Muñoz, C.M.; Fuentes, E.; Fernández-López, J.; Sendra, E.; Sayas, E.; Navarro, C.; Pérez-Alvarez, J.A. Effect of tiger nut fibre on quality characteristics of pork burger. *Meat Sci.* **2010**, *85*, 70–76. [CrossRef] [PubMed]
25. Ghaderi-Ghahfarokhi, M.; Barzegar, M.; Sahari, M.A.; Azizi, M.H. Nanoencapsulation Approach to Improve Antimicrobial and Antioxidant Activity of Thyme Essential Oil in Beef Burgers During Refrigerated Storage. *Food Bioprocess Technol.* **2016**, *9*, 1187–1201. [CrossRef]
26. de Carvalho, F.A.L.; Lorenzo, J.M.; Pateiro, M.; Bermúdez, R.; Purriños, L.; Trindade, M. Effect of guarana (*Paullinia cupana*) seed and pitanga (*Eugenia uniflora* L.) leaf extracts on lamb burgers with fat replacement by chia oil emulsion during shelf life storage at 2 °C. *Food Res. Int.* **2019**, *125*, 108554. [CrossRef]
27. Summo, C.; De Angelis, D.; Difonzo, G.; Caponio, F.; Pasqualone, A. Effectiveness of Oat-Hull-Based Ingredient as Fat Replacer to Produce Low Fat Burger with High Beta-Glucans Content. *Foods* **2020**, *9*, 1057. [CrossRef]
28. Gök, V.; Akkaya, L.; Obuz, E.; Bulut, S. Effect of ground poppy seed as a fat replacer on meat burgers. *Meat Sci.* **2011**, *89*, 400–404. [CrossRef]
29. Lucas González, R.; Roldán-Verdu, A.; Sayas-Barberá, E.; Fernández-López, J.; Pérez-Álvarez, J.A.; Viuda-Martos, M. Assessment of emulsion gels formulated with chestnut (*Castanea sativa* M.) flour and chia (*Salvia hispanica* L) oil as partial fat replacers in pork burger formulation. *J. Sci. Food Agric.* **2019**, *100*, 1265–1273. [CrossRef]

30. Afshari, R.; Hosseini, H.; Khaneghah, A.M.; Khaksar, R. Physico-chemical properties of functional low-fat beef burgers: Fatty acid profile modification. *LWT* **2017**, *78*, 325–331. [CrossRef]
31. Moghtadaei, M.; Soltanizadeh, N.; Goli, S.A.H.; Sharifimehr, S. Physicochemical properties of beef burger after partial incorporation of ethylcellulose oleogel instead of animal fat. *J. Food Sci. Technol.* **2021**, *58*, 4775–4784. [CrossRef] [PubMed]
32. Vargas-Ramella, M.; Munekata, P.E.S.; Pateiro, M.; Franco, D.; Campagnol, P.C.B.; Tomasevic, I.; Domínguez, R.; Lorenzo, J.M. Physicochemical Composition and Nutritional Properties of Deer Burger Enhanced with Healthier Oils. *Foods* **2020**, *9*, 571. [CrossRef] [PubMed]
33. Gómez-Estaca, J.; Pintado, T.; Jiménez-Colmenero, F.; Cofrades, S. The effect of household storage and cooking practices on quality attributes of pork burgers formulated with PUFA- and curcumin-loaded oleogels as healthy fat substitutes. *LWT* **2020**, *119*, 108909. [CrossRef]
34. Youssef, M.K.; Barbut, S. Effects of protein level and fat/oil on emulsion stability, texture, microstructure and color of meat batters. *Meat Sci.* **2009**, *82*, 228–233. [CrossRef] [PubMed]
35. Moghtadaei, M.; Soltanizadeh, N.; Goli, S.A.H. Production of sesame oil oleogels based on beeswax and application as partial substitutes of animal fat in beef burger. *Food Res. Int.* **2018**, *108*, 368–377. [CrossRef]
36. Ganhão, R.; Morcuende, D.; Estévez, M. Protein oxidation in emulsified cooked burger patties with added fruit extracts: Influence on colour and texture deterioration during chill storage. *Meat Sci.* **2010**, *83*, 402–409. [CrossRef]
37. Patinho, I.; Selani, M.M.; Saldaña, E.; Bortoluzzi, A.C.T.; Rios-Mera, J.D.; da Silva, C.M.; Kushida, M.M.; Contreras-Castillo, C.J. Agaricus bisporus mushroom as partial fat replacer improves the sensory quality maintaining the instrumental characteristics of beef burger. *Meat Sci.* **2020**, *172*, 108307. [CrossRef]
38. Zinina, O.; Merenkova, S.; Galimov, D.; Okuskhanova, E.; Rebezov, M.; Khayrullin, M.; Anichkina, O. Effects of Microbial Transglutaminase on Technological, Rheological, and Microstructural Indicators of Minced Meat with the Addition of Plant Raw Materials. *Int. J. Food Sci.* **2020**, *2020*, 1–11. [CrossRef]
39. Sharefiabadi, E.; Nacak, B.; Serdaroğlu, M. Use of linseed and coconut flours in chicken patties as gluten free extenders. *IOP Conf. Ser. Earth Environ. Sci.* **2021**, *854*, 012086. [CrossRef]
40. Al-Mrazeeq, K.M.; Al-Abdullah, B.M.; Al-Ismail, K.M. Evaluation of some sensory properties and cooking loss of different burger formulations. *Ital. J. Food Sci.* **2010**, *22*, 134–142.
41. Salcedo-Sandoval, L.; Cofrades, S.; Ruiz-Capillas, C.; Jiménez-Colmenero, F. Effect of cooking method on the fatty acid content of reduced-fat and PUFA-enriched pork patties formulated with a konjac-based oil bulking system. *Meat Sci.* **2014**, *98*, 795–803. [CrossRef] [PubMed]
42. Heck, R.T.; Fagundes, M.B.; Cichoski, A.J.; de Menezes, C.R.; Barin, J.S.; Lorenzo, J.M.; Wagner, R.; Campagnol, P.C.B. Volatile compounds and sensory profile of burgers with 50% fat replacement by microparticles of chia oil enriched with rosemary. *Meat Sci.* **2019**, *148*, 164–170. [CrossRef] [PubMed]
43. Watanabe, A.; Kamada, G.; Imanari, M.; Shiba, N.; Yonai, M.; Muramoto, T. Effect of aging on volatile compounds in cooked beef. *Meat Sci.* **2015**, *107*, 12–19. [CrossRef] [PubMed]
44. Gardner, K.; Legako, J.F. Volatile flavor compounds vary by beef product type and degree of doneness. *J. Anim. Sci.* **2018**, *96*, 4238–4250. [CrossRef]
45. He, J.; Liu, H.; Balamurugan, S.; Shao, S. Fatty acids and volatile flavor compounds in commercial plant-based burgers. *J. Food Sci.* **2021**, *86*, 293–305. [CrossRef]
46. Rutkowska, J.; Antoniewska, A.; Martinez-Pineda, M.; Nawirska-Olszańska, A.; Zbikowska, A.; Baranowski, D. Black Chokeberry Fruit Polyphenols: A Valuable Addition to Reduce Lipid Oxidation of Muffins Containing Xylitol. *Antioxidants* **2020**, *9*, 394. [CrossRef]
47. Barros, J.C.; Munekata, P.E.S.; de Carvalho, F.A.L.; Pateiro, M.; Barba, F.J.; Domínguez, R.; Trindade, M.A.; Lorenzo, J.M. Use of tiger nut (*Cyperus esculentus* L.) oil emulsion as animal fat replacement in beef burgers. *Foods* **2020**, *9*, 44. [CrossRef]
48. Sikora, M.; Adamczyk, G.; Krystyjan, M.; Dobosz, A.; Tomasik, P.; Berski, W.; Lukasiewicz, M.; Izak, P. Thixotropic properties of normal potato starch depending on the degree of the granules pasting. *Carbohydr. Polym.* **2015**, *121*, 254–264. [CrossRef]
49. Półtorak, A.; Wyrwisz, J.; Moczkowska, M.; Marcinkowska-Lesiak, M. The impact of aging process on the components of texture of beef from different production systems. *Postępy Tech. Przetwórstw. Spożywczego* **2014**, *2*, 112–119.
50. Grau, R.; Hamm, R. Eine einfache Methode zur Bestimmung der Wasserbindung im Muskel. *Die Naturwissenschaften* **1953**, *40*, 29–30. [CrossRef]
51. Hanula, M.; Pogorzelska-Nowicka, E.; Pogorzelski, G.; Szpicer, A.; Wojtasik-Kalinowska, I.; Wierzbicka, A.; Półtorak, A. Active Packaging of Button Mushrooms with Zeolite and Açai Extract as an Innovative Method of Extending Its Shelf Life. *Agriculture* **2021**, *11*, 653. [CrossRef]
52. Ablay, Ö.D.; Özdikicierler, O.; Gümüşkesen, A.S. Optimization of Ultrasound-Assisted Alkali Neutralization in the Refining of Safflower Oil to Minimize the Loss of Bioactive Compounds. *Eur. J. Lipid Sci. Technol.* **2021**, *123*, 2100004. [CrossRef]
53. Singleton, V.L.; Rossi, J.A. Colorimetry of total phenolics with phosphomolybdic-phosphotungstic acid reagents. *Am. J. Enol. Viticult.* **1965**, *16*, 144–158.
54. Belwal, T.; Dhyani, P.; Bhatt, I.D.; Rawal, S.R.; Pande, V. Optimization extraction conditions for improving phenolic content and antioxidant activity in Berberis asiatica fruits using response surface methodology (RSM). *Food Chem.* **2016**, *207*, 115–124. [CrossRef] [PubMed]

55. Brodowska, M.; Guzek, D.; Kołota, A.; Głąbska, D.; Górska-Horczyczak, E.; Wojtasik-Kalinowska, I.; Weirzbicka, A. Effect of diet on oxidation and profile of volatile compounds of pork after freezing storage. *J. Food Nutr. Res.* **2016**, *55*, 40–47.
56. Wojtasik-Kalinowska, I.; Guzek, D.; Brodowska, M.; Godziszewska, J.; Górska-Horczyczak, E.; Pogorzelska-Nowicka, E.; Sakowska, A.; Gantner, M.; Wierzbicka, A. The effect of addition of Nigella sativa L. oil on the quality and shelf life of pork patties. *J. Food Process. Preserv.* **2017**, *41*, e13294. [CrossRef]
57. Ulbricht, T.L.V.; Southgate, D.A.T. Coronary heart disease: Seven dietary factors. *Lancet* **1991**, *338*, 985–992. [CrossRef]
58. Fernández, M.; Ordóñez, J.A.; Cambero, I.; Santos, C.; Pin, C.; de la Hoz, L. Fatty acid compositions of selected varieties of Spanish dry ham related to their nutritional implications. *Food Chem.* **2007**, *101*, 107–112. [CrossRef]
59. Górska-Horczyczak, E.; Wojtasik-Kalinowska, I.; Wierzbicka, A. Supplemental linseed oil and antioxidants affect fatty acid composition, oxidation and colour stability of frozen pork. *S. Afr. J. Anim. Sci.* **2020**, *50*, 253–263. [CrossRef]

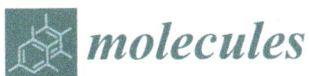

Article

Influence of Agronomic Practice on Total Phenols, Carotenoids, Chlorophylls Content, and Biological Activities in Dry Herbs Water Macerates

Kalina Sikorska-Zimny [1,2,*], Paweł Lisiecki [2,3], Weronika Gonciarz [4], Magdalena Szemraj [3], Maja Ambroziak [2,†], Olga Suska [2,†], Oliwia Turkot [2,†], Małgorzata Stanowska [2,†], Krzysztof P. Rutkowski [1], Magdalena Chmiela [4] and Wojciech Mielicki [2,5]

Citation: Sikorska-Zimny, K.; Lisiecki, P.; Gonciarz, W.; Szemraj, M.; Ambroziak, M.; Suska, O.; Turkot, O.; Stanowska, M.; Rutkowski, K.P.; Chmiela, M.; et al. Influence of Agronomic Practice on Total Phenols, Carotenoids, Chlorophylls Content, and Biological Activities in Dry Herbs Water Macerates. *Molecules* **2021**, *26*, 1047. https://doi.org/10.3390/molecules26041047

Academic Editors: Jan Oszmianski and Sabina Lachowicz

Received: 26 January 2021
Accepted: 12 February 2021
Published: 17 February 2021

Publisher's Note: MDPI stays neutral with regard to jurisdictional claims in published maps and institutional affiliations.

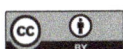

Copyright: © 2021 by the authors. Licensee MDPI, Basel, Switzerland. This article is an open access article distributed under the terms and conditions of the Creative Commons Attribution (CC BY) license (https://creativecommons.org/licenses/by/4.0/).

[1] Skierniewice, Fruit and Vegetables Storage and Processing Department, Division of Fruit and Vegetable Storage and Postharvest Physiology, Research Institute of Horticulture, Pomologiczna 13a Street, 96-100 Skierniewice, Poland; krzysztof.rutkowski@inhort.pl
[2] Stefan Batory State University, Batorego 64c Street, 96-100 Skierniewice, Poland; pawel.lisiecki@umed.lodz.pl (P.L.); majaambroziak98@gmail.com (M.A.); olgasuska98@gmail.com (O.S.); oliwia4811@wp.pl (O.T.); gosia.stanowska@op.pl (M.S.); wojciech.mielicki@umed.lodz.pl (W.M.)
[3] Department of Pharmaceutical Microbiology and Microbiological Diagnostics, The Medical University of Łódź, Pomorska 137 Street, 90-235 Lodz, Poland; magdalena.szemraj@umed.lodz.pl
[4] Department of Immunology and Infectious Biology, Faculty of Biology and Environment Protection, The University of Łódź, Banacha 12/16 Street, 90-237 Lodz, Poland; weronika.gonciarz@biol.uni.lodz.pl (W.G.); magdalena.chmiela@biol.uni.lodz.pl (M.C.)
[5] Department of Pharmaceutical Biochemistry and Molecular Diagnostics, The Medical University of Łódź, Muszyńskiego 1 Street, 90-151 Lodz, Poland
* Correspondence: kalinasikorskazimny@gmail.com or kalina.sikorska@inhort.pl; Tel.: +48-53-4800-418
† Students of Dietitian Majority of Stefan, Batory State University, Skierniewice, Poland; PUSB Dietitian Circle.

Abstract: Oregano (*Origanum vulgare* L.) and thyme (*Thymus vulgaris* L.) have long been known for their organoleptic properties. Both plants are widely used in cuisine worldwide in fresh and dried form and as a pharmaceutical raw material. The study aimed to assess if the type of cultivation influenced chosen chemical parameters (total polyphenols by Folin-Ciocalteu method; carotenoids and chlorophyll content by Lichtenthaler method), antimicrobial activity (with chosen reference microbial strains) and shaped cytotoxicity (with L929 mouse fibroblasts cell line) in water macerates of dry oregano and thyme. Polyphenols content and antimicrobial activity were higher in water macerates obtained from conventional cultivation (independently from herb species), unlike the pigments in a higher amount in macerates from organic herbs cultivation. Among all tested macerates stronger antimicrobial properties (effective in inhibiting the growth of *Pseudomonas aeruginosa*, *Bacillus cereus* and *Salmonella enteritidis*) and higher cytotoxicity (abilities to diminish the growth of L929 fibroblasts cytotoxicity) characterized the conventionally cultivated thyme macerate.

Keywords: thyme; oregano; dry herbs; polyphenols; chlorophyll; carotenoids; microbial; cytotoxicity

1. Introduction

Oregano (*Origanum vulgare* L., also known as wild marjoram), and thyme (*Thymus vulgaris* L.) are popular and widely used in cuisines and the cosmetic industry. Oregano and thyme are native species of the Mediterranean region [1,2] although they became popular herbs in the Baltic Sea region as well [3–5]. Due to their chemical composition, both herbs are willingly used in the cuisines and medicine/herbal medicine and cosmetics industries.

The properties of the oregano are connected not only with its flavor and scent, but this plant also supports the digestive system (secretion of gastric juices and bile), respiratory system (helps with catarrh of the upper respiratory tract), has a relaxing and expectorant effect, but also has antifungal and bactericidal properties [1,3]. Some of these pro-health properties are the result of the antioxidant effect of oregano [6]. This effect is related to the presence of numbers of compounds such as phenolic acids, flavonoids, and essential oils like sabinene, carvacrol, geranial, terpineol, linalool or cymene [1]. The concentration of these compounds is shaped not only by the variety and the environmental conditions of the plant during growth (greater exposure to sun, rain, the season of picking the plant) but also by the type of cultivation (organic, conventional), the geographical position but also by the method of oil extraction [6]. The beneficial antioxidant effect is a derivative of the (variable) composition, and therefore these properties will also be influenced by the factors mentioned. Antimicrobial activity of oregano is connected with compounds like carvacrol, thymol, γ-terpinene, and p-cymene [1], Faleiro et al. estimated the concentration as 33% for thymol, 26% for γ-terpinene and 11% for p-cymene [7].

Thyme in the cuisine is used as a spice for meat, potato, and mushroom dishes. The healing properties of thyme focus on the respiratory system's effect; hence thyme is used in cough syrups, expectorants, and soothing throat irritations, in the form of ointments, drops used in the case of upper respiratory tract catarrh [8]. Thyme is also used in dental prophylaxis as a toothpaste component and liquids for teeth cleaning and oral care (also in endodontics, during disinfecting root canals) [9]. Thyme, similar to oregano, is used against digestive problems and has antibacterial, antifungal, and antiviral properties [6]. These effects are, inter alia, a derivative of the presence of thymol and carvacrol in thyme. These antioxidant compounds (phenolic derivatives) are present in thyme in large amounts: about 18–80% and 1–20% (for thymol and carvacrol, respectively) [10,11]. Two of these phenolic compounds (carvacrol and thymol) have strong antimicrobial activity against both bacteria and fungi, therefore, are considered to be useful as future fighting agents against drug-resistant microbial [12]. Detailed examination pointed on carvacrol with high anti-*Listeria monocytogenes* properties [13], experiments conducted by Rota et al. showed that carvacrol and thymol had a high inhibitory effect against the Gram-positive *L. monocytogenes* and *S. aureus*, the Gram-negative *S. enteritidis*, *E. coli O157:H7*, *Yersinia enterocolitica*, and *Shigella flexneri* [14].

Different factors have been demonstrated to influence the content of the biologically active compounds, such as technological process, cultivation method, climatic conditions or variety. Among them technological processes such as drying increase the herbs' availability on the market throughout the year, thereby not tied to climatic and cultivation conditions [15]. It enables transport over long distances, thus increasing the availability of these herbs on the market. Moreover, drying, by limiting the water content, helps to inhibit the growth of microorganisms on the product [16]. It needs to be remembered that the drying process changes the chemical composition of plants [15].

Other factors that influence the content of the biologically active compounds in plants are cultivation method, climatic conditions, variety, therefor content of, e.g., polyphenols may differ in published articles [17].

As mentioned before, oregano and thyme possess antioxidant properties connected with the presence of polyphenols compounds like phenolics: acids, diterpenes; flavonoids and volatile oils [18]. These broad group of secondary metabolites of plants are present in flowers, fruits, leaves, stems, roots, and tubers. The antioxidant properties of polyphenols are connected with the ability to scavenge free radicals, counteract lipid peroxidation, and reduced enzymes' activity [17]. Polyphenols are sensitive for high temperatures; therefore, the drying process reduces their plant tissue content [19]. Consumers' important factors during shopping are the color of dried spices, preferably intensive green (most similar to fresh plant) and less popular discolored in grey shades [20]. The color of a dried green plant is related to the content of chlorophyll and carotenoids. These pigments decompose during the technological procedures of drying herbs; therefore, except for visual evaluation of herbs color, the chemical analysis of chlorophylls and carotenoid content is useful.

The cultivation method influences all the features mentioned above. They compare organic and conventional method points on differentials in the usage of synthetic substances during and before plant growth. Organic cultivation method prohibits the use of synthetic plant protection products and fertilizers, which are substituted with pheromone traps, plant extracts and sticky boards (as a substitute of synthetic plant protection products) or manure (of different origin) and compost (as a substitute of synthetic fertilizers) [21,22]. Organically cultivated herbs are expected to be richer in bioactive compound due to elicitation phenomenon: "this process induces a defense response in a plant and leads to several biochemical processes resulting from which numerous groups of secondary metabolites are produced" [23].

The possibility to use both spices in cuisines is connected with their usage in the water solution. Therefore, important is to conduct an experiment with water macerates (of oregano and thyme) and examine their chemical and biological properties to evaluate the pro-healthy values.

The authors focused on determining the content of chosen compounds in water macerates of oregano and thyme, obtained from organic and conventional cultivation, its cytotoxicity, and the assessment of their impact on microorganisms' development.

2. Results

2.1. Chemical Composition

2.1.1. Polyphenols

The highest content of total polyphenols was determined in conventionally cultivated thyme (0.42 mg GAE/mL sample) and the lowest in "organic" oregano (0.20 mg GAE/mL sample). Total polyphenols content in water macerates for both herbs were higher in conventional cultivations of oregano and thyme; significant differences were obtained in "organic" oregano comparing to other samples. There were no significant differences among the thyme samples (Table 1).

Table 1. The chosen chemical compounds are determined in water macerates of dry oregano and thyme cultivated in conventional (CONV) and organically (ORG).

Herb	Cultivation Type	Polyphenols		Chlorophyll a		Chlorophyll b		Carotenoids	
		mg GAE/mL Sample		µg/1 mL Sample					
oregano	ORG	0.20	a	7.81	cd	12.32	cd	2.07	bcd
	CONV	0.36	bc	4.84	ab	7.21	ab	1.03	abcd
thyme	ORG	0.40	bcd	7.35	cd	11.40	cd	1.67	abc
	CONV	0.42	cd	2.96	ab	4.56	ab	0.76	abc

According to Duncan's test, the means in columns followed by the same letters are not significantly different at $p = 0.05$.

2.1.2. Chlorophyll and Carotenoids

Oregano had a higher content of chlorophyll (a and b) than thyme. The highest chlorophyll a and b content was determined in "organic" oregano (7.81 µg/mL and 12.23 µg/mL of macerates, for chlorophyll a and b, respectively), the lowest in "conventional" thyme (2.96 µg/mL and 4.56 µg/mL of macerates, for chlorophyll a and b, respectively). Chlorophylls (a and b) were significantly higher in organically cultivated herbs (for both species).

Carotenoids were in higher amount in macerates of organically cultivated herbs (2.07 and 1.67 µg/mL for oregano and thyme, respectively) than a conventional one (1.03 and 0.76 µg/mL for oregano and thyme, respectively).

The determined results (higher content of pigments in organic herbs) were not noticeable during the preparation (Figures 1 and 2) of macerates, where colors of organic and conventional cultivated, dry plants were similar.

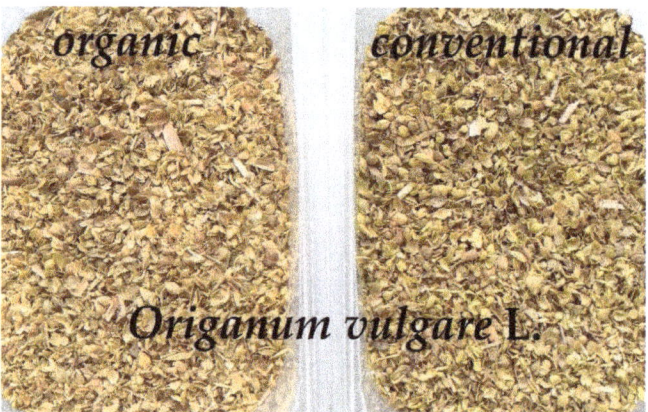

Figure 1. Comparison of colors of dry oregano from organic and conventional cultivation.

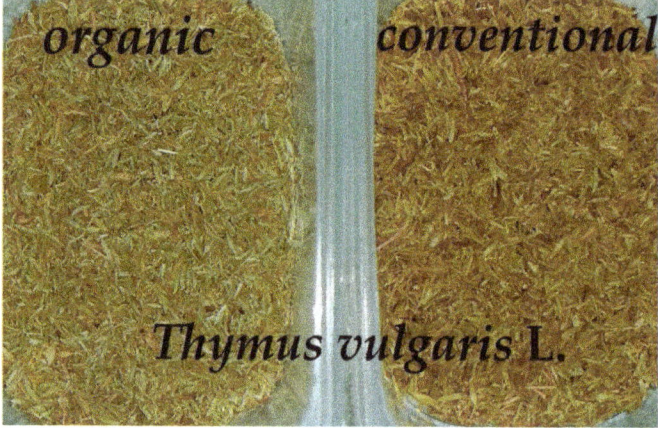

Figure 2. Comparison of colors of dry thyme from organic and conventional cultivation.

2.2. Antimicrobial Activity

The effects of the water macerates of both herbs on tested standard microbial are presented in Table 2. Four strains of Gram-negative bacteria and five strains of Gram-positive bacteria were used in the research. The experiment was repeated triplicate, and the results were consistent.

The macerates of both herbs obtained from organic cultivation did not exhibit antibacterial activity against standard strains of Gram-negative bacteria MIC/MBC > 50 mg/mL (Table 2). Oregano macerate obtained from conventional cultivation exhibited weak activity against *E. coli* and *Salmonella* Enteritidis (MIC/MBC = 50 mg/mL) and moderate activity against *P. aeruginosa* with MIC/MBC= 12.5 mg/mL. Thyme macerate received from conventional cultivation had been effective in inhibiting the growth of *S. enteritidis* (MIC/MBC = 12.5 mg/mL). The highest sensitivity to the conventional thyme macerate showed the tested strains of *P. aeruginosa* (MIC/MBC = 0.626 mg/mL).

Table 2. Determined values of MIC and MBC for tested water macerates in relation to standard microorganisms.

Microorganisms	Water Macerates				Antimicrobial Reference Standard *	
	Thyme CONV	Thyme ORG	Oregano CONV	Oregano ORG	Gentamicin	Fluconazole
	MIC/MBC (mg/mL)				MIC/MBC (µg/mL)	
Gram-Positive Bacteria						
Staphylococcus aureus ATCC 25923	12.5/12.5	>50/>50	6.25/6.25	50/50	0.5	nt
Enterococcus faecalis ATCC 29212	25/25	>50/>50	25/25	>50/>50	16	nt
Bacillus cereus PCM 1948	6.25/6.25	12.5/12.5	3.125/3.125	6.25/6.25	0.25	nt
Bacillus subtilis ATCC 6635	25/25	50/50	6.25/6.25	25/25	0.25	nt
Listeria monocytogenes PCM 2191	50/50	50/50	25/25	25/25	0.25	nt
Gram-Negative Bacteria						
Escherichia coli ATCC 25922	>50/>50	>50/>50	50/50	>50/>50	2	nt
Pseudomonas aeruginosa ATCC 27853	0.625/0.625	>50/>50	12.5/12.5	>50/>50	2	nt
Shigella flexneri ATCC 12022	50/50	>50/>50	>50/>50	>50/>50	nd ^	nt
Salmonella Enteritidis ZMF 279	12.5/12.5	>50	50/50	>50/>50	0.25	nt
Fungi						
Candida albicans ATCC 10241	>50/>50	>50/>50	>50/>50	>50/>50	nt	5/>5
Aspergillus brasiliensis ATCC 16404	>50/>50	>50/>50	>50/>50	>50/>50	nt	5/>5

* Gentamicin—broad-spectrum antibiotic, fluconazole—antifungal chemotherapeutic; ^ not detection; nt—the activity of fluconazole (against bacteria) and gentamicin (against fungi) have not been tested.

Both macerates obtained from organic herbs were less active in inhibiting the growth of all the tested strains of Gram-positive bacteria, excluding *L. monocytogenes*, compare to conventional macerates (Table 2). The bactericidal effect of thyme conventional macerate against *S. aureus* was achieved at the concentration of 12.5 mg/mL, against *E. faecalis* and *B. subtilis* at 25 mg/mL. Thyme organic macerate was active against *B. subtilis* at concentration 25 mg/mL and did not inhibit the growth of *S. aureus* and *E. faecalis* (MIC/MBC > 50 mg/mL). The thyme and oregano macerates obtained from herbs cultivation in organic and conventional condition demonstrated weak activity against *L. monocytogenes* with MIC/MBC values, 50 mg/mL, and 25 mg/mL, respectively.

The "organic" oregano macerate was not active against *E. faecalis* (MIC/MBC > 50 mg/mL), but oregano conventional macerate was effective at concentration 25 mg/mL. The highest inhibitory effect on the tested strains of *S. aureus* and *B. subtilis* showed the oregano conventional macerate, resulting in MIC/MBC 3.125 mg/mL and 6.25 mg/mL, respectively (Table 2). The oregano organic macerate demonstrated activity against *S. aureus* and *B. subtilis* in higher concentrations with MIC/MBC 6.25 mg/mL and 25 mg/mL, respectively.

The highest sensitivity of conventional oregano and thyme macerates demonstrated Bacillus cereus' strain, resulting in MIC/MBC 3.125 mg/mL and 6.25 mg/mL, respectively. The thyme and oregano organic macerates showed the same effect at twofold higher concentrations, 6.25 mg/mL, and 12.5 mg/mL, respectively.

The macerates' antifungal activity was tested against two fungal strains—*C. albicans* (yeast fungus) and *A. brasiliensis* (mould fungus). None of the tested macerates and those obtained from herbs cultivation in organic and conventional conditions did not inhibit the fungal strains' growth ((MIC/MBC > 50 mg/mL).

The tested macerates' antibacterial activity was lower than the activity of gentamicin or fluconazole used as the antimicrobial reference standard.

The "conventional" thyme in the highest concentration of 50; 25 mg/mL and 12.5 significantly diminished the growth of L929 fibroblasts (43–71% of dead cells) (Figure 3), while thyme "organic" did not show cytotoxic activity at any of the tested concentrations (Figure 3). Moreover, "organic" thyme significantly increased the ability of L929 cells to reduce MTT within the range 5–50 mg/mL compare to extract isolated from thyme "conventional" (Figure 3).

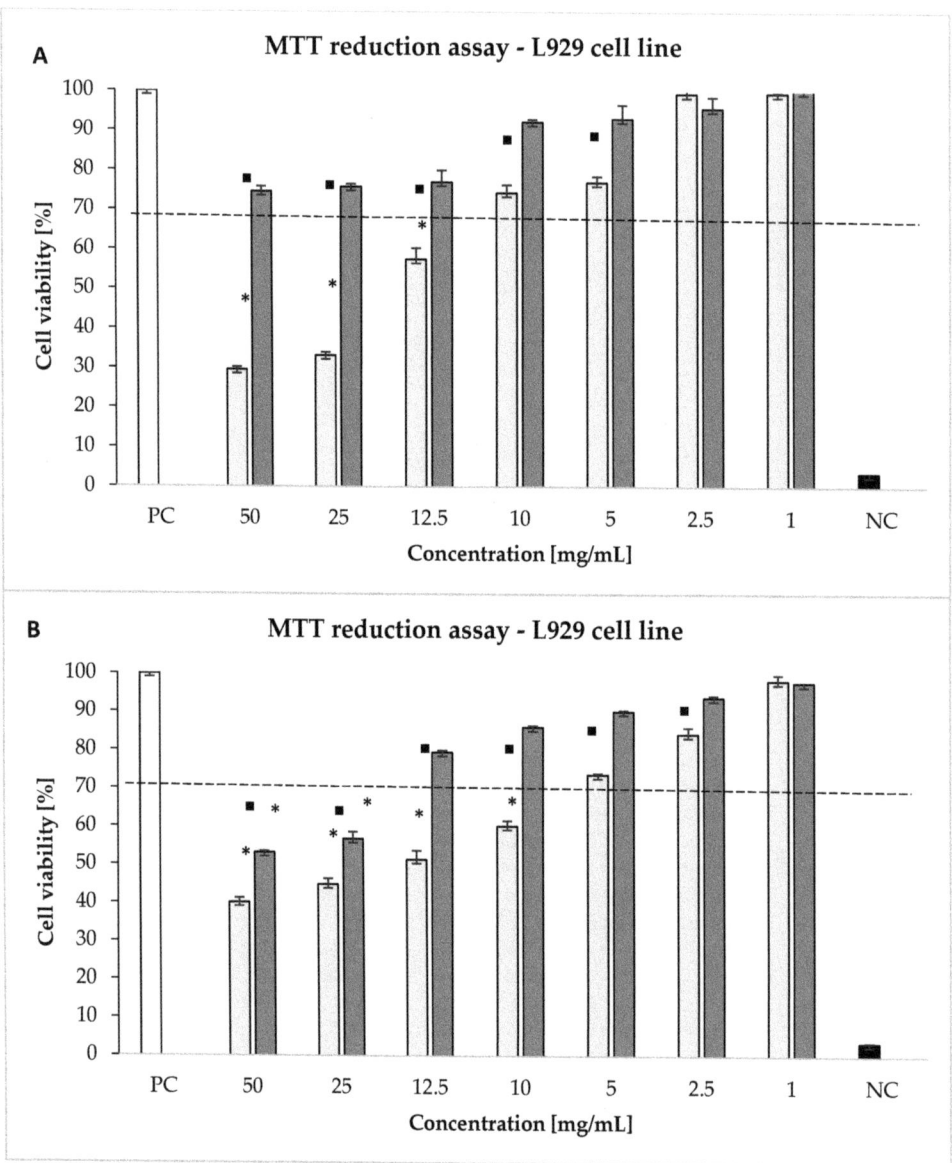

Figure 3. Cytotoxic effect of plants extracts: (**A**) thyme, (**B**) oregano towards L929 cells. The cytotoxicity was assessed by MTT [(3-(4,5-dimethylthiazol-2-yl)-2,5-diphenyltetrazolium bromide)] reduction assay. The cell viability was calculated for four experiments, including three repeats for each compound. Complete RMPI-1640 medium (cRPMI) was used as a positive control (PC) of cell viability (100% viable cells) and 0.03% H_2O_2 as a negative control (NC) of cell viability (100% dead inactive cells). Statistical significance: * $p < 0.05$; * untreated cells vs cells treated with tested plants extracts "conventional" extract (light grey bars) vs "organic" extract (dark grey bars).

Oregano "conventional" has a stronger inhibitory effect on L929 cell metabolic activity at range concentrations 10–50 mg/mL (40–60% of dead cells), while thyme "organic" in the highest concentration 50 and 25 mg/mL significantly diminished the growth of L929 fibroblasts (44–47% of dead cells) (Figure 3). Furthermore, oregano "organic" significantly increased the ability of L929 cells to reduce MTT within the range 50–2.5 mg/mL compare to extract isolated from oregano "conventional" (Figure 3).

3. Discussion

According to the authors' best knowledge, there was no conducted analysis of organic and conventional cultivated oregano and thyme water macerates (not infusions). Available in literature are results over chemical analysis of herbs infusion dedicated as beverages (melissa, mint) or macerates based on other solution (methanol, ethanol), mostly used as a solvent in the method of extraction or infusions (pouring with hot water).

In conducted analysis higher polyphenol content was determined in thyme than in oregano that stands according to values obtained by Dragland et al. which determined 45 mmol/100 g and 63.7 mmol/100 g for oregano and thyme respectively in commercial cultivation [24]. Moreover, Vallverdú-Queralt et al. determined total polyphenols in dried oregano and thyme at the level of 2.23 and 3.36 mg GAE/g DW for oregano and thyme, respectively [25]. Jałoszyński determined polyphenols in dry oregano at the level: 63.96–168.87 mg GAE/100 g, where the lower content is similar to obtained in presented work (calculate on DM herbs) [19]. Taghipour et al. determined thyme's polyphenols at a level of 30 mg GAE/g DM that is similar to values obtained in presented work [26]. It also needs to be highlighted that phenolic losses during drying of herbs can reach 50% (dependently of temperature and drying method). Generally, the compound degrades at a higher level with higher temperature applied [19].

Although determined higher polyphenols content in macerates for conventional cultivation stands against the work of Matłok et al., who determined the much higher bioactive potential of dry oregano cultivated with organic fertilizers comparing to conventional cultivation [27]. However, Lv et al. compared peppermint and cinnamon cultivated organically and conventionally and determined in both herbs higher total phenolic content in conventionally cultivated herbs [28].

Still, there is no clear explanation of higher polyphenol content in a specific type of plant cultivation (sometimes higher in organic, sometimes in conventional). Some authors divide polyphenols (into soluble and hydrolysable), where soluble are more stable during processing (cooking) [29], although there are still no data available about polyphenols profiles in dry herbs, together with water macerates. Moreover, the water content of fresh plant might decrease polyphenols content, since the drying process of high-water content must undergo a more extended drying time procedure, or higher temperature must be applied. In any case, both factors are reducing polyphenols content in the final product.

Chlorophylls play an important role in the photosynthetic membranes, where they are present usually in a ratio of 3:1 [30], although this content can be shaped by the growth conditions and environmental factors [31,32]. Chlorophyll a and b differ in a side chain's composition, which for chlorophyll a its methyl group and chlorophyll b its aldehyde group.

Matłok et al. pointed on a strict correlation between chlorophylls content and carotenoids in foliar plants due to general biosynthetic pathways in the plants' chloroplasts [27]. Therefore, the higher content of pigments involved in photosynthesis is related to higher carotenoid content (beta carotene) [21].

In the experiment over water macerates of herbs from organic and conventional cultivation, higher content of chlorophylls and carotenoids were determined in organic cultivation, which is opposite to Hallmann et al. [21]. Although Onofrei et al. pointed on a higher content of pigments presents in organically cultivated thyme and oregano [33]. It needs to be added that Hallmann et al. refer to lower content only of beta-carotene, and in the conducted experiment, the authors were determining the total carotenoids content [21]. Simultaneously Halmann et al. [21] pointed to the fact of a higher content of lutein and zeaxanthin (belonging to carotenoids) in organically cultivated herbs comparing to conventional one and in case of thyme major carotenoid is zeaxanthin [34].

Onofrei et al. explained the higher content of pigments in herbs cultivated with organic fertilizers by the possible improvement in the availability of nutrients caused by these fertilizers, and thus enhancing the metabolic pathways (e.g., photosynthesis) synthesis of several plant secondary compounds [33]. According to Skubij and Dzida, over the influence of organic fertilizers on the plants' chemical compounds [35]. The other factor influencing carotenoid content is UV radiation that also increases antioxidant content [21,27].

Manukyan determined higher content of chlorophyll a and b in thyme at a level of 0.03–0.052 mg/g and 0.13–0.21 mg/g, (for chlorophyll a and b, respectively) [34]. Tzima et al. obtained the lower results: 88.6 mg/100 g DM for chlorophyll a, and 24.00 mg/100 g DM for chlorophyll b [36].

Kulbat-Warycha et al. determined similar to presented in work content of chlorophyll a in oregano but lower chlorophyll b and higher of total carotenoids (0.009 g/L; 0.002 g/L and 0.004 g/L FW for chlorophyll a, b, and carotenoids, respectively) [37].

Antimicrobial activity of water macerates was higher in conventional cultivated herbs. The obtained results go along with higher polyphenols content determined in these macerates. The highest antimicrobial activity (of "conventional" thyme) was determined against *Bacillus cereus*, which is especially important in dry herbs. These products may have a high number of bacteria and molds, which in favorable conditions, can quickly develop [38]. Research of Fogele et al. and Boer et al. pointed on a high level of *Bacillus cereus* determined in dry spices [38,39]. Boer et al. determined antimicrobial activity of 2% water macerates and pointed of weak or non-antimicrobial abilities of most of examined herbs solutions (rosemary, basil, ginger, sage) [38]. Other investigation showed that 20% cold water oregano extract was effective against the strains of *P. aeruginasa* and *K. pneumoniae* [40]. Our study demonstrated the highest antibacterial effect of thyme water macerate obtained from conventional cultivation against the strains of *P. aeruginosa*. This opportunistic human pathogen was found to contaminate herbal plants and spices caused by the unsafe collection, drying, preparation or storage [41].

Quadir et al. examined antimicrobial activity of chosen herbal extracts, but they have not confirmed any activity of thyme extract against *B. subtilis*, explanation to this fact may be connected with used solution concentrate (1:10) [42]. Our investigation shows that "conventional" oregano macerate exhibited moderate activity against *B. subtilis*.

Our study demonstrated that water macerates of oregano obtained from the conventional method of cultivation had been effective in inhibiting the growth of *S. aureus*. Other studies also pointed to a high activity oregano water extract against this microorganism [43]. *S. aureus* is most commonly isolated from dry herbs [41].

Research is connecting herbs' antimicrobial ability with the presence of phenols that can precipitate proteins (or react with cells by sulfhydryl groups of proteins causing unavailability of the substrate) and inhibit microorganisms' enzymes [44,45].

Plant extracts including thyme and oregano have been used in the traditional medicine for the treatment of several respiratory diseases like asthma and bronchitis [46] as well as other pathologic processes, thanks to several properties such as antiseptic, antispasmodic, antitussive, antimicrobial, antifungal, antioxidative, and antiviral [47,48]. Our study showed that extract isolated from thyme "organic" does not show cytotoxic activity according to ISO 10993-5 in all concentrations used in this study (1–50 mg/mL) whereas the activity of extract isolated from thyme "conventional" was below the cytotoxicity norm in the range 12.5–50 mg/mL. Similar results were observed in the study by de Oliveira et al. [49]. They showed that the *T. vulgaris* extract at 25, 50 and 100 mg/mL provided cell viability above 50% to RAW 264.7, FMM-1, MCF−7 and HeLa cell line [49]. New plant extracts are also tested for antioxidant activity in conjunction with the modulation of the inflammatory response. For example, Loizzo et al. examined different oregano's oils varieties inhibition of NO production in the murine monocytic macrophage cell line

RAW 264.7, obtaining an IC50 value of 66.4 µg/mL and >200 µg/mL for *O. ehrenbergii* and *O. syriacum*, respectively [50]. The antioxidant activity of our preparations with the use of gastric epithelial cells is planned to be tested in the context of minimizing the risk of epithelial damage and the development of an inflammatory reaction. Plant preparations with a cytotoxic effect against cancer cells are extremely valuable. Jamali et al. show that thymol induced toxicity, apoptosis, and cell cycle arrest in MDA-MB231 BC cells [51]. Our study shows that oregano extracts have strong cytotoxic activity against L929 fibroblasts. Oregano extracts: ethyl acetate and ethanol extracts from leaves also have reported the cytotoxicity activity against human breast cancer cells (MCF7) [52]. On the other hand, carvacrol, the major component of oregano, showed antimutagenic activity, which seems to be mainly linked to the induction of mitochondrial dysfunction [53,54].

4. Materials and Methods

4.1. Macerates Preparation

Dried oregano and thyme were bought in a local shop. Both types of herbs (organic and conventional cultivated) were obtained from the same manufacturer. Thyme and oregano (conventional and organic, separately) were soaked with distilled water (1:5) and left for five days for the maceration process. The extracts were filtered through a cellulose filter (fine pore, 0.45 µm) and then subjected to further analysis.

4.2. Chemical Analysis

4.2.1. The Content of Polyphenols

The Folin-Ciocalteu assay was carried out according to the method described by Singleton and Rossi (1965) [55]. The results were expressed as mg/mL of the sample as gallic acid. Measurements were conducted in six replicates; absorbance was measured at 750 nm against the blank sample.

4.2.2. The Content of Chlorophylls and Carotenoids

Carotenoids and chlorophyll a and b were determined according to Lichtenthaler (1983) spectrophotometric method, with the extraction of 80% acetone and absorbance measured at 470, 646, 663 nm [30].

4.3. Microbial Analysis

4.3.1. Microbial Strains and Culture Conditions

Reference microbial strains were obtained from the American Type Culture Collection (ATCC), including *Staphylococcus aureus* ATCC 25923, *Enterococcus faecalis* ATCC 29212, *Bacillus subtilis* ATCC 6635, *Escherichia coli* ATCC 25922, *Pseudomonas aeruginosa* ATCC 27833 and *Shigella flexneri* ATCC 12022. The *Listeria monocytogenes* PCM 2191 and *Bacillus cereus* PCM 1948 strains were taken from the Polish Collection of Microorganisms (PCM). One bacterial strain *Salmonella* Enteritidis ZMF 279 was derived from the collection of the Department of Pharmaceutical Microbiology and Diagnostic Microbiology, Medical University of Lodz. Two fungal strains were also used: *Candida albicans* ATCC 10231 and *Aspergillus brasiliensis* ATCC 16404. All tested microorganisms were stored at −80 °C in 15% glycerol stocks. Before the investigation, the bacterial strains were transferred to Mueller-Hinton agar medium (Oxoid, Thermo Fisher Scientific, Waltham, MA, USA) and cultured overnight at 37 °C. Fungal strains were transferred on Sabouraud agar medium (Oxoid, Thermo Fisher Scientific, Waltham, MA, USA) and cultured for two days at 30 °C.

4.3.2. Antimicrobial Assay

Before the investigation, the extracts were concentrated to 100 mg/mL by lyophilization. The antimicrobial activity of extracts was assessed according to their minimum inhibitory concentrations (MIC), and minimum bactericidal/fungicidal concentrations (MBC) expressed in mg/mL. According to the European Committee on Antimicrobial Susceptibility recommendations, antibacterial and antifungal activities were determined using the broth microdilution method [56]. The Mueller-Hinton broth (pH~7.2) (Oxoid, Thermo Fisher Scientific, Waltham, MA, USA) was used for bacteria. Liquid medium RPMI-1640 (w/o red phenol, pH~7.2) (Sigma-Aldrich, Darmstad, Germany) was used for the fungal strains. Two-fold series dilutions of extract in the growth medium were performed in 96-well sterile microtiter plates (Kartell Labware, Noviglio, Italy) in concentrations ranging from 50 to 0.09 mg/mL. The MIC values were defined as the lowest extract concentrations with no bacterial growth after the incubation. The MBCs were determined by seeding 5 µL from all clear MIC wells onto Mueller-Hinton agar plates (Oxoid, Thermo Fisher Scientific, Waltham, MA, USA) (bacterial strains) or Sabouraud agar medium (Oxoid, Thermo Fisher Scientific, Waltham, MA, USA) (fungal strains). MBC was defined as the lowest concentration that killed 99.9% of the final inocula after 24 h incubation at 37 °C (bacterial strains) or 48 h at 30 °C (fungal strains). The antimicrobial tests were performed in triplicate. Gentamicin and fluconazole were used as an antimicrobial reference standard.

4.4. Cytotoxicity Studies

4.4.1. In Vitro Cell Culture

According to the ISO (International Organization for Standardization, 2009) norm 10993-5 (Biological evaluation of medical devices—Part 5: Tests for in vitro cytotoxicity), testing of cytotoxicity was performed using L929 mouse fibroblasts (LGC Standards, Middlesex, UK). The cells were maintained under standard conditions (37 °C, 5% CO_2) in compelled culture medium (cRPMI-1640 medium supplemented with 10% fetal bovine serum (FBS) and antibiotics: 100 U/mL penicillin and 100 µg/mL streptomycin) Sigma-Aldrich (Darmstad, Germany) as previously described [57]. Before being used in the cytotoxicity assay, the cells' viability was assessed by excluding trypan blue dye and was in the range of 93–95%.

4.4.2. Measurements of Cellular Metabolic Activity and Global Growth Inhibition

The metabolic activity of the L929 cells was tested after application of water extracts obtained from dried plants. Cells in culture medium were seeded in 96-well plates (2×10^5 cells/well) for 24 h at 37 °C, 5% CO_2. The tested extracts were diluted in cRPMI-1640 medium in concentrations of 50; 25; 12.5; 10; 5; 2.5 and 1 mg/mL, added to the cells (100 µL/well), and incubated under standard conditions for 24 h. Following incubation, the cell monolayers were carefully screened using light microscopy, as recommended by ISO norm 10993-5, to evaluate cell morphology. Cell metabolic activity was estimated by measuring the ability of cells to reduce MTT [(3-(4,5-dimethylthiazol-2-yl)-2,5-diphenyltetrazolium bromide)], which is one of the tests recommended by the Food and Drug Administration (FDA) and ISO as previously described [57].

4.5. Statistical Analysis

Statistical analysis over chemical parameters was performed with Duncan's test ($p = 0.05$). Obtained results are presented results are shown as the mean value of six replications. The statistical significance of the cytotoxicity results was determined by Kruskal-Wallis test ($p < 0.05$). Data are presented as mean values ± SD. For statistical analysis, the STATISTICA 12 and 13 PL software was used (Stat Soft, Kraków, Poland).

5. Conclusions

Many commonly used antibiotics are becoming useless due to the increasing resistance of pathogens. For this reason, there is an urgent need to search for new antimicrobial, anti-inflammatory and pro-regenerative drugs with high biocompatibility and targeted activity. Plant biocomponents with well-characterized properties and good biocompatibility are good candidates for developing new drugs, medicinal food, or dietary supplements. A significant impact on such formulations expected therapeutic value is the plant's breeding conditions, limiting the content of potentially toxic compounds, or determining an active biological substance's content.

Water macerates of oregano and thyme are a valuable solution. Dependently, they can be a good source of polyphenols and have good antimicrobial abilities (conventional) and are rich in pigments (organic). It is worth pointing that "conventional" thyme macerate exhibited strong activity against the strains of *P. aeruginosa*. This opportunistic pathogen alleged to cause gastroenteritis in humans if ingested in large numbers. Can be isolated from soil and water and is commonly associated with spoilage of food such as eggs, cured meats, fish, and milk and cosmetic.

Thyme "conventional" macerates diminished the growth of L929 fibroblasts cytotoxicity, and "organic" oregano increased the ability of L929 cells to reduce MTT. Cultivation type had shaped influence on the ability of L929 cells to reduce MTT—both organic herbs macerates had significant higher abilities to increase this property; however, conventional cultivated herbs (water macerates) had higher antimicrobial activity and higher polyphenols content. Extracts, isolated from ecological plant cultures, may be used in higher concentrations in formulations for medical use due to their lower cytotoxic activity. This allows achieving a higher concentration of biologically active substances while maintaining biological safety, and faster achievement of the therapeutic and cosmetic effect.

Author Contributions: Conceptualization: K.S.-Z.; methodology: K.S.-Z., P.L., W.G., M.C., M.S. (Magdalena Szemraj); validation: K.S.-Z., W.G.; chemical analysis: K.S.-Z., M.A., O.S., O.T., M.S. (Małgorzata Stanowska); microbial analysis and description: P.L., M.S. (Magdalena Szemraj); cytotoxicity analysis and description: W.G., M.C.; writing—original draft preparation: K.S.-Z.; review and editing: W.G., P.L., M.C., K.P.R., W.M.; supervision: K.S.-Z.; funding acquisition: K.S.-Z., K.P.R., W.M., P.L., M.C. All authors have read and agreed to the published version of the manuscript.

Funding: Microbial analysis were partially supported financially by the Department of Pharmaceutical Microbiology and Microbiological Diagnostics (503/3- 012-03/503-31-001), Faculty of Pharmacy, Medical University of Lodz, Poland.

Institutional Review Board Statement: Faculty of Biology and Environmental Protection University of Lodz, Poland, fulfills the statutory conditions for conducting research on cell lines in accordance with the European Union low.

Informed Consent Statement: Not applicable.

Data Availability Statement: The data presented in this study are available on request from the corresponding author.

Conflicts of Interest: The authors declare no conflict of interest.

Sample Availability: Not available.

References

1. Wogiatzi, E.; Gougoulias, N.; Papachatzis, A.; Vagelas, I.; Chouliaras, N. Greek Oregano Essential Oils Production, Phytotoxicity and Antifungal Activity. *Biotech. Biotechnoll. Equip.* **2009**, *23*, 1150–1152. [CrossRef]
2. Stahl-Biskup, E.; Venskutonis, R.P. Thyme. In *Handbook of Herbs and Spices*; Peter, K.V., Ed.; Woodhead Publishing: Sawston, UK, 2012; pp. 499–525.
3. Sivicka, I.; Adamovičs, A.; Žukauska, I. Research of oregano *(Origanum vulgare* L.) inflorescence's parameters. In Proceedings of the Annual 18th International Scientific Conference "Research for Rural Development", Latvia University of Agriculture, Jelgava, Latvia, 16–18 May 2012; Volume 1, pp. 56–60.
4. Mäkinen, S.M.; Pääkkönen, K.K. Processing, effects and use of oregano and marjoram in foodstuffs and in food preparation. In *Oregano: The genera Origanum and Lippia*; Kintzios, S.E., Ed.; Taylor and Francis: London, UK, 2002; Volume 25, pp. 217–233.
5. Ložienė, K. Selection of fecund and chemically valuable clones of thyme (Thymus) species growing wild in Lithuania. *Ind. Crop. Prod.* **2009**, *29*, 502–508. [CrossRef]
6. Sakkas, H.; Papadopoulou, C. Antimicrobial Activity of Basil, Oregano, and Thyme Essential Oils. *J. Microb. Biotech.* **2017**, *27*, 429–438. [CrossRef]
7. Faleiro, L.; Miguel, G.; Gomes, S.; Costa, L.; Venâncio, F.; Teixeira, A.; Figueiredo, A.C.; Barroso, J.G.; Pedro, L.G. Antibacterial and Antioxidant Activities of Essential Oils Isolated from *Thymbra capitata* L. (Cav.) and *Origanum vulgare* L. *J. Agric. Food Chem.* **2005**, *53*, 8162–8168. [CrossRef]

8. Nabissi, M.; Marinelli, O.; Morelli, M.B.; Nicotra, G.; Iannarelli, R.; Amantini, C.; Maggi, F. Thyme extract increases mucociliary-beating frequency in primary cell lines from chronic obstructive pulmonary disease patients. *Biomed. Pharm.* **2018**, *105*, 1248–1253. [CrossRef]
9. Damtie, D.; Mekonnen, Y. Antibacterial activity of essential oils from Ethiopian thyme (*Thymus serrulatus* and *Thymus schimperi*) against tooth decay bacteria. *PLoS ONE* **2020**, *15*, e0239775. [CrossRef]
10. Kędzia, A.; Dera-Tomaszewska, B.; Ziółkowska-Klinkosz, M.; Kędzia, A.W.; Kochańska, B.; Gębska, A. Activity of thyme oil (Oleum Thymi) against aerobic bacteria. *Post Fitoter.* **2012**, *2*, 67–71.
11. Tellez-Monzón, L.A.; Nolazco-Cama, D.M. Estudio de la composición química del aceite esencial de orégano (*Origanum vulgare* spp.) de Tacna. *Ing. Ind.* **2017**, *35*, 195–205.
12. Sim, J.X.F.; Khazandi, M.; Chan, W.Y.; Trott, D.J.; Deo, P. Antimicrobial activity of thyme oil, oregano oil, thymol and carvacrol against sensitive and resistant microbial isolates from dogs with otitis externa. *Vet. Dermat.* **2019**, *30*, 524. [CrossRef]
13. Yamazaki, K.; Yamamoto, T.; Kawai, Y.; Inoue, N. Enhancement of antilisterial activity of essential oil constituents by nisin and diglycerol fatty acid ester. *Food Microbiol.* **2004**, *21*, 283–289. [CrossRef]
14. Rota, C.; Carraminana, J.J.; Burillo, J.; Herrera, A. In vitro antimicrobial activity of essential oils from aromatic plants against selected foodborne pathogens. *J. Food Protect.* **2004**, *67*, 1252–1256. [CrossRef]
15. Dorozko, J.; Kunkulberga, D.; Sivicka, I.; Kruma, Z. The influence of various drying methods on the quality of edible flower petals. FOODBALT 2019. In Proceedings of the 13th Baltic Conference on Food Science and Technology "Food, Nutrition, Well-Being", Latvia University of Life Sciences and Technologies, Jelgava, Latvia, 2–3 May 2019; Volume 1, pp. 182–187.
16. Moreira, M.D.R.; Ponce, A.; Del Valle, C.E.; Roura, S.I. Edible coatings on fresh squash slices: Effect of film drying temperature on the nutritional and microbiological quality. *J. Food Proc. Preserv.* **2009**, *33*, 226–236. [CrossRef]
17. Kalwa, K.; Wyrostek, J. Ocena zawartości związków biologicznie aktywnych oraz zawartość i skład olejku eterycznego w melisie lekarskiej (*Melissa officinalis* L.). *Post Nauk Technol. Przem Rol-Spoż* **2018**, *73*, 54–65.
18. Kapadiya, D.B.; Dabhi, B.K.; Aparnathi, K.D. Spices and Herbs as a Source of Natural Antioxidants. *Food Int. J. Curr. Microbiol. App. Sci.* **2016**, *5*, 280–288. [CrossRef]
19. Jałoszyński, K.; Figiel, A.; Wojdyło, A. Drying kinetics and antioxidant activity of oregano. *Acta Agroph.* **2008**, *11*, 81–90.
20. Embuscado, M.E. Spices and herbs: Natural sources of antioxidants–a mini-review. *J. Funct. Foods.* **2015**, *18*, 811–819. [CrossRef]
21. Hallmann, E.; Sabała, P. Organic and Conventional Herbs Quality Reflected by Their Antioxidant Compounds Concentration. *Appl. Sci.* **2020**, *10*, 3468. [CrossRef]
22. Burnett, S.E.; Mattson, N.S.; Williams, K.A. Substrates, and fertilisers for organic container production of herbs, vegetables, and herbaceous ornamental plants grown in greenhouses in the United States. *Sci. Hortic.* **2016**, *208*, 111–119. [CrossRef]
23. Matłok, N.; Gorzelany, J.; Stępień, A.E.; Figiel, A.; Balawejder, M. Effect of Fertilization in Selected Phytometric Features and Contents of Bioactive Compounds in Dry Matter of Two Varieties of Basil (*Ocimum basilicum* L.). *Sustainability* **2019**, *11*, 6590. [CrossRef]
24. Dragland, S.; Senoo, H.; Wake, K.; Holte, K.; Blomhoff, R. Several Culinary and Medicinal Herbs Are Important Sources of Dietary Antioxidants. *J. Nutr.* **2003**, *133*, 1286–1290. [CrossRef]
25. Vallverdú-Queralt, A.; Regueiro, J.; Martínez-Huélamo, M.; Alvarenga, J.F.R.; Leal, L.N.; Lamuela-Raventos, R.M. A comprehensive study on the phenolic profile of widely used culinary herbs and spices: Rosemary, thyme, oregano, cinnamon, cumin, and bay. *Food Chem.* **2014**, *154*, 299–307. [CrossRef]
26. Taghipour, S.; Rahimi, A.; Zartoshti, M.R.; Arslan, Y. The effect of micronutrients on antioxidant properties of thyme (*Thymus vulgaris* L.) under humic acid using condition. *YYU J. Agric. Sci.* **2017**, *27*, 589–600.
27. Matłok, N.; Stępień, A.E.; Gorzelany, J.; Wojnarowska-Nowak, R.; Balawejder, M. Effects of Organic and Mineral Fertilization on Yield and Selected Quality Parameters for Dried Herbs of Two Varieties of Oregano (*Origanum vulgare* L.). *Appl. Sci.* **2020**, *10*, 5503.
28. Lv, J.; Huang, H.; Yu, L.; Whent, M.; Niu, Y.; Shi, H.; Yu, L.L. Phenolic composition and nutraceutical properties of organic and conventional cinnamon and peppermint. *Food Chem.* **2012**, *132*, 1442–1450. [CrossRef]
29. Faller, A.L.K.; Fialho, E. The antioxidant capacity and polyphenol content of organic and conventional retail vegetables after domestic cooking. *Food Rese. Int.* **2009**, *42*, 210–215. [CrossRef]
30. Lichtenthaler, H.K.; Wellburn, A.R. Determinations of total carotenoids and chlorophylls A and B of leaf extracts in different solvents. *Biochem. Soc. Trans.* **1983**, *11*, 591–592. [CrossRef]
31. Garousi, F.; Veres, S.; Bódi, É.; Várallyay, S.; Kovács, B. Role of selenite and selenate uptake by maise plants in chlorophyll A and B content. *Int. J. Biol. Biomol. Agric. Food Biot. Eng.* **2015**, *9*, 625–668.
32. Chen, B.H.; Chen, Y.Y. Stability of chlorophylls and carotenoids in sweet potato leaves during microwave cooking. *J. Agric. Food Chem.* **1993**, *41*, 1315–1320. [CrossRef]
33. Onofrei, V.; Burducea, M.; Lobiuc, A.; Teliban, G.C.; Ranghiuc, G.; Robu, T. Influence of organic foliar fertilisation on antioxidant activity and content of polyphenols in *Ocimum basilicum* L. *Acta Pol. Pharm.* **2017**, *74*, 611–615.
34. Manukyan, A. Secondary metabolites and their antioxidant capacity of Caucasian endemic thyme (*Thymus transcaucasicus* Ronn.) as affected by environmental stress. *J. Appl. Res. Med. Arom. Plants* **2019**, *13*, 100209. [CrossRef]
35. Skubij, N.; Dzida, K. Effect of natural fertilisation and the type of substrate on the biological value of the thyme herb (*Thymus vulgaris* L.). *Acta Sci. Pol. Hortorum. Cultus* **2016**, *15*, 291–304.

36. Tzima, K.; Brunton, N.P.; Rai, D.K. Evaluation of the impact of chlorophyll removal techniques on polyphenols in rosemary and thyme by-products. *J. Food Biochem.* **2020**, *44*, e13148. [CrossRef] [PubMed]
37. Kulbat-Warycha, K.; Georgiadou, E.C.; Mańkowska, D.; Smolińska, B.; Fotopoulos, V.; Leszczyńska, J. Response to stress and allergen production caused by metal ions (Ni, Cu and Zn) in oregano (*Origanum vulgare* L.) plants. *J. Biotechnol.* **2020**, *324*, 171–182. [CrossRef] [PubMed]
38. De Boer, E.; Spiegelenberg, W.M.; Janssen, F.W. Microbiology of spices and herbs. *Antonie van Leeuwenhoek* **1985**, *51*, 435–438. [CrossRef]
39. Fogele, B.; Granta, R.; Valciņa, O.; Bērziņš, A. Occurrence and diversity of Bacillus cereus and moulds in spices and herbs. *Food Control* **2018**, *83*, 69–74. [CrossRef]
40. Bankova, R.; Popova, T.P. Antimicrobial Activity in vitro of Aqueous Extracts of Oregano (*Origanum vulgare* L.) and Thyme (*Thymus vulgaris* L.). *Int. J. Curr. Microbiol. Appl. Sci.* **2017**, *6*, 1–12. [CrossRef]
41. de Sousa Lima, C.M.; Fujishima, M.A.T.; de Paula Lima, B.; Mastroianni, P.C.; Fábio, F.; de Sousa, O.; Oliveira da Silva, J. Microbial contamination in herbal medicines: A serious health hazard to elderly consumers. *BMC Complement. Med. Ther.* **2020**, *20*, 1–9. [CrossRef]
42. Quadir, M.; Shahzadi, S.K.; Bashir, A.; Munir, A.; Shahzad, S. Evaluation of phenolic compounds and antioxidant and antimicrobial activities of some common herbs. *Int. J. Anal. Chem.* **2017**, *2017*, 1–6. [CrossRef]
43. Kandasamy, M.; Nasimuddin, S.; Gnanadesikan, S.; Nithyalakshmi, J.; Vennimalai, S. Antibacterial activity of aqueous infusion and decoction of dried leaves of oregano (*Origanum vulgare*) on clinical bacterial isolates. *Indian J. Microbiol. Res.* **2017**, *4*, 442–447.
44. Shan, B.; Cai, Y.-Z.; Brooks, J.D.; Corke, H. The in vitroantibacterial activity of dietary spice and medicinal herb extracts. *Int. J. Food Microb.* **2007**, *117*, 112–119. [CrossRef]
45. Al-Alzoreky, N.S. Antimicrobial activity of pomegranate (*Punica granatum* L.) fruit peels. *Int. J. Food Microbiol.* **2009**, *34*, 244–248. [CrossRef] [PubMed]
46. Alonso, J.R. *Tratado de Fitomedicina. Bases Clínicas y Farmacológicas*; Isis Ediciones SRL: Buenos Aires, Brazil, 1998; pp. 1–1039.
47. Soliman, K.M.; Badeaa, R.I. Effect of oil extracted from some medicinal plants on different mycotoxigenic fungi. *Food Chem. Toxicol.* **2002**, *40*, 1669–1675. [CrossRef]
48. Bukovská, A.; Cikos, S.; Juhás, S.; Il'ková, G.; Rehák, P.; Koppel, J. Effects of a combination of thyme and oregano essential oils on TNBS-induced colitis in mice. *Mediat. Inflamm.* **2007**, *2007*, 23296. [CrossRef]
49. de Oliveira, J.R.; de Jesus Viegas, D.; Martins, A.P.R.; Carvalho, C.A.T.; Soares, C.P.; Camargo, S.E.A.; de Oliveira, L.D. Thymus vulgaris L. extract has antimicrobial and anti-inflammatory effects in the absence of cytotoxicity and genotoxicity. *Arch. Oral Biol.* **2017**, *82*, 271–279. [CrossRef]
50. Loizzo, M.R.; Menichini, F.; Conforti, F.; Tundis, R.; Bonesi, M.; Saab, A.M.; Statti, G.A.; de Cindio, B.; Houghton, P.J.; Menichini, F.; et al. Chemical analysis, antioxidant, anti-inflammatory and anticholinesterase activities of Origanum ehrenbergii Boiss and *Origanum syriacum* L. essential oils. *Food Chem.* **2009**, *117*, 174–180. [CrossRef]
51. Jamali, T.; Kavoosi, G.; Safavi, M.; Ardestani, S.K. In-vitro evaluation of apoptotic effect of OEO and thymol in 2D and 3D cell cultures and the study of their interaction mode with DNA. *Sci. Rep.* **2018**, *25*, 15787. [CrossRef]
52. El-Babili, F.; Bouajila, J.; Souchard, J.P.; Bertrand, C.; Bellvert, F.; Fouraste, I.; Moulis, C.; Valentin, A. Oregano: Chemical analysis and evaluation of its antimalarial, antioxidant, and cytotoxic activities. *J. Food Sci.* **2011**, *76*, 512–518. [CrossRef]
53. Bakkali, F.; Averbeck, S.; Averbeck, D.; Zhiri, A.; Baudoux, D.; Idaomar, M. Antigenotoxic effects of three essential oils in diploid yeast Saccharomyces cerevisiae after treatments with UVC radiation, 8-MOP plus UVA and MMS. *Mut. Res.* **2006**, *606*, 27–28. [CrossRef] [PubMed]
54. Mezzoug, N.; Elhadri, A.; Dallouh, A.; Amkiss, S.; Skali, S.; Abrini, J.; Zhiri, A.; Baudoux, D.; Diallo, B.; El Jaziri, M. Investigation of the mutagenic and antimutagenic effects of Origanum compactum essential oil and some of its constituents. *Mutat. Res. Genet. Toxicol. Environ.* **2007**, *629*, 100–110. [CrossRef] [PubMed]
55. Singleton, V.L.; Rossi, J.A. Colorimetry of total phenolics with phosphomolybdic-phosphotungstic acid reagents. *Am. J. Enol. Vitic.* **1965**, *16*, 144–158.
56. European Committee on Antimicrobial Susceptibility Testing (EUCAST) 2020. MIC Determination of Non-Fastidious and Fastidious Organisms. EUCAST Version 6. Available online: https://www.eucast.org/ast_of_bacteria/mic_determination/?no_cache=1 (accessed on 21 December 2020).
57. Kamizela, A.; Gawdzik, B.; Urbaniak, M.; Lechowicz, Ł.; Białońska, A.; Kutniewska, S.E.; Chmiela, M. New γ-Halo-δ-lactones and δ-Hydroxy-γ-lactones with Strong Cytotoxic Activity. *Molecules* **2019**, *24*, 1875. [CrossRef] [PubMed]

MDPI
St. Alban-Anlage 66
4052 Basel
Switzerland
Tel. +41 61 683 77 34
Fax +41 61 302 89 18
www.mdpi.com

Molecules Editorial Office
E-mail: molecules@mdpi.com
www.mdpi.com/journal/molecules

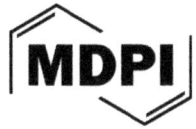